4/1/2023

"fingerprinting" – could this be done w/ the rules? would that be interesting – yes useful?...

Drug Discovery Research: A Comprehensive Overview

Drug Discovery Research: A Comprehensive Overview

Editor: Graham Craig

MURPHY & MOORE
www.murphy-moorepublishing.com

www.murphy-moorepublishing.com

MURPHY & MOORE

Cataloging-in-Publication Data

Drug discovery research : a comprehensive overview / edited by Graham Craig.
p. cm.
Includes bibliographical references and index.
ISBN 978-1-63987-169-8
1. Drugs--Design. 2. Drug development. 3. Drugs--Research. 4. Pharmaceutical chemistry. I. Craig, Graham.
RS420 .D78 2022
615.19--dc23

Murphy & Moore Publishing,
1 Rockefeller Plaza,
New York City, NY 10020, USA

ISBN 978-1-63987-169-8 (Hardback)

Contents

Preface

The main aim of this book is to educate learners and enhance their research focus by presenting diverse topics covering this vast field. This is an advanced book which compiles significant studies by distinguished experts in the area of analysis. This book addresses successive solutions to the challenges arising in the area of application, along with it; the book provides scope for future developments.

The process which is involved in discovering new candidate medications is termed as drug discovery. It lies at the intersection of the fields of pharmacology, biotechnology and medicine. The process of drug discovery consists of identifying screening hits, medicinal chemistry, and increasing the selectivity, oral bioavailability, potency and affinity of the drug through optimization. Finding a drug for a particular disease makes use of a method which is termed as high-throughput screening. This involves testing a vast collection of chemicals for their capability to affect a target area. The selectivity of the compounds in relation to their determined targets is also studied since the molecule should affect only the intended target, not other related targets. This book is compiled in such a manner, that it will provide in-depth knowledge about the science and business of drug discovery. The ever growing need of advanced technology is the reason that has fueled the research in this field in recent times. This book will serve as a reference to a broad spectrum of readers.

It was a great honour to edit this book, though there were challenges, as it involved a lot of communication and networking between me and the editorial team. However, the end result was this all-inclusive book covering diverse themes in the field.

Finally, it is important to acknowledge the efforts of the contributors for their excellent chapters, through which a wide variety of issues have been addressed. I would also like to thank my colleagues for their valuable feedback during the making of this book.

Editor

1

Chemical Similarity Networks for Drug Discovery

Yu-Chen Lo and Jorge Z. Torres

Abstract

Chemical similarity networks are an emerging area of interest in medicinal chemistry, chemical biology, and systems chemoinformatics that are currently being applied to drug target prediction, drug repurposing, and drug discovery in the new paradigm of poly-pharmacology and systems biology. In this chapter, we discuss the network-based drug target identification and discovery framework called chemical similarity network analysis pull-down (CSNAP) and its applications. We highlight the utility of CSNAP in identifying novel antimitotic drugs and their targets through practical case studies.

Keywords: drug discovery, chemical similarity networks, target identification

1. Introduction

Chemical similarity is an important concept in drug discovery used to identify compounds with similar bioactivities based on structural similarity between two ligands [1, 2]. Once a lead compound has been discovered from a chemical screen, a drug designer can design a series of structural analogues with improved pharmaceutical properties. The fundamental principle behind similarity-based drug discovery is the "chemical similarity principle," which states that if two molecules share similar structures, then they will likely have similar bioactivities. While there are exceptions, correlation between chemical structure and compound activities has been well established in medicinal chemistry [3]. Consequently, determining whether two molecules are structurally similar is a prerequisite for similarity-based drug discovery. At a rudimentary level, the similarity between two ligands can be easily discerned through visual inspection by identifying common functional groups, structural motifs, or substructures. However, human intervention is often subjective and not suitable for large-scale analysis.

Thus, applying computational algorithms for unbiased chemical similarity comparison and database searching is essential for a successful drug discovery campaign.

Several computational chemical similarity search algorithms have been developed [1, 4, 5]. The most commonly used approaches use chemical substructure fingerprints. Non-hashed structural fingerprints such as MACCS keys or Obabel FP3 fingerprints detect predefined substructures or functional group patterns in a molecule by mapping common chemical motifs into binary arrays known as structural keys. To compare the chemical similarity between two molecules, each molecule is converted into a binary series of 0 and 1, indicating the absence and presence of a particular substructure. On the other hand, chemical hashed fingerprints such as Daylight fingerprints or Obabel FP2 fingerprints use path information derived from molecular graphs to compare chemical structures [4]. While path-based fingerprints usually confer higher specificity, structural fingerprints can nevertheless be useful for detecting hits with distinct chemical scaffolds. Once the chemical fingerprints have been determined in a chemical search and the molecules have been converted to appropriate data representations, the next step is to evaluate the chemical similarity using a distance metric. Common distance measures include Euclidean, Manhattan, and Mahalanobis metrics, which have been widely applied in chemoinformatics and bioinformatics applications [6]. However, in the case of binary chemical fingerprints, the simplest and most direct distance measure is the Tanimoto index. Tanimoto metrics calculate the fraction of shared bits between chemical fingerprints in the range of 0–1. Although there is no universal Tanimoto index cutoff (Tc) to determine whether two molecules are sufficiently similar, a Tc value of 0.7 is a reasonable starting point for most chemical searches. Alternatively, statistical scores such as a *Z*-score can also be calculated based on the overall Tc score distribution [7].

In addition to 2D fingerprints, 3D chemical similarity fingerprints have also been developed. 3D chemical similarity fingerprints utilize the 3D structural information of the ligands such as molecular shape, pharmacophore points, or molecular interaction fields (MIF) for structural similarity comparison. Although 3D chemical similarity comparison can often capture structural features essential for protein-ligand binding, 3D alignment algorithms often require extensive optimization procedures to maximize the overlapped volume and are computationally intensive. Alternatively, nonalignment methods based on chemical descriptors such as GETAWAY or 3D-MoRSE descriptors can also be used [8, 9]. The 3D chemical descriptor is capable of capturing 3D ligand properties from 2D information and may improve computational time. However, substantial postvalidation may be required to confirm 3D structural similarity.

2. Network-based target prediction and drug discovery

The application of chemical similarity searches for ligand bioactivity prediction has recently gained substantial interest [10]. Due to the high failure rate of many new chemical entities (NCE) in the late stage of clinical trials, understanding on- and off-target binding of a drug to predict mechanisms of action and adverse reactions has become crucial for drug discovery programs [11]. If the chemical structure of a compound is known, then it is possible to predict compound bioactivities based on the chemical similarity methods described previously. Drug targets can be inferred from bioactivity databases with annotated targets sharing the highest similarity to the target molecules. Many public bioactivity databases are freely available and can be applied to this application including ChEMBL, PubChem, DrugBank, and Binding Database to name a few [12–14].

The simplest approach for drug target inference is by a simple chemical similarity search where the target of a query compound is inferred from the annotated ligand sharing the highest chemical similarity (**Figure 1**). However, there are several limitations to this approach. First, target information for the reference molecules may be incomplete; thus, target inference from a single molecular entity can miss potential targets from molecules sharing lower chemical similarity. Likewise, pair-wise target predictions may not provide consistent predictions for a group of structurally similar ligands. Second, chemical similarity values are not effective at ranking on and off targets and do not consider the structure-activity relationship (SAR) of congeneric series. Most importantly, simple ligand-based searches cannot be applied to analyzing large numbers of ligands such as the unannotated hits from a chemical screen. To circumvent this shortcoming, we recently proposed a new network target inference approach based on chemical similarity networks called chemical similarity network analysis pull-down (CSNAP) [15].

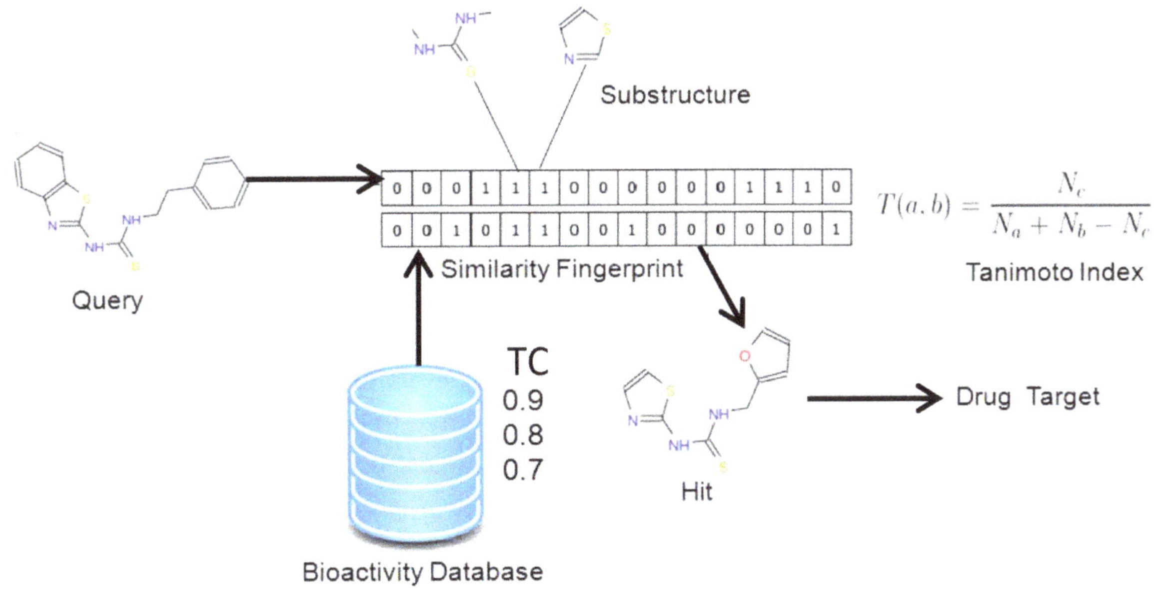

Figure 1. Chemical similarity search using 2D chemical fingerprints.

CSNAP uses a network-based algorithm to predict drug targets and does not rely on absolute chemical similarity values. It utilizes a scoring function (*S*-score) to find the consensus targets of a ligand in its nearest neighbors in a chemical similarity network, which is similar to that used to predict protein functions in a protein-protein interaction (PPI) network [16]. CSNAP is compatible with publicly available bioactivity databases, and we routinely use the ChEMBL database, which is one of the largest bioactivity databases that contains more than 1 million compounds with known target annotations. The original CSNAP algorithm applies 2D Obabel chemical similarity fingerprints (FP2, FP3, FP4, and MACCS) for target predictions. More recently, we developed CSNAP3D that combines 2D and 3D chemical search algorithms to improve the chemical search space [17]. CSNAP3D uses a fast 2D chemical similarity search using either FP2 or FP3 fingerprints to identify sets of hit molecules from large compound databases, and hit molecules are rescored using a combination of 3D similarity descriptors based on a combination of shape and pharmacophore. From our benchmark studies, we found that the CSNAP computational framework was highly accurate and was capable of analyzing large compound sets with diverse chemical structures. Consistently, the CSNAP application has been recently extended for large-scale metabolite analysis [18]. We have made the CSNAP algorithm freely available as the CSNAP web and it can be accessed at http://services.mbi.ucla.edu/CSNAP/.

3. CSNAP implementation

3.1. Chemical similarity network algorithms

Mathematically, a chemical similarity network can be considered as a graph G (V, E) where the vertex V represents compounds and the edge E represents chemical similarity and connects two compounds if they share a chemical similarity above an arbitrary threshold [19]. The CSNAP algorithm is performed in three steps: (1) chemical similarity database search, (2) chemical similarity network construction, and (3) drug target scoring and inference.

3.1.1. Chemical similarity search

Chemical similarity searching is the first step in the CSNAP algorithm (**Figure 2A**). The chemical similarity comparisons are performed using various 2D Obabel fingerprints including FP2, FP3, MACCS, and others. Query compounds prepared in SMILES or SDF formats are used as inputs to the CSNAP program. The compounds are searched sequentially against the ChEMBL database. To identify the ChEMBL compounds most similar to the query, the relative chemical similarity score is quantified by a Z-value relative to the distribution of the top 100 chemical similarity values. The ChEMBL compounds with a Z-score >2.5 are selected and serve as the annotated compounds for target inference in the next step.

3.1.2. Chemical similarity network construction

To generate chemical similarity networks, pair-wise chemical similarity values are evaluated between every pair of compounds. A network edge is established between two ligands whenever their similarity value is above a predefined threshold (>0.7) (**Figure 2B**). When large compound data sets are analyzed by the CSNAP algorithm, structurally diverse compounds are partitioned into subnetworks of distinct chemical scaffolds, known as "chemotypes." The chemical similarity networks can be used to estimate the chemical diversity of input structures at this stage.

3.1.3. Drug target scoring and inference

CSNAP infers drug targets using consensus statistics. Specifically, drug targets in the first neighbor of the query are identified and ranked based on their target annotation frequency (**Figure 2C**). A consensus score called an *S*-score is used to rank the probability that the predicted target will interact with the query ligand (**Figure 2D**). There are several advantages of using this network-based scoring function. First, the *S*-score eliminates the possibility of missing target information from the nearest neighbor and considers all possible targets within the same congeneric series. Second, since the drug target is inferred from the target consensus and is in agreement with the observed structure-activity relationship, the robustness of the prediction increases substantially. From our benchmark studies, we showed that this network-based target inference approach improves the prediction success rate over traditional approaches that use simple chemical searches [15].

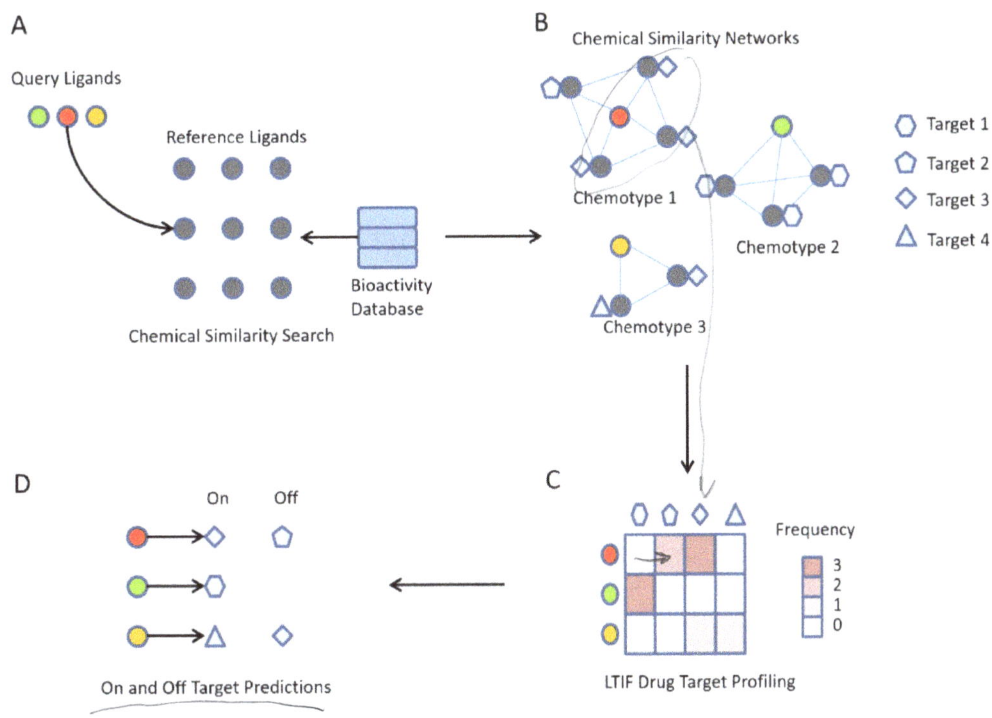

Figure 2. Chemical similarity network analysis pull-down (CSNAP) algorithm for large-scale drug target prediction. (A) Two-dimensional chemical search of three query ligands (green, red, and yellow) identified nine reference compounds from the bioactivity database. (B) Chemical similarity networks clustered compounds into subnetworks corresponding to three major chemotypes. Note that reference compounds interact with four distinct targets. (C) An *S*-score based on consensus statistics is applied to rank the most probable target based on the target annotation frequency of the first-order neighbor targets. (D) On and off targets are differentiated by ranking the predicted *S*-scores.

3.2. Case study: CSNAP web server for automated drug target prediction

To reduce concept to practice, we constructed a CSNAP web server for large-scale target prediction and drug discovery. The CSNAP web includes a front-end graphical user interface (GUI) that provides user interaction and output visualization, while target prediction is performed at the back-end by running the CSNAP algorithm.

3.2.1. CSNAP web input

The CSNAP web server accepts two ligand input formats: SDF and SMILES, which are two of the most commonly used molecular formats that handle large compound databases. In addition, a JME molecular editor is also included, which can be used to convert a chemical structure to a SMILES string on the fly (**Figure 3A**). Several chemical fingerprints are provided to perform chemical comparisons during the search and network clustering steps, including Obabel FP2, FP3, PF4, and MACCS fingerprints (**Figure 3B**). Obabel FP2 fingerprints use a path-based algorithm and are more specific than FP3, FP4, and MACCS that utilize a predefined set of substructures for chemical searches. On the other hand, when structural analogues are not available in the chemical database, FP3 can instead be used to search structurally distinct chemicals with similar bioactivities. To perform chemical searches, the chemical similarity cutoff needs to be defined. Here, CSNAP web supports a combination of absolute cutoff based on Tanimoto coefficient ($Tc > 0.7$) and relative chemical similarity cutoff based on a Z-score. From our experience, the default option using a *Z*-score cutoff of 2.5 will be optimal for most initial CSNAP predictions.

Once the query ligands and chemical search parameters have been defined, the CSNAP algorithm will search the ChEMBL compound activity database to identify structurally similar compounds for target inference (**Figure 3B**). The ChEMBL database assigns targets to a compound based on the level of target specificity (confidence score). Similarly, the compounds are also classified based on the assay type from which they are derived, including biochemical, functional, or ADMET assays. These database parameters will also need to be selected to perform the CSNAP analysis.

3.2.2. CSNAP web output

The CSNAP output page consists of three main panels: (1) chemical similarity networks, (2) chemical structure information, and (3) ligand-target interaction fingerprint (LTIF) (**Figure 3C**).

3.2.3. Chemical similarity networks

The chemical similarity networks panel displays the generated chemical networks using the CSNAP algorithm based on input ligands. The chemical similarity network connects query (red) and annotated ligands (gray) from the ChEMBL database, and the targets are inferred using consensus statistics. For large compound sets, the number of generated chemical clusters can be used to estimate the chemical diversity of the sets. To retrieve additional information regarding a specific ligand, the user can click on the node and the relevant information will be displayed in the chemical structure information panel.

3.2.4. Chemical structure information

The chemical structure information panel displays the chemical information selected from the chemical similarity network panel. The panel consists of several columns that include chemical structure information (chemical ID, chemical structure, SMILES string, InChI key) and the predicted target information (target name and UniProt ID). In the ChEMBL prediction column, the predicted targets of each compound are ranked by the *S*-score.

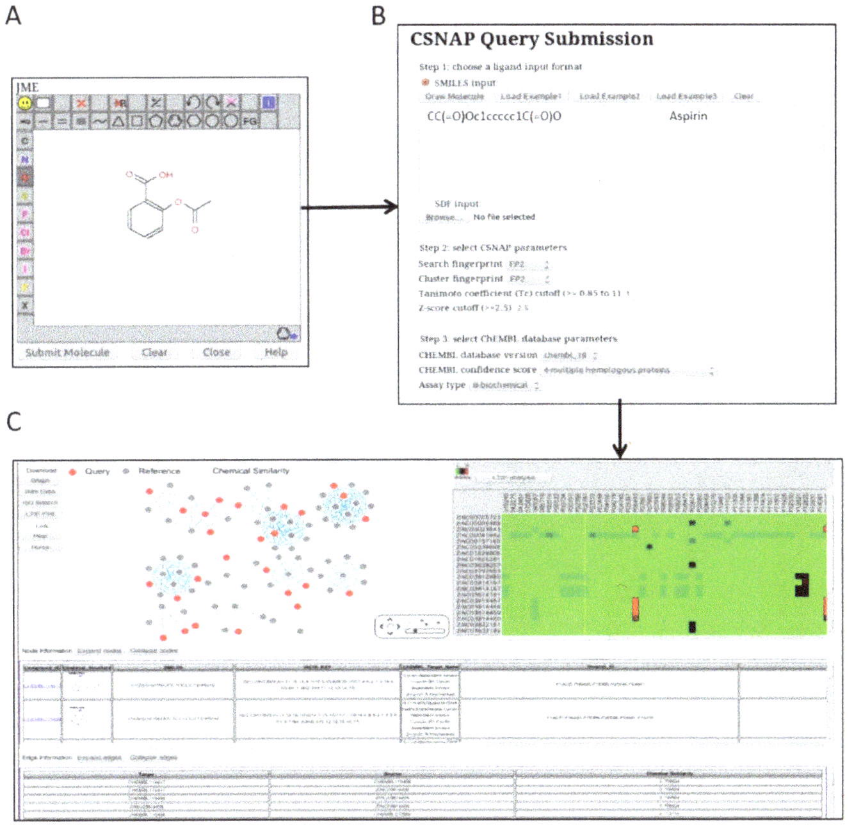

Figure 3. Drug target prediction using the CSNAP web server: (A) construct a query molecule using the JME molecular editor. (B) The molecule is converted to a SMILES string and entered into the CSNAP query submission page. (C) The CSNAP output page consists of three main panels: (1) the chemical similarity network, (2) the chemical structure information, and (3) the ligand-target interaction fingerprint (LTIF).

3.2.5. Ligand-target interaction fingerprint (LTIF)

To analyze the results from large-scale target prediction searches, the ligand-target interaction fingerprint (LTIF) is provided in the CSNAP web output. The LTIF panel displays the predicted *S*-score of each compound mapped against the predicted targets, and the color intensity of the LTIF heatmap is correlated with the *S*-score values. The LTIF can be used to infer compounds sharing similar target binding profiles, which may have similar bioactivity. By clicking on the LTIF button at the top of the LTIF panel, a separate window is created that shows the target spectrum and Gene Ontology (GO) term search derived from the LTIF analysis.

3.2.6. Target spectrum and Gene Ontology (GO) search

To further differentiate primary targets from off-targets in the LTIF, the CSNAP web also computes a target spectrum, by summing the *S*-score ($\sum S$) of all analyzed compounds for each target column (**Figure 4**). For a single compound analysis, the highest peak corresponds to the primary target. Similarly, for multi-ligand analysis, the highest peak corresponds to the most abundant target in the set. To determine the functional role of the predicted targets, the Gene Ontology (GO) search result is also provided (**Figure 4**). GO is a popular bioinformatics tool that maps genes into functions based on controlled vocabulary (GO terms) and has been widely used for pathway analysis of functional genomic data [20]. Here, CSNAP web incorporates a GO search in target predictions as a strategy for posttarget selection and validation. The GO terms can be used to further select relevant targets in a cell-based or phenotype-based screen based on the knowledge of anticipated molecular etiology including cellular components, molecular functions, and biological process. Smaller subsets of targets can then be filtered for additional experimental validation.

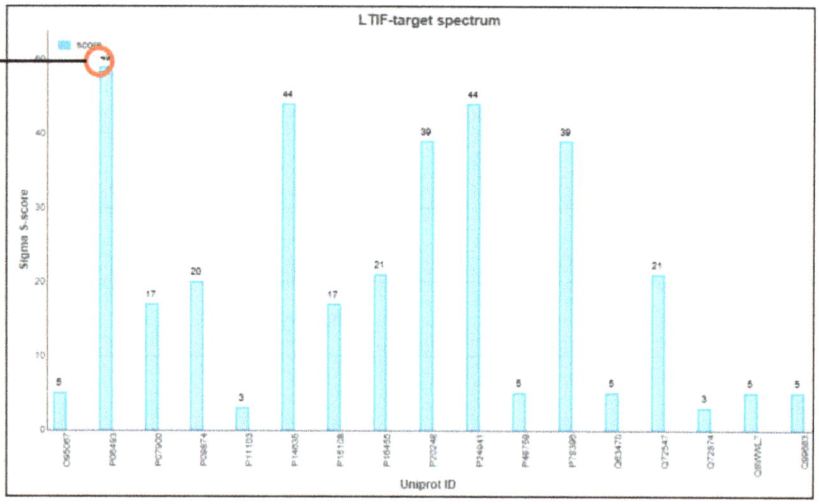

ID	Symbol	GO ID	Aspect	GO Name	Reference
O95067	CCNB2	GO:0000079	Process	regulation of cyclin-dependent protein serine/threonine kinase activity	GO_REF:0000002
O95067	CCNB2	GO:0000086	Process	G2/M transition of mitotic cell cycle	Reactome:REACT_2203
O95067	CCNB2	GO:0000278	Process	mitotic cell cycle	Reactome:REACT_152
O95067	CCNB2	GO:0001701	Process	in utero embryonic development	GO_REF:0000019
O95067	CCNB2	GO:0005515	Function	protein binding	PMID:15232106
O95067	CCNB2	GO:0005515	Function	protein binding	PMID:17408621
O95067	CCNB2	GO:0005515	Function	protein binding	PMID:23455922
O95067	CCNB2	GO:0005634	Component	nucleus	GO_REF:0000002
O95067	CCNB2	GO:0005654	Component	nucleoplasm	Reactome:REACT_169151
O95067	CCNB2	GO:0005654	Component	nucleoplasm	Reactome:REACT_169321
O95067	CCNB2	GO:0005813	Component	centrosome	PMID:21399614
O95067	CCNB2	GO:0005829	Component	cytosol	Reactome:REACT_147793
O95067	CCNB2	GO:0005829	Component	cytosol	Reactome:REACT_150414
O95067	CCNB2	GO:0005829	Component	cytosol	Reactome:REACT_150454
O95067	CCNB2	GO:0005829	Component	cytosol	Reactome:REACT_160217
O95067	CCNB2	GO:0005829	Component	cytosol	Reactome:REACT_163651
O95067	CCNB2	GO:0005829	Component	cytosol	Reactome:REACT_169293
O95067	CCNB2	GO:0005829	Component	cytosol	Reactome:REACT_6216
O95067	CCNB2	GO:0005829	Component	cytosol	Reactome:REACT_6217
O95067	CCNB2	GO:0005829	Component	cytosol	Reactome:REACT_852
O95067	CCNB2	GO:0007049	Process	cell cycle	GO_REF:0000037
O95067	CCNB2	GO:0007067	Process	mitotic nuclear division	GO_REF:0000037
O95067	CCNB2	GO:0007077	Process	mitotic nuclear envelope disassembly	Reactome:REACT_160255
O95067	CCNB2	GO:0015630	Component	microtubule cytoskeleton	GO_REF:0000054
O95067	CCNB2	GO:0016020	Component	membrane	GO_REF:0000019

Figure 4. Posttarget validation using Gene Ontology (GO) analysis in the CSNAP web. (Top) Target spectrum. (Bottom) GO search results.

4. Application of CSNAP for drug target prediction and discovery

4.1. CSNAP validation

The CSNAP algorithm was validated using 206 known drugs from the directory of useful decoy (DUD) set [21]. The benchmark set included 46 angiotensin-converting enzyme (ACE), 47 cyclin-dependent kinase 2 (CDK2), 23 heat-shock protein 90 (HSP90), 34 HIV reverse-transcriptase (HIVRT), 25 HMG-CoA reductase (HMGA), and 31 poly [ADP-ribose] polymerase (PARP) inhibitors. Using the default search criteria (fingerprint: FP2, Tc = 1, *Z*-score = 2.5), we evaluated the ability of the CSNAP algorithm to accurately predict the designated targets of each compound based on the *S*-score rankings. CSNAP analysis of the 206 compounds showed that the chemical similarity network clustered the drugs into distinct subnetworks, corresponding to diverse chemical scaffolds (chemotypes) (**Figure 5**). For a given subnetwork, the *S*-score was further used to predict the drug target of each compound based on their network connectivity with the reference ligands. The prediction results were then compared with those obtained by the similarity ensemble approach (SEA) [22]. The CSNAP algorithm gave an overall 80–94% true-positive prediction rate (TPR) in comparison with SEA (63–75%) based on the top 1, top 5, and top 10 ranking of target predictions. In particular, CSNAP substantially improved the target prediction rate for promiscuous ligands such as CDK2 and ACE inhibitors (92 and 96%) compared to the SEA approach (30 and 65%) (**Figure 6**).

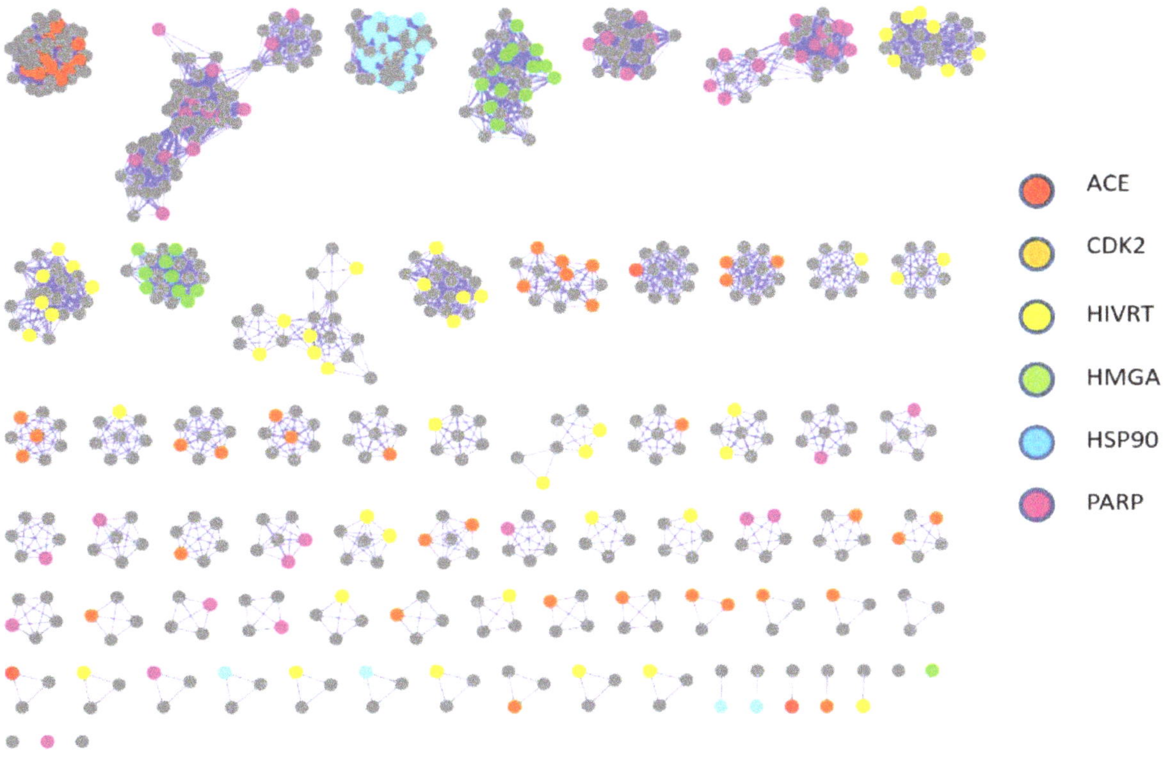

Figure 5. CSNAP2D clustering of 206 benchmark compounds consisting of six known drug classes from the directory of useful decoy (DUD) set.

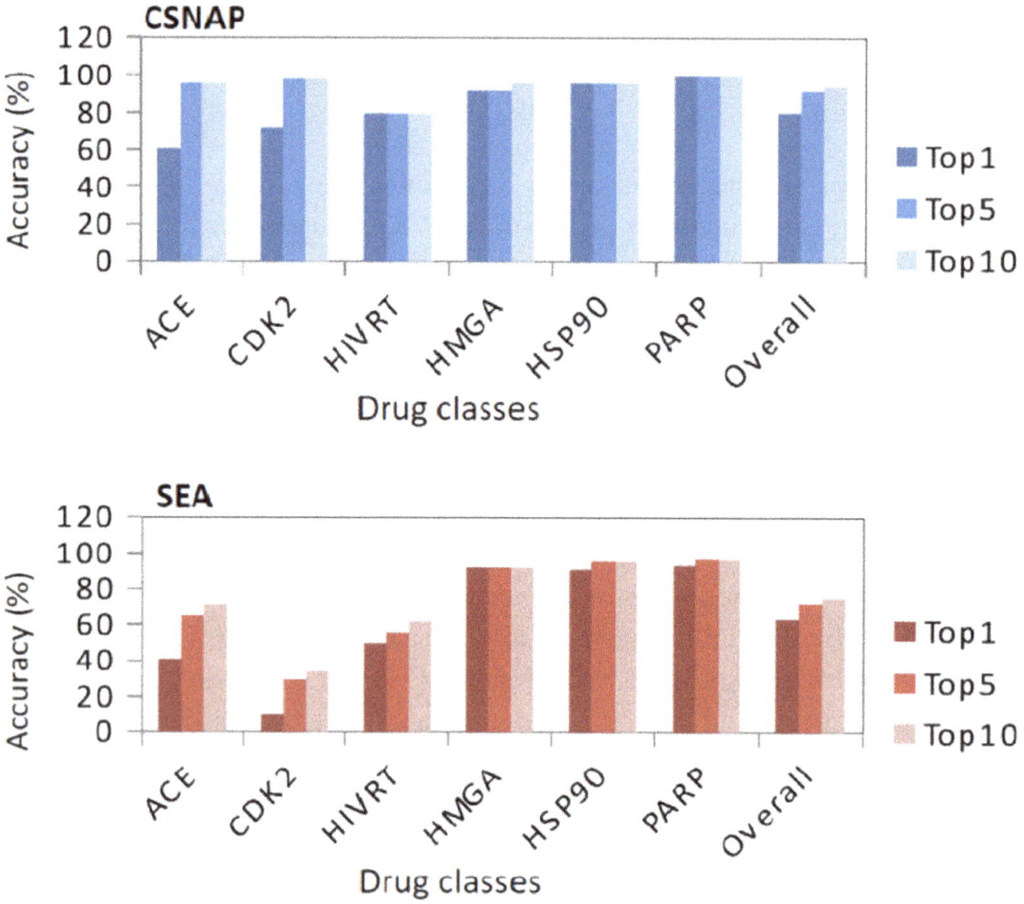

Figure 6. Performance comparison between CSNAP and SEA. CSNAP achieved improved prediction accuracy (TPR) for promiscuous drug classes like ACE, CDK2, and HIVRT inhibitors.

4.2. Target prediction of hits from an antimitotic chemical screen

We applied the CSNAP algorithm to predict the drug targets of a set of 212 compounds that were inhibitors of cell division [23]. CSNAP clustering of the mitotic compounds resulted into 85 chemical similarity subnetworks (**Figure 7A**). To identify the most common targets within the set, we applied the LTIF analysis. The target spectrum derived from the LTIF revealed four broad classes of mitotic targets including fatty acid desaturases (SCD, SCD1, and FADS2), ABL1 kinase, non-receptor-type tyrosine phosphatases (PTPN7, PTPN12, PTPN22, PTPRC, and ACP1), and beta tubulins. In particular, the target spectrum showed that beta tubulin had the largest peak height and was the most prominent protein target for the mitotic compounds. Further analysis showed that 51 compounds were associated with tubulin-targeting chemotypes. The predicted drug targets were validated by comparing siRNA-treated and drug-treated mitotic phenotypes in cell culture using immunofluorescence microscopy. In addition, *in vitro* tubulin polymerization assays were used to determine the effects of these compounds on microtubule formation. Among the 51 tested compounds, 31 compounds showed a perturbation of microtubule polymerization >25%, and thus, the CSNAP algorithm achieved a prediction accuracy of >70%.

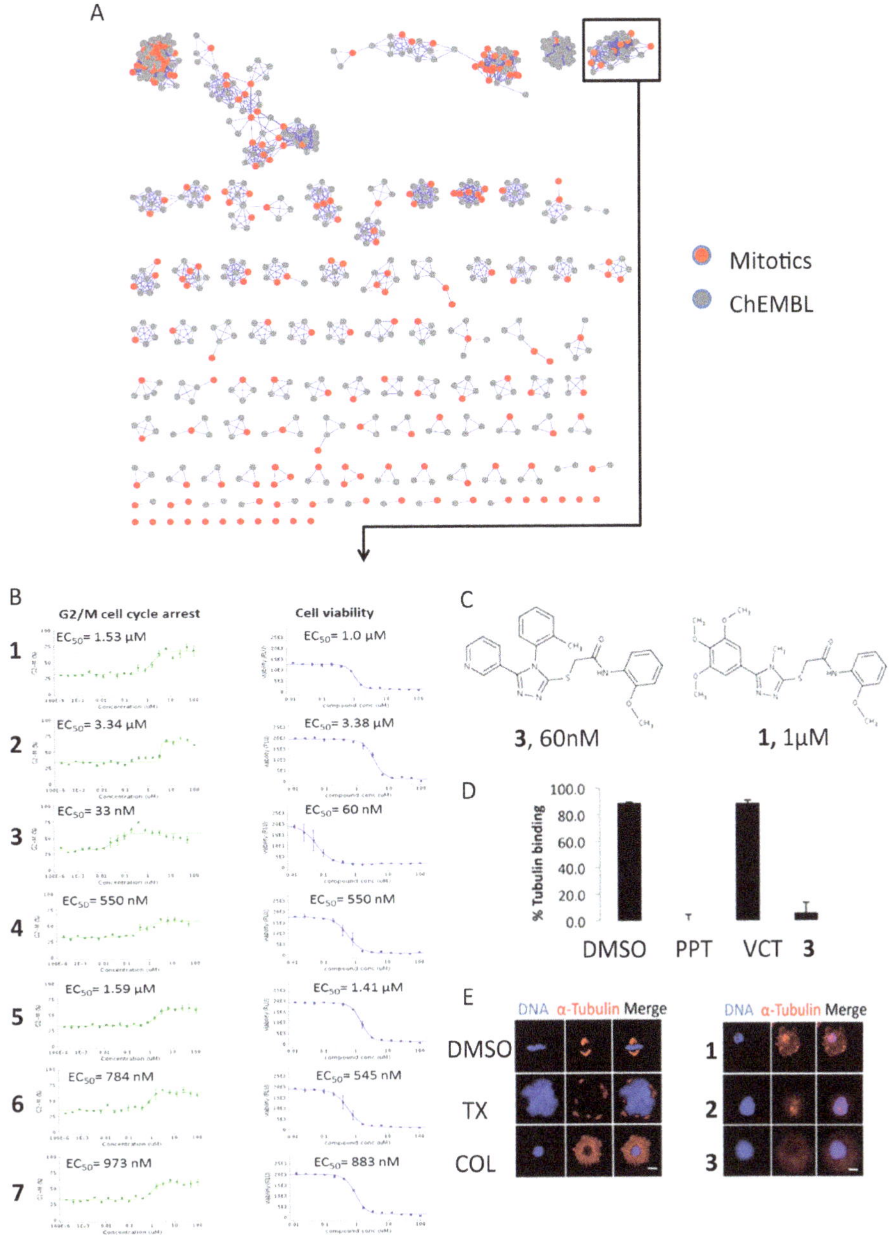

Figure 7. Discovery of novel tubulin-targeting drugs (compounds **1–7**). (A) CSNAP analysis of 212 mitotic drugs identified seven novel tubulin destabilizing compounds. (B) The compounds induced a G2/M cell cycle arrest and decreased cell viability in cell-based assays. (C) Discovery of compound **3** as the most potent compound in the series. (D) A mass spectrometry-based competition assay was used to show that compound **3** and podophyllotoxin (PPT) competed for binding to tubulin in contrast to vincristine (VCT). (E) Compound-treated (**1–3**) and colchicine-treated (COL) cells displayed a tubulin destabilizing effect in comparison with the tubulin stabilizing effect of taxol (TX).

4.3. Discovery of novel tubulin-targeting antimitotics

Using a negative selection strategy, we identified seven novel tubulin-targeting agents that were active in our tubulin polymerization assay but had not been associated with known tubulin chemotypes (**Figure 7A**). The seven compounds were analogues of phenyl-sulfanyl-thiazol-acetamide scaffolds that exhibit various degrees of tubulin destabilizing effects through a mechanism similar to that of the tubulin destabilizing agent colchicine. The most potent compound, compound **3**, in the series exhibited a cytotoxic effect in the nano-molar range (EC_{50}: G2/M = 33 nM; EC_{50}: cell death = 60 nM) when evaluated in cell viability and G2/M arrest assays (**Figure 7B, C**) [15]. The predicted mechanism was validated using a mass spectrometry-based competition assay where both the selected analogues and podophyllotoxin, a known colchicine site binder, competed for binding to tubulin in contrast to the negative control vincristine that interacted with a distant site in beta tubulin (**Figure 7D**) [24]. Likewise, both compound-treated and colchicine-treated cells displayed a tubulin destabilizing phenotype, characterized by rapid shortening of microtubule length and the disappearance of microtubule polymer mass (**Figure 7E**).

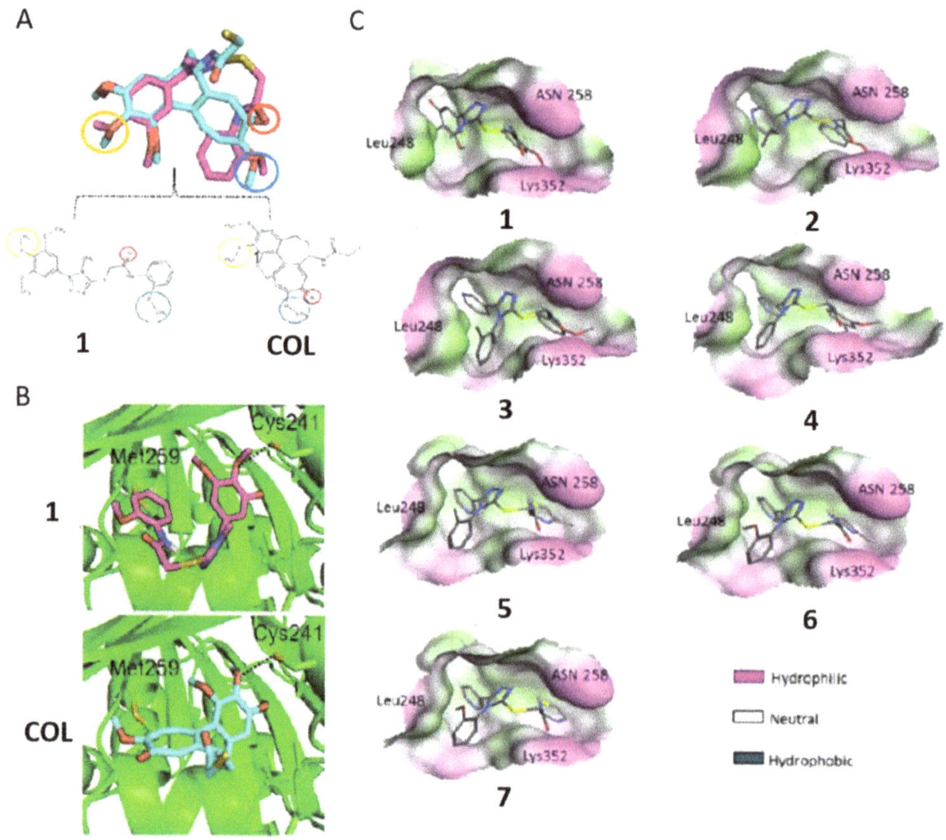

Figure 8. Binding mechanism of a novel tubulin destabilizing chemotype (compounds **1–7**). (A) Pharmacophore alignment between compound **1** and colchicine (COL) showed a consensus pharmacophore. (B) Docking of compound **1** in the colchicine site using the tubulin crystal structure (PDB code: 1SA0) revealed colchicine-like interactions with critical residues (Met259, Cys241). (C) Docking of the seven analogues into the colchicine site showed similar interactions.

4.4. Characterization of novel tubulin-targeting antimitotics

To investigate how the novel antimitotics interacted with beta tubulin, we performed structural alignments between compound **6** and colchicine and identified a consensus pharmacophore between the two molecules (**Figure 8A**). Further docking of compound **6** into the colchicine binding site also showed that both compound **6** and colchicine interacted with common residues, including the 2 and 10 methoxy groups and 9-keto group that interacted with Met259 and Cys241 of beta tubulin, respectively (**Figure 8B**). Similarly, all seven analogues docked into the same site through similar interactions. Interestingly, the elucidated binding modes could be used to explain the observed SAR. For example, the increased potency of compound **7** and **8** in comparison with **6** could be attributed to the hydrophilic interactions between the *N*-propyl and *N*-phenyl groups with Leu248 and Lys352 within the subpockets of the colchicine binding site (**Figure 8C**).

5. CSNAP3D: a 3D upgrade to the CSNAP approach

Chemical similarity searches based on 2D chemical structures have several limitations. First, compounds with distinct scaffolds can exhibit similar bioactivity due to "scaffold hopping" by interacting with a common receptor [25, 26]. Second, although 2D fingerprints based on substructure or fragment searches have the potential to detect scaffold hopping, the scaffold enrichment rate is low. Furthermore, 2D searches do not capture essential features of protein-ligand interactions in three-dimensional space. Consequently, 3D chemical searches based on the three-dimensional information of the ligands will offer additional opportunities to discover novel compounds.

5.1. 3D chemical similarity search

The most common approach to compare ligand similarity in 3D is by shape superposition, which maximizes the Gaussian volume overlap between two ligands [27]. Alternatively, ligand alignments that use molecular interaction field (MIF) or pharmacophore have also been proposed [28, 29]. These approaches take into account the shared chemical features arranged in three-dimensional space. To identify the optimal 3D chemical descriptors, we performed an unbiased screen of diverse 3D chemical descriptors based on molecular shapes or pharmacophores. Using 206 benchmark compounds from the DUD set, we tested the ability of each 3D descriptor to enrich class-specific scaffolds ranked by respective similarity scores. The lowest energy conformer of each ligand was generated using the MOE program. The results showed that 3D chemical descriptors using a combination of shape and pharmacophore features achieved the highest enrichment rate and ligand alignment accuracy compared to those based on shape or pharmacophore alone. This observation agrees with our current understanding that shape complementary and chemical matching are essential for the protein-ligand binding process.

We subsequently developed a 3D chemical similarity search method called "ShapeAlign" that utilized two open-source softwares: "Shape-it" and "Align-it" [30]. Similar to the combo score implemented in the ROCS program, the ShapeAlign algorithm also used a combination of shape and pharmacophore for 3D chemical searches. However, ShapeAlign incorporated a 2D fingerprint similarity score as an integral part of the searching process. Given a ligand with a pre-generated 3D conformation, the ShapeAlign algorithm first detects ligands from the chemical database with the highest shape matching evaluated by a shape Tanimoto index. The hit molecules are then aligned and rescored according to the degree of pharmacophore matching using the Align-it program.

5.2. Drug target prediction using CSNAP3D

We incorporated the "ShapeAlign" algorithm into our CSNAP program called "CSNAP3D" to cluster chemical structures and predict drug targets based on 3D ligand similarity. To evaluate CSNAP3D performance, we assessed the average true-positive rate (TPR) and false-positive rate (FPR) of predicting drug targets for the 206 benchmark compounds. The result showed that CSNAP3D achieved a TPR of >95% at 0.85 Tanimoto cutoff in comparison with other 2D target prediction approaches including CSNAP2D, SEA, and PASS approaches [17]. A comparison of CSNAP3D and CSNAP2D generated networks showed that diverse 2D scaffold subnetworks were clustered into smaller subsets of 3D chemical networks, suggesting that CSNAP3D could be used to identify scaffold hopping ligands not identifiable by conventional 2D methods (**Figure 9**).

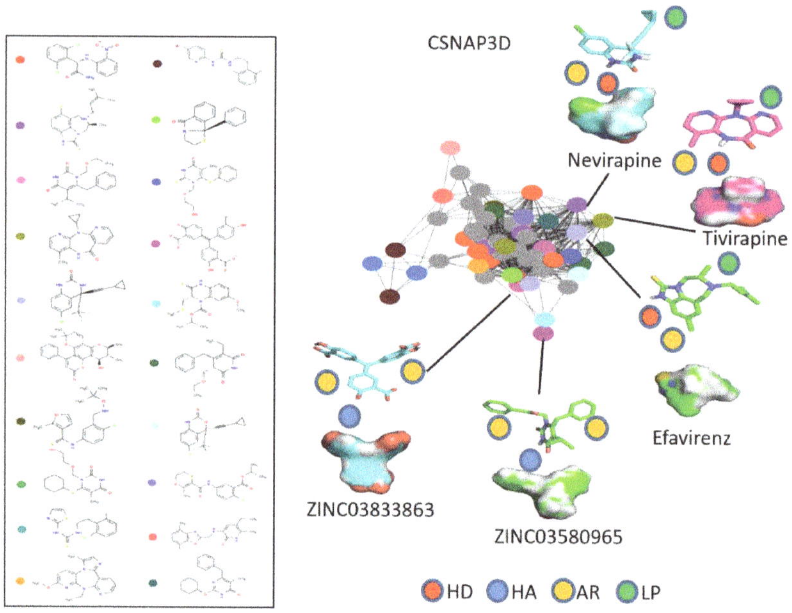

Figure 9. CSNAP3D clustered 34 distinct HIVRT NNRTI chemotypes into a shape-based chemical similarity network. The figure shows that many NNRTIs are scaffold hopping ligands to a common nucleotidyltransferase binding site. The 3D alignment between ligands was based on molecular shape and pharmacophore points (HD: hydrogen donor, HA: hydrogen acceptor, AR: aromatic, LP: lipophilic).

5.2.1. Target prediction of HIVRT inhibitors

As further validation, we presented a case study of predicting targets for a set of HIVRT inhibitors using the CSNAP3D algorithm. HIVRT inhibitors can be classified as nucleoside-based analogues (NRTIs) or non-nucleoside-based analogues (NNRTIs) [31]. In particular, NNRTIs have been difficult drug classes for computational dug target prediction due to the chemical diversity of the drug classes where many compounds are scaffold hopping ligands that bind to a common nucleotidyltransferase binding site. Although 3D ligand-based target predictions that use either the alignment or nonalignment methods have been attempted, many of these approaches yielded low predictability. Here, we applied CSNAP3D to predict the drug targets of 34 structurally diverse HIVRT NNRTIs and compared the prediction results with the CSNAP2D approach (**Figure 9**). Initial 2D chemical similarity network analysis clustered the 34 NNRTIs into 20 structurally diverse chemical similarity scaffolds. Further LTIF analysis, by mapping target prediction *S*-scores to the heatmap, showed that more than 20 compounds did not have a prediction. The NNRTIs were similarly analyzed by the CSNAP3D program using the ShapeAlign algorithm. In contrast, all the 34 ligands were clustered by CSNAP3D into a single shape-based chemical similarity network, suggesting that many NNRTIs are scaffold hopping ligands to a common binding site. LTIF analysis showed that 33 of NNRTIs were correctly predicted, thus achieving a TPR of >97%. In particular, 3D chemical similarity networks correctly identify three FDA-approved NNRTIs, namely efavirenz, nevirapine, and tivirapine whose structure alignment agreed with previous crystal structures and SAR studies (**Figure 9**). In addition, several novel scaffold hopping pairs were also identified (**Figure 9**).

5.2.2. Discovery of novel taxol scaffold hopping ligands

Taxol (paclitaxel) is a well-known anticancer natural product derived from the Yew tree, whose antiproliferative effect was first discovered in 1960s from an NCI anticancer drug screening campaign [32]. Taxol has since been found to be effective for treating a wide range of cancers including ovarian, breast, lung, bladder, prostate, melanoma, esophageal, and other solid tumors. However, the efficacy of taxol has been limited by severe side effects, toxicity, and synthetic feasibility. Thus, identification of low-weight taxol mimetics with more tolerable drug profiles is critical. While several taxol mimetics have been discovered including Synstab B and GS-164, both discovered by chemical screening, their binding mechanisms have remained undetermined [33, 34].

Here, we sought a rational approach to discover taxol mimetics using the CSNAP3D algorithm based on our existing structural knowledge of the original taxol molecule. CSNAP3D analysis of the 212 mitotic compounds from a chemical screen identified 42 potential taxol mimetics linked to 30 taxol structural conformers. Seven predicted taxol mimetics were found to be true positives with a >25% fold change in optical density when tested in tubulin polymerization assays *in vitro* and four compounds shared a consensus chemotype by co-localizing within one chemical similarity subnetwork. The structural alignment of the four selected molecules with taxol showed that they shared a similar T-shape conformation despite a simpler scaffold (**Figure 10A**). Docking studies showed that the increase in microtubule polymerization activity could be attributed to the phenyl moiety of these ligands, which was capable of forming a pi–pi stacking interaction with the critical residue His229 within the taxane site (**Figure 10B**). Three of the compounds demonstrated cytotoxic and antimitotic effects in cell culture with a potency <5 μM. Similarly, all the compounds displayed a similar tubulin stabilizing phenotype, characterized by microtubule aster formation in immunofluorescence microscopy studies (**Figure 10C**).

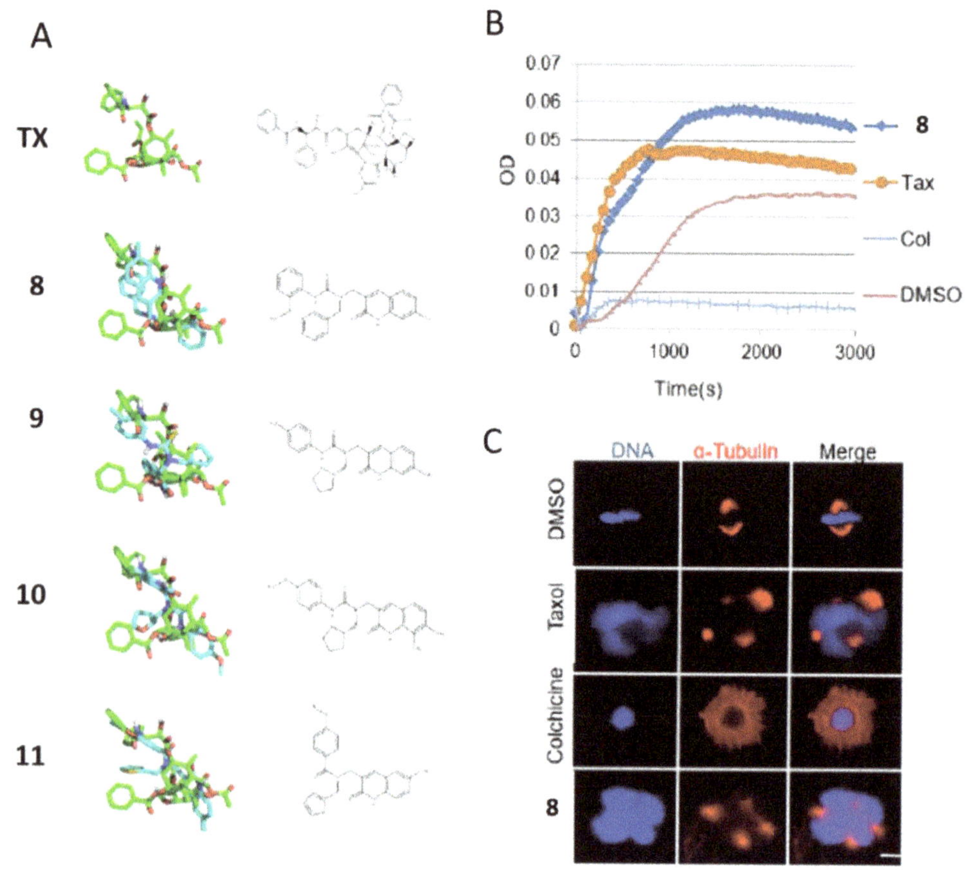

Figure 10. Structure-based discovery of taxol mimetics. (A) CSNAP3D analysis of 212 mitotic compounds from a cell-based screen identified four low molecular weight taxol (TX) mimetic analogues. (B) Compound **8** **(8)** demonstrated a fast tubulin polymerization rate at 50 μM similar to taxol (Tax) at 5 μM in comparison with colchicine (Col). (C) Compound **8** displayed a tubulin stabilizing phenotype, characterized by microtubule aster formation in immunofluorescence microscopy studies.

6. Conclusions and future directions

Chemical similarity is an important concept in medicinal chemistry and drug discovery to identify similar compounds with improved bioactivities. Here, we have expanded on this concept to chemical similarity network theory, where descriptive network statistics and graph topology can be applied to large-scale analysis of chemical diversity, bioactivities, and target identification. To demonstrate the utility of this approach, we have implemented the CSNAP algorithm, which can be used for large-scale compound analysis and target predictions. Analogous to protein function prediction in PPI networks, we applied consensus statistics to identify the common targets of each query ligand. We showed that this scoring function outperforms several target prediction methods based on simple chemical similarity searches. To address the challenge of scaffold hopping, where structurally diverse ligands can potentially interact with a common receptor, we developed the CSNAP3D algorithm as a CSNAP extension. CSNAP3D searches chemical structure using the "ShapeAlign" protocol, which utilizes a combination of shape and pharmacophore descriptors. We found that CSNAP3D improves target prediction, particularly for challenging drug classes such as HIVRT NNRTIs that showed high structural diversity and are scaffold hopping ligands. Finally, we successfully applied CSNAP3D to rationally discover low molecular weight taxol mimetics, which exhibit a taxol-like anticancer mechanism and potentially possess improved transport and pharmacokinetic properties than its natural counterpart.

The current CSNAP framework can be extended in several directions. For instance, consensus scoring can be expanded by considering higher-order neighbors, which has been demonstrated to improve prediction accuracy in PPI networks. Similarly, graph theoretical approaches based on maximum network flow and other global optimization approaches can be applied for target assignments [35]. To improve posttarget validation, high throughput functional genomics data can be incorporated to aid in the identification of critical targets relevant to a disease pathway. One example is multiplayer network approaches that integrate drug, target, and annotation interaction networks to enhance target predictions and validations [36]. While CSNAP3D has substantially improved the predictability of CSNAP2D, the algorithm is limited to receptors with bound ligands and the ligand alignment is based on the lowest energy conformer. This shortcoming can be circumvented by considering multi-conformer networks that correlate ligand conformation with target specificities. Likewise, pseudo-ligands generated as the mirror image of an orphan receptor can be considered for receptor deorphanization.

In conclusion, chemical similarity networks are an emerging field in ligand-based drug discovery where the collective properties of a ligand can be easily dissected using descriptive network statistics and graph topology. Here, we presented a new network-based approach for drug discovery and target identification called chemical similarity network analysis pull-down (CSNAP) and a new CSNAP framework called CSNAP3D. The CSNAP computational framework represents a new concept in computational drug discovery with practical application in target identification and drug discovery. We anticipate that the CSNAP approach will stimulate further work in systems and network-based drug discovery that will aid in the discovery of novel drugs for the treatment of cancer and other important diseases.

Author details

Yu-Chen Lo[1] and Jorge Z. Torres[2*]

*Address all correspondence to: torres@chem.ucla.edu

1 Department of Bioengineering, Stanford University, Stanford, CA, USA

2 Department of Chemistry and Biochemistry, University of California, Los Angeles, CA, USA

References

[1] Yan X, Liao C, Liu Z, Hagler AT, Gu Q, Xu J. Chemical structure similarity search for ligand-based virtual screening: methods and computational resources. Current Drug Targets. 2015, Vol. 16, 1p.

[2] Willett P. Chemoinformatics—similarity and diversity in chemical libraries. Current Opinion in Biotechnology. 2000;11(1):85–8.

[3] Maggiora G, Vogt M, Stumpfe D, Bajorath J. Molecular similarity in medicinal chemistry. Journal of Medicinal Chemistry. 2014;57(8):3186–204.

[4] Faulon J-L, Bender A. Handbook of chemoinformatics algorithms. Boca Raton, FL: Chapman & Hall/CRC; 2010. xii, 440 p.

[5] Gasteiger J. Handbook of chemoinformatics: from data to knowledge. Weinheim: Wiley-VCH; 2003.

[6] Lee JK. Statistical bioinformatics: a guide for life and biomedical science researchers. Hoboken, NJ: Wiley-Blackwell; 2010. xiv, 350 p., 20 p. of plates p.

[7] Baldi P, Benz RW. BLASTing small molecules--statistics and extreme statistics of chemical similarity scores. Bioinformatics. 2008;24(13):i357–65.

[8] Consonni V, Todeschini R, Pavan M, Gramatica P. Structure/response correlations and similarity/diversity analysis by GETAWAY descriptors. 2. Application of the novel 3D molecular descriptors to QSAR/QSPR studies. Journal of Chemical Information and Computer Science. 2002;42(3):693–705.

[9] Devinyak O, Havrylyuk D, Lesyk R. 3D-MoRSE descriptors explained. Journal of Molecular Graphics and Modelling. 2014;54:194–203.

[10] Hopkins AL. Network pharmacology. Nature Biotechnology. 2007;25(10):1110–1.

[11] Lounkine E, Keiser MJ, Whitebread S, Mikhailov D, Hamon J, Jenkins JL, et al. Large-scale prediction and testing of drug activity on side-effect targets. Nature. 2012;486(7403):361–7.

[12] Gaulton A, Bellis LJ, Bento AP, Chambers J, Davies M, Hersey A, et al. ChEMBL: a large-scale bioactivity database for drug discovery. Nucleic Acids Research. 2012;40(Database issue):D1100–7.

[13] Li Q, Cheng T, Wang Y, Bryant SH. PubChem as a public resource for drug discovery. Drug Discovery Today. 2010;15(23–24):1052–7.

[14] Wishart DS, Knox C, Guo AC, Shrivastava S, Hassanali M, Stothard P, et al. DrugBank: a comprehensive resource for in silico drug discovery and exploration. Nucleic Acids Research. 2006;34(Database issue):D668–72.

[15] Lo YC, Senese S, Li CM, Hu Q, Huang Y, Damoiseaux R, et al. Large-scale chemical similarity networks for target profiling of compounds identified in cell-based chemical screens. PLoS Computational Biology. 2015;11(3):e1004153.

[16] Schwikowski B, Uetz P, Fields S. A network of protein-protein interactions in yeast. Nature Biotechnology. 2000;18(12):1257–61.

[17] Lo YC, Senese S, Damoiseaux R, Torres JZ. 3D chemical similarity networks for structure-based target prediction and Scaffold hopping. ACS Chemical Biology. 2016;11(8):2244–53.

[18] Aretz I, Meierhofer D. Advantages and pitfalls of mass spectrometry based metabolome profiling in systems biology. International Journal of Molecular Sciences. 2016;17:632.

[19] Kolaczyk ED. Statistical analysis of network data: methods and models. New York; London: Springer; 2009. xii, 386 p.

[20] Ashburner M, Ball CA, Blake JA, Botstein D, Butler H, Cherry JM, et al. Gene ontology: tool for the unification of biology. The Gene Ontology Consortium. Nature Genetics. 2000;25(1):25–9.

[21] Mysinger MM, Carchia M, Irwin JJ, Shoichet BK. Directory of useful decoys, enhanced (DUD-E): better ligands and decoys for better benchmarking. Journal of Medicinal Chemistry. 2012;55(14):6582–94.

[22] Keiser MJ, Roth BL, Armbruster BN, Ernsberger P, Irwin JJ, Shoichet BK. Relating protein pharmacology by ligand chemistry. Nature Biotechnology. 2007;25(2):197–206.

[23] Senese S, Lo YC, Huang D, Zangle TA, Gholkar AA, Robert L, et al. Chemical dissection of the cell cycle: probes for cell biology and anti-cancer drug development. Cell Death & Disease. 2014;5:e1462.

[24] Li CM, Lu Y, Ahn S, Narayanan R, Miller DD, Dalton JT. Competitive mass spectrometry binding assay for characterization of three binding sites of tubulin. Journal of Mass Spectrometry. 2010;45(10):1160–6.

[25] Schneider G, Neidhart W, Giller T, Schmid G. "Scaffold-Hopping" by topological pharmacophore search: a contribution to virtual screening. Angewandte Chemie, International Edition in English. 1999;38(19):2894–6.

[26] Sun H, Tawa G, Wallqvist A. Classification of scaffold-hopping approaches. Drug Discovery Today. 2012;17(7–8):310–24.

[27] Yan X, Li J, Liu Z, Zheng M, Ge H, Xu J. Enhancing molecular shape comparison by weighted Gaussian functions. Journal of Chemical Information and Modeling. 2013;53(8):1967–78.

[28] Cruciani G. Molecular interaction fields: applications in drug discovery and ADME prediction. Weinheim: Wiley-VCH; 2006. xviii, 307 p.

[29] Liu X, Ouyang S, Yu B, Liu Y, Huang K, Gong J, et al. PharmMapper server: a web server for potential drug target identification using pharmacophore mapping approach. Nucleic Acids Research. 2010;38(Web Server issue):W609–14.

[30] Taminau J, Thijs G, De Winter H. Pharao: pharmacophore alignment and optimization. Journal of Molecular Graphics and Modelling. 2008;27(2):161–9.

[31] Zhan P, Chen X, Li D, Fang Z, De Clercq E, Liu X. HIV-1 NNRTIs: structural diversity, pharmacophore similarity, and implications for drug design. Medicinal Research Reviews. 2013;33(Suppl 1):E1–72.

[32] Renneberg R. Biotech History: Yew trees, paclitaxel synthesis and fungi. Biotechnology Journal. 2007;2(10):1207–9.

[33] Haggarty SJ, Mayer TU, Miyamoto DT, Fathi R, King RW, Mitchison TJ, et al. Dissecting cellular processes using small molecules: identification of colchicine-like, taxol-like and other small molecules that perturb mitosis. Chemistry & Biology. 2000;7(4):275–86.

[34] Shintani Y, Tanaka T, Nozaki Y. GS-164, a small synthetic compound, stimulates tubulin polymerization by a similar mechanism to that of taxol. Cancer Chemotherapy and Pharmacology. 1997;40(6):513–20.

[35] Jungnickel D. Graphs, networks, and algorithms. Fourth edition. ed. Heidelberg; New York: Springer; 2013. xx, 675 p.

[36] Berenstein AJ, Magarinos MP, Chernomoretz A, Aguero F. A multilayer network approach for guiding drug repositioning in neglected diseases. PLoS Neglected Tropical Diseases. 2016;10(1):e0004300.

2

Pharmacologic Interventions for Preventing Chondrocyte Apoptosis in Rheumatoid Arthritis and Osteoarthritis

Charles J. Malemud

Abstract

Chronic inflammation drives the progression of rheumatoid arthritis (RA) and osteoarthritis (OA) to synovial joint failure. The inflammatory state in both musculoskeletal diseases is associated with significantly elevated levels of pro-inflammatory cytokines in joint synovial fluid, which is best exemplified by increases in interleukin-1β (IL-1β), IL-6, IL-17, tumor necrosis factor-α, among others, as well as increased activity of soluble mediators such as nitric oxide and certain growth factors including vascular endothelial growth factor and fibroblast growth factor. The multitude of these factors activate chondrocyte signal transduction pathways resulting in programmed cell death, otherwise known as apoptosis as well as compromising chondrocyte autophagy. Importantly, chondrocyte apoptosis causes a loss of articular cartilage vitality which dampens cartilage repair mechanisms because at present, the possibility that chondrocyte progenitor cells could replace those differentiated chondrocytes lost via apoptosis remains debatable. Certain pharmacologic interventions which have been proven to induce apoptosis in various cancer cell studies *in vitro* suggest the possibility that drugs could be developed to specifically suppress or completely inhibit chondrocyte apoptosis in RA and OA cartilage. This review supports that contention and indicates that apoptosis can be inhibited by identifying novel cellular targets which promote apoptosis and autophagy.

Keywords: apoptosis, chondrocyte, osteoarthritis, rheumatoid arthritis, signal transduction

1. Introduction

Controlled cell death otherwise known as programmed cell death or apoptosis constitutes a critical event which is germane to the normal development of the immune system, the appropriate integration of cells within tissues and organs and organ homeostasis [1–7]. However, the aberrant frequency of apoptotic cells can compromise normal tissue architecture and, in doing so, contribute to the loss of cell vitality [8–10]. This is especially the case in explaining the loss of chondrocyte viability in arthritic conditions of synovial joints, such as rheumatoid arthritis (RA) and osteoarthritis (OA).

Significant progress has been achieved over the previous decade or so in furthering our understanding of the cellular and molecular events that trigger the increased frequency of chondrocyte apoptosis in RA and OA [11–16]. These advances include (1) an appreciation that the significant increase in the levels of pro-inflammatory cytokines in synovial fluid from RA and OA patients also can induce chondrocyte apoptosis *in vitro* [17–21]; (2) that the elevated frequency of chondrocyte apoptosis by these cytokines is deregulated by altered signal transduction which can involve continuous activation of stress-activated/mitogen-activated protein kinases (SAPK/MAPK) [22–25], the Janus kinase/Signal Transducers and Activators of Transcription (JAK/STAT) pathway [26–31], the phosphatidylinositide-3-kinase/Akt/mammalian target of rapamycin (PI3K/Akt/mTOR) pathway [32–36], and other protein kinase pathways [37–40]; (3) that specific co-factors are capable of regulating the activation of these signaling pathways [41–44]; and (4) that micro-RNAs (mi-RNAs) can regulate the activity of these co-factors and, in this manner, control the induction of apoptosis via these signaling pathways [45–48].

Furthermore, the increased frequency of chondrocyte apoptosis now confirmed in guinea pig OA cartilage [49] as well as human RA and OA articular cartilage [50–53] presents a particularly onerous scenario for the survival of synovial joints under these conditions. Although a population of chondroprogenitor cells was identified in several studies of adult normal and diseased articular cartilage [54–56], significant repair of damaged articular cartilage in RA and OA by these cells is effete. This effect on cartilage repair may result from elevated levels of pro-inflammatory cytokines such as IL-17, which was recently shown to inhibit the chondrocyte maturation lineage emanating from progenitor cells in RA [57]. Therefore, even if chondrocyte precursor cells exist in adult articular cartilage which could potentially become authentic chondrocytes lost from articular cartilage via apoptosis or chondrocytes lost via diffusion of cartilage extracellular matrix fragments into synovial fluid, the reduction in chondrocyte vitality via apoptosis would be a challenging event to overcome, especially in a synovial joint microenvironment replete with pro-inflammatory cytokines.

In this chapter, we have systematically examined the mechanistic underpinning for identifying novel targets in order to suppress or even inhibit chondrocyte apoptosis in RA and OA. However, the scenario in RA, in particular, is even more complex than in OA because in the context of devising therapeutic strategies designed to inhibit chondrocyte apoptosis in RA, one must also take into account the fact that in the hyperplastic RA synovial tissue, comprised of activated synoviocytes, immune cells, macrophages and other inflammatory cells are generally considered to be relatively "apoptosis-resistant" [58, 59]. Thus, this characteristic of the RA joint ensures a plentiful source of immune-mediated cells and non-immune inflammatory cells which drive the progression of RA. It is also likely that at some time during the course of the progression of OA, immune-mediated inflammation may also cause a similar chronic inflammatory microenvironment, as found in RA, to arise and persist in OA synovial tissue [55] resulting, in part, in an increased frequency of apoptotic chondrocytes [60].

2. Compelling evidence that many factors relevant to RA and OA promote or induce chondrocyte apoptosis *in vitro*

Analyses of synovial fluids and sera from RA and OA patients with active disease showed that these samples contained significantly elevated levels of various pro-inflammatory cytokines and growth factors when compared to a control group [52–68]. Of note, incubation of rat [69], non-arthritic or human chondrocytes from OA cartilage [70–76] or immortalized lines of human chondrocytes [77] with physiological levels of these cytokines, growth factors (e.g., VEGF and FGF) or additional soluble mediators (e.g., nitric oxide) were shown to induce apoptosis, which was accompanied by activation of SAPK/MAPK, JAK/STAT or PI3K/Akt/mTor signaling in these cells [78–81]. In addition, mediators of inflammation, including prostaglandin E_2 and neuropeptides (e.g., Substance P), are also implicated in perpetuating chronic inflammation [38]. The induction of apoptosis was also shown to be related to altered levels of various down-regulators of apoptosis. These included BCL-2-like protein-11 (Bim) [18], B-cell lymphoma-2 (Bcl-2) [75], cell-derived inhibitors of apoptosis proteins (IAPs) [81–84] and Suppressor of Cytokine Synthesis (SOCS) [85, 86]. Furthermore, alterations in the functions of mitochondria [87] and endoplasmic reticulum (ER) [88–91] related to cell stress, the generation of reactive oxygen species [92] and the recently described advanced oxidation protein products [93] with respect to their capacity to induce apoptosis were reported as well. Taken together, these results provided compelling evidence that pro-inflammatory cytokines, growth factors and soluble mediators germane to the progression of RA and OA are responsible for inducing chondrocyte apoptosis in these conditions.

3. The relationship between apoptosis and autophagy

A recent review of RA pathogenesis by Angelotti et al. [94] emphasized the view that numerous cells comprising the innate immune system, including macrophages, dendritic cells, mast cells, natural killer cells and neutrophils as well as T-cells and B-cells, regulators of adaptive immunity, are primarily responsible for perpetuating the state of chronic inflammation through their capacity to alter the survival of resident synovial fibroblasts. It is also likely that such cell combinations are also involved in the progression of OA as well, as evidenced by the skewing of cartilage homeostasis toward catabolism, and the loss of chondrocyte vitality via the induction of apoptosis [95–97]. However, it was previously shown that the classical apoptosis cascade can be activated by various pro-inflammatory cytokines, and certain growth factors, chemokines, chemokine receptors (**Table 1**) and other interleukins, including

IL-8 (CXCL8) and adhesion molecules [64]. Thus, these factors are likely to be the most influential in inducing apoptosis pathway RA. However, a non-classical form of apoptosis, termed, "chondroptosis" is just as likely to be activated in OA. In that regard, "chondroptosis" involves an increase in the number of ER and Golgi apparatus reflecting an increase in protein synthesis that accompanies the loss of viable chondrocytes [98].

Furthermore, changes in the number of viable articular chondrocytes in experimentally induced arthritis [99], human RA [100], and OA are almost certainly associated with the autophagic-mediated cell death of chondrocytes [101–105], which occurs in concert with the activation of the extrinsic apoptosis pathway, the latter mediated by Tumor necrosis Factor-Related Apoptosis-Inducing Ligand (TRAIL), Death Receptor-5 (DR5) and caspase-3 [106, 107]. In that regard, it was noteworthy that Huang et al. [108] reported that exogenous leptin promoted chondrocyte apoptosis while inhibiting chondrocyte autophagy via the up-regulation of lysyl oxidase-like 3 (LOXL3). Thus, in their study [108], overexpression of LOXL3 inhibited chondrocyte autophagy by activating mechanistic target of rapamycin complex-1 (mTORC1) [36]. In contrast, cartilage-specific

Cytokine, chemokine, chemokine receptors and growth factors	Reference
IL-17, IL-18BP	[62]
IL-17, IL-20, IL-21	[63]
IL-7	[64]
IL-12/IL-23	[64]
IL-15/IL-16	[64]
IL-17/IL-18	[64]
IL-19/-20/-21	[64]
IL-32	[64]
VEGF[1]; TGF-β_1[2]; Leptin; FGF[3]	[64–66]
CXCR3; CXCR4,-5; CXCR-1,-5,-6; IL-8; MIP-1α[4]; GRO-α[5](CXCL1); GRO-$\beta\gamma$[6]; MCP-1[7]; RANTES[8]; Eotaxin-1	[65, 68]
IL-6	[64, 67, 68]
TNF-α	[64, 67, 69]
IL-1β	[64]

[1]Vascular endothelial growth factor.
[2]Transforming growth factor-β_1.
[3]Fibroblast growth factor.
[4]Macrophage inflammatory protein-1 (CCL3).
[5]Growth-related oncogene-α.
[6]GRO-$\beta\gamma$.
[7]Monocyte chemotactic protein-1.
[8]Regulated on activation, normal T-cell expressed and secreted.

Table 1. Cytokines, chemokines, chemokine receptors and growth factors in RA and OA.

deletion of mTOR resulted in the up-regulation of autophagy [102]. Autophagy protected mouse cartilage from degeneration [109]. Autophagy was also shown to protect chondrocytes from glucocorticoid-induced apoptosis via reactive oxygen species, Akt and FOXO3 signaling [110] as well as from advanced glycation end-product-induced apoptosis which was accompanied by lower levels of MMP-3 and MMP-13 in rat chondrocyte cultures [111].

4. Do micro-RNAs play a critical role in chondrocyte apoptosis?

Micro-RNAs (miRs) are critical mediators of mRNA degradation as well acting as repressors of translation. MiRs have been implicated in the development of skeletal long bones via their multiple effects on osteogenesis [112]. However, recent evidence has also improved the recognized role of miRs in RA pathology as a result of evidence that many miRs including miR-16, miR-146a/b, miR-150, miR-155 and miR-223 are over-expressed both in the peripheral circulation of RA patients and in the RA synovial joint [113], although other miRs relevant to RA, such as miR-21, miR-125a, miR-223, and miR-451 are principally found to be at elevated levels in the plasma and sera of RA patients.

Additional evidence has been presented to show that several of these miRs also regulate apoptosis. For example, the level of the pro-apoptotic protein, Bim, was increased when activated T-cells were incubated with a repressor of miR-148a resulting in an increase in the Th1 apoptotic response [114]. Thus, accumulating evidence showed that both the immune cells and chondrocyte apoptotic and autophagic response can be manipulated by either experimental overexpression or repression of various miRs which are relevant to OA [115] and RA [116] pathophysiology.

The results of numerous studies have confirmed the role of specific miRs as directly affecting apoptosis or indirectly affecting apoptosis through their activity on other molecules that regulate chondrocyte apoptosis. For example, mIR-146a was reported to be over-expressed in OA [117]. In that regard, mIR-146a was shown to promote human OA chondrocyte proliferation and to inhibit apoptosis by targeting tumor necrosis factor receptor-associated factor 6 (TRAF6) via NF-κB [118, 119]. By contrast, mIR-146a was also shown to target IL-1β, to induce VEGF production, and to promote rat chondrocyte apoptosis via Smad4 [120]. On the other hand, silencing of miR-34a inhibited rat chondrocyte apoptosis [121], whereas overexpression of mIR-34a promoted apoptosis in normal human chondrocytes by targeting SIRT1/p53 signaling [122], although other evidences indicated that miR-34a was increased in intervertebral disc degeneration and was associated with an elevated frequency of apoptotic cartilage end plate chondrocytes [123]. In another study, glycerol-3-phosphate dehydrogenase 1-like protein was shown to be a target for mIR-181a, which is deregulated in OA wherein human chondrocyte apoptosis was increased [124]. In yet another study, phosphatase and tensin homolog deleted on chromosome 10 (PTEN) [36] was identified as the target for mIR-181 whereby mIR-181 up-regulated the expression of proteins associated with apoptosis, including caspase-3 and PARP. However, mIR-181 also up-regulated MMP-2 (gelatinase A; 72 kDa gelatinase) and MMP-9 (gelatinase B; 92 kDa gelatinase) [125] which are two MMPs directly relevant to cartilage matrix protein degradation in arthritis [126].

Of note, several miRs were identified as potential targets for inducing chondrocyte survival and therefore could be considered anti-apoptosis factors; these included mIR-98 [127–129], mIR-9 [130], mIR-15a-5p [131], mIR-142-3p [132] and mIR-502-5p [133]. Additional mIRs, exemplified by miR-195 [134], mIR-139 [135], mIR-29b-3p [136], mIR-488-3p [137] and mIR-203 [138] could very well be included in this group. For example, by employing the C28/I2 line of immortalized human chondrocytes, Zhao et al. [138] showed that knockdown of mIR-203 targeting the myeloid cell leukemia-1 (MCL-1) protein activated Wnt/β-catenin and JAK/STAT signaling promoted chondrocyte survival.

To summarize this section, gaining a further understanding of how to manipulate specific mIRs to achieve increased or decreased synthesis of specific targets known to influence chondrocyte apoptosis may signal the next major advance in targeted OA and RA therapy designed to promote chondrocyte survival.

5. Pharmacologic interventions designed to specifically inhibit chondrocyte apoptosis

5.1. Signal transduction pathways

Lewis and Malemud [82] previously reviewed several potential pharmacologic strategies designed to limit the loss of chondrocyte vitality via apoptosis. These included, targeting x-linked inhibitor of apoptosis (XIAP), tumor necrosis factor-like weak inducer of apoptosis (TWEAK), TRAIL, decoy-receptor-3 (DcR3), tumor necrosis factor receptor protein-like molecules, p53 up-regulated modulator of apoptosis (PUMA), and apoptosis-signal-regulating kinases. In that regard, we proposed several interventional strategies which we acknowledged involved developing a deeper understanding of which signal transduction pathways were altered in RA and OA chondrocytes [19, 28, 36, 77, 82, 106]. For example, XIAP, an inhibitor of activated caspase-9, and caspases-3 and -7 [82] was also shown to interact with mitogen-activated protein kinase kinase 2 (MEKK2) [139]. The interaction between XIAP and MEKK2 resulted in a biphasic activation of NF-κB, a known downstream effector of TNF-α-mediated apoptosis. This finding is relevant to the regulation of chondrocyte apoptosis in both RA and OA primarily because XIAP is a well-known inhibitor of apoptosis protein-3 (IAP3) [140]. In fact, we had previously shown that recombinant human TNF-α (rhTNF-α) induced human chondrocyte apoptosis via activation of p38, JNK1/2 and STAT3 [72], whereas apoptosis of the immortalized human chondrocyte line, C-28/I2 induced by rhTNF-α, but not by rhIL-6, was dependent on upstream MEK1/2 [77]. Therefore, we posit that in order to consider using potential drug interventions that alter the activation of various signaling pathways it will be useful to consider what we know about how alterations in receptor-mediated signaling pathways (reviewed in [19]) may influence apoptosis.

Activation of SAPK/MAPK signaling is most often associated with induction of chondrocyte apoptosis. Thus, induction of rabbit articular chondrocyte apoptosis by the nitric oxide (NO) donor sodium nitroprusside (SNP) was linked to inhibition of c-Jun-amino-terminal kinase (JNK) by virtue of the finding that the JNK small molecule inhibitor (SMI) SP600125, reduced the frequency of apoptotic chondrocytes along with NO-induced NF-κB, p53 and caspase-3 [141]. IL-1β, another potent inducer of chondrocyte apoptosis, was also shown to be JNK-dependent as both chemical inhibitors of JNK as well as RNA interference with Bim, the latter up-regulated by IL-1β, were shown to be phosphorylated-JNK-dependent [142]. In other studies, chondrocyte apoptosis was again linked to IL-1β-induced activation of p38 kinase [143–145], along with JNK [145], and MMP-3 gene expression with IL-1β negatively regulating chondrocyte autophagy [145]. Of note, AG490, a pan-JAK SMI significantly reduced leptin-induced chondrocyte apoptosis *in vitro* as well as reducing STAT3 phosphorylation, reactive oxygen species, MMP-13 and B-cell lymphoma 2-associated X protein [146]. Interestingly, Li et al. [147] showed that the PI3K/NF-κB pathway was activated by TNF-α in human chondrocytes. However, the effect of leptin did not involve mTOR, suggesting that newly developed small molecule mTOR inhibitors (reviewed in [36]) might not be useful for neutralizing activated PI3K/NF-κB in response to leptin-induced apoptosis.

Several attempts to employ various compounds and/or natural products to inhibit chondrocyte apoptosis have taken advantage of various findings related to the role of these compounds and natural products in many of the aforementioned signal transduction pathways. For example, IL-1β-induced chondrocyte apoptosis was inhibited by oligomeric proanthocyanidin, a water-soluble plant polyphenolic compound [148]. Thus, the over-expression of peroxiredoxin 4 (PRDX4), a member of the PRDX family (a molecule essential for scavenging free radicals and reducing reactive oxygen species) reduced IL-1β-induced rat chondrocyte apoptosis [149]. Importantly, AZD5363, an inhibitor of Akt activation also reduced the apoptosis protective effect of PRDX4. In another aspect, chondrocyte apoptosis induced by IL-1β not only involved reduced Bcl-2 levels, activated (i.e., phosphorylated) Akt, and activated PRAS40, a proline-rich 40 kDa Akt substrate and an inhibitor of mTORC1 kinase activity, but was also linked to increasing the levels of Bax, and activated caspase-3/-9 [149].

Shikonin, a compound with anti-tumor, anti-inflammatory, anti-viral and pharmacological efficacy significantly inhibited apoptosis by decreasing IL-1β, TNF-α and inducible NO synthase (iNOS) in rats with experimentally induced OA [150]. The effect of shikonin in this animal model of OA was accompanied not only by reduced caspase-3 and cyclooxygenase-2 activity but also by increased activation of Akt, indicating a prominent role for PI3K/Akt signaling in this rat model of OA. Finally, a few novel targets, including protein kinase R-like endoplasmic reticulum kinase and activating transcription factor 6, were identified as potent regulators of chondrocyte apoptosis *in vitro* and *in vivo* [151], although the precise signaling mechanisms attributed to these molecules have yet to be completely established.

5.2. Additional potential targets related to apoptosis

Several experimental studies, of note, have focused on several cellular components which may eventually become suitable pharmacologic targets for altering chondrocyte apoptosis and/or autophagy in osteoarthritis (**Table 2**). However, the results of these mainly *in vitro* studies point out why it will be necessary to determine the underlying mechanisms regarding how these factors work to inhibit apoptosis. Thus, only after successful evaluation in animal models of RA and OA, can we envision that these targets could eventually be employed in a clinical setting.

Factor	Target	Reference
HIF-1α/HIF-2α[1]	HIF-1α—SOX9; HIF-2α—Fas	[152]
Integrin-β1	G1T1[2]	[153]
IGFBP-3[3]	Nur77[4]	[154]
SGBT[5]	Caspase-3/Hsp70[6]	[155]
UCP4[7]	ROS[8]	[156]
DEL1[9]	Caspase-3/Caspase-7	[157]
Rela[10]	Pik3r1[11]	[158]
Beclin[12]	Bcl-2; Bcl-2 associated X	[159]
AST[13]	LC3-II/I[14]; P62/SQSTM1[15]	[160]
AQP-1[16]	Caspase-3	[161]
Mt1/Mt2[17]	ROS[8]	[162]
Sirt1[18]	Bcl-2; Bax	[163]

[1]Hypoxia-inducible factor-1α/-2α.
[2]G-protein-coupled receptor kinase interacting protein-1.
[3]Insulin-like growth factor-1 binding protein-3.
[4]Nerve growth factor 1B.
[5]Small glutamine-rich tetratricopeptide repeat-containing β.
[6]Heat shock protein-70.
[7]Uncoupling protein-4.
[8]Reactive oxygen species.
[9]Developmental endothelial locus-1.
[10]RelA/p65 of NF-κB complex.
[11]Pik3r1 encodes a p85α regulatory protein that is a subunit of phosphatidylinositol 3-kinase (PI3K).
[12]Beclin-1, a product of the *BECN1* gene is a mammalian ortholog of the yeast autophagy-related gene 6 (Atg6) and BEC-1 in the *C. elegans* nematode.
[13]Astragaloside IV.
[14]Microtubule-associated protein 1A/1B-light chain-I/II.
[15]P62/sequestosome-1.
[16]Aquaporin-1.
[17]Metallothionein-1/metallothionein-2.
[18]Silent information regulation of transcription 1.

Table 2. Cellular factors that regulate chondrocyte apoptosis and/or autophagy *in vitro*.

6. Conclusions and future perspectives

It is now generally agreed upon by many investigators that a chronic state of inflammation is, in part, responsible for driving and perpetuating the progression of RA (reviewed in [94]) and OA (reviewed in [58, 164]). Moreover, additional recent evidence has indicated that both apoptosis and an altered state of autophagy are critical events in chronic musculoskeletal disorders, such as RA and OA [60, 102–105, 164–167]. Although the loss of chondrocyte vitality is a common pathological finding in RA and OA, cellular mechanisms that result in synovial fibroblast and immune-cell-mediated "apoptosis-resistance," such as those that were found to underlie B-cell activity in RA [168–171], aids in distinguishing between the fundamental underpinning responsible for bony abnormalities in the two conditions. However, equally important is that the increased frequency of apoptotic chondrocytes in both RA and OA constitutes a major contributor to inefficient cartilage repair and synovial joint failure. We contend that any pharmacologic strategies designed to simultaneously target the "apoptosis-resistance" in the RA hyperplastic synovial tissue and the elevated frequency of chondrocyte apoptosis would be an onerous undertaking. So for the present, concentrating on developing agents that suppress or inhibit chondrocyte apoptosis might be the initial way to proceed. For example, the current literature on this subject has already indicated that certain drugs used in the medical therapy of RA suppress chondrocyte apoptosis *in vitro*. In that regard, the drug sulphasalazine, commonly employed in combination with methotrexate, for treating RA [172] was found to inhibit rabbit chondrocyte apoptosis induced by SNP [173]. In this study, the reduced frequency of chondrocyte apoptosis was accompanied by an increase in phosphorylated p38 kinase and ERK1/2 expression compared to treatment of chondrocytes with SNP alone.

Another area worthy of consideration is to employ *in vitro* studies to, in effect, rule out for further considerations for developing drugs for treating potential targets of chondrocyte apoptosis. A suitable example of this strategy was a recent finding by Nasi et al. [174] that the NALP3 inflammasome (reviewed in [175]) was not involved in chondrocyte apoptosis characteristic of several alterations in cartilage characteristically found in a murine menisectomy model of OA. Although alterations in the structure of articular cartilage such as cartilage destruction, synovial inflammation, cell death and calcification were seen in this OA animal model, a deficiency in IL-1α had no impact on these features. Importantly, deficiencies in IL-1β and NALP3 actually resulted in an enhancement of cartilage damage in this OA animal model.

The suppression or more favorably the complete inhibition of chondrocyte apoptosis in RA and OA using pharmacologic interventional strategies would be a laudable achievement in the continuing search for novel disease-modifying-anti-rheumatic drugs. A variety of potential novel targets have now been identified during the previous 3 years that at least employing cancer cells induces the frequency of apoptosis. Thus, targets have been identified to induce apoptosis in these cancers and therefore, may be eventually exploited for blocking chondrocyte apoptosis. For example, the activity of 2,5-dihydroxy-3-undecyl-1,4 benzoquinone, 6 g, also known as embelin was reviewed [82] as an inducer of apoptosis in inflammatory breast cancer cells and pancreatic cancer cells. Embelin was also shown to block the transcription of several gene products relevant to tumor cell survival, proliferation, invasiveness and metastatic cancer cell proliferation. Of note, treatment with non-toxic concentrations of embelin could also sensitize cultured malignant glioma to TRAIL-induced apoptosis [176]. Lewis and Malemud [82] reviewed the findings showing that embelin blocked the activation of NF-κB, RANKL and, STAT3, the latter finding demonstrating "proof-of-principle" that STAT3-activated transcription could also be employed to probe the extent to which this signaling pathway was required for maintaining chondrocyte survival *in vitro* [177]. In that regard, these pre-clinical results may provide a suitable platform for exploiting the overall objective of preventing synovial joint failure in RA and OA through the maintenance of normal articular chondrocyte viability and cartilage integrity.

Acknowledgements

The results of experimental studies cited in Refs. [70, 72, 77, 80] were supported in part by grants from the National Institutes of Health, Takeda Pharmaceuticals of North America and Genentech/Roche Group.

Author details

Charles J. Malemud

Address all correspondence to: cjm4@cwru.edu

Department of Medicine, Division of Rheumatic Diseases, Case Western Reserve University School of Medicine/University Hospitals Cleveland Medical Center, Cleveland, Ohio, USA

References

[1] Reed JC. Bcl-2 and the regulation of programmed cell death. Journal of Cell Biology. 1994;**124**:1-6. PMCID: PMC2119888

[2] Ashkenazi A, Dixit M. Death receptors: Signaling and modulation. Science. 1998;**281**:1305-1308. PMID: 9721089

[3] Opferman JT, Letia A, Beard C, et al. Development and maintenance of B and T lymphocytes requires antiapoptotic MCL-1. Nature. 2003;**426**:671-676. DOI: 10.1038/nature02067

[4] Schultz DR, Harrington WJ Jr. Apoptosis: Programmed cell death at a molecular level. Seminars in Arthritis & Rheumatism. 2003;**32**:345-369. DOI: 10.1053/sarh.2003.50005

[5] Starr TK, Jameson SC, Hogquist KA. Positive and negative selection of T cells. Annual Review of Immunology. 2003;**21**:139-176. DOI: 10.1146/annurev.immunol.21.120601.141107

[6] Hernandez JB, Newton RH, Walsh CM. Life and death in the thymus—Cell death signaling during T cell development. Current Opinion in Cell Biology. 2010;**22**:865-871. DOI: 10.1016/j.ceb.2010.08.003

[7] Malemud CJ. Immunotherapies and rheumatoid arthritis-introduction. Journal of Clinical and Cellular Immunology. 2013;**S6**:e001

[8] Wolfer A, Wilson A, Nemir M, et al. Inactivation of Notch1 impairs VDJβ rearrangement and allows pre-TCR-independent survival of early αβ lineage thymocytes. Immunity. 2002;**16**:869-879. PMID: 12121668

[9] Schultzke JD, Bojarski C, Zeissig S, et al. Disrupted barrier function through epithelial cell apoptosis. Annals of the New York Academy of Sciences. 2006;**1072**:288-299. DOI: 10.1196/annals.1326.027

[10] Beug ST, Cheung HH, LaCasse EC, et al. Modulation of immune signaling by inhibitors of apoptosis. Trends in Immunology. 2012;**33**:535-545. DOI: 10.1016/j.it.2012.06.004

[11] Liu H, Pope RM. Apoptosis in rheumatoid arthritis: Friend or foe. Rheumatic Disease Clinics of North America. 2004;**30**:603-625. DOI: 10.1016/j.rdc.2004.04.010

[12] Malemud CJ, Gillespie HJ. The role of apoptosis in arthritis. Current Rheumatology Reviews. 2005;**1**:131-142

[13] Korb A, Pavenstädt H, Pap T. Cell death in rheumatoid arthritis. Apoptosis. 2009;**14**:447-454. DOI: 10.1007/s10495-009-0317-y

[14] Kim HA, Blanco FJ. Cell death and apoptosis in osteoarthritis. Current Drug Targets. 2007;**8**:333-345. PMID: 17305511

[15] Del Carlo M Jr, Loesser RF. Cell death in osteoarthritis. Current Rheumatology Reports. 2008;**10**:37-42. PMID: 18457610

[16] Zamli Z, Sharif M. Chondrocyte apoptosis: A cause or consequence of osteoarthritis. International Journal of Rheumatic Diseases. 2011;**14**:159-166. DOI: 10.1111/j.1756-185X.2011.01618.x

[17] Cope AP, Schultze-Koops H, Aringer AM. The central role of T cells in rheumatoid arthritis. Clinical and Experimental Rheumatology. 2007;**5**(Suppl 46):S4-S11. PMID: 17977483

[18] Hutcheson J, Perlman H. Apoptotic regulators and RA. Current Rheumatology Reviews. 2008;**4**:254-258

[19] Malemud CJ. Recent advances in neutralizing the IL-6 pathway in arthritis. Open Access Rheumatology: Research and Reviews. 2009;**1**:133-150. PMID: 27789987

[20] Charlier E, Relic B, Deroyer C, et al. Insights on the mechanisms of chondrocyte death in osteoarthritis. International Journal of Molecular Sciences. 2016;**17**. pii. E2146. DOI: 10.3390.ijms17122146

[21] Wu L, Liu Z. The molecular mechanisms of preventing apoptosis of cartilage chondrocyte to target osteoarthritis. Future Medicinal Chemistry. 2017;**9**:537-540. DOI: 10.4155/fmc-2017-0034

[22] Kühn K, Shikhman AR, Lotz M. Role of nitric acid, reactive oxygen species, and 38 MAP kinase in the regulation of human chondrocyte apoptosis. Journal of Cellular Physiology. 2003;**197**:379-387. DOI: 10.1002/jcp.10372

[23] Deng Y, Ren X, Yang L, et al. A JNK-dependent pathway is required for TNF-α-induced apoptosis. Cell. 2003;**115**:61-70 14532003

[24] Asquith DL, McInnes IB. Emerging cytokine targets in rheumatoid arthritis. Current Opinion in Rheumatology. 2007;**19**:246-251. DOI: 10.1097/BOR.0b013e3280eed78c

[25] Wisler BA, Dennis JE, Malemud CJ. New organ-specific pharmacological strategies interfering with signal pathways in inflammatory disorders/autoimmune disorders. Current Signal Transduction Therapy. 2011;**6**:279-291

[26] Ivashkiv LB, Xu X. Signaling by STATs. Arthritis Research & Therapy. 2004;**6**:159-168. DOI: 10.1186/ar1197

[27] Kaplan MH. STAT4: A critical regulator of inflammation *in vivo*. Immunologic Research. 2005;**31**:231-242. DOI: 10.1385/IR:31:3:231

[28] Malemud CJ, Pearlman E. Targeting JAK/STAT signaling pathway in inflammatory diseases. Current Signal Transduction Therapy. 2009;**4**:201-221

[29] Stark GR, Darnell JE Jr. The JAK-STAT pathway at 20. Immunity. 2012;**36**:503-514. DOI: 10.1016/j.immuni.2012.03.013

[30] Rani A, Murphy JJ. STAT5 in cancer and immunity. Journal of Interferon Cytokine Research. 2016;**36**:226-237. DOI: 10.1089/jir.2015.0054

[31] Malemud CJ. Negative regulators of JAK/STAT signaling in rheumatoid arthritis and osteoarthritis. International Journal of Molecular Sciences. 2017;**18**. pii: E484. DOI: 10.3390/ijms18030484

[32] Choy E. Understanding the dynamics: Pathways involved in the pathogenesis of rheumatoid arthritis. Rheumatology (Oxford, England). 2012;**51**(Suppl 5):v3-v11. DOI: 10.1093/rheumatology/kes113

[33] Banham-Hall E, Clatworthy MR, Okkenhaug K. The therapeutic potential for PI3K inhibitors in autoimmune rheumatic diseases. Open Rheumatology. 2012;**6**:245-258. DOI: 10.2174/1874312901206010245

[34] Nagai S, Kurebayashi Y, Koyasu S. Role of PI3K/Akt and mTOR complexes in Th17 differentiation. Annals of the New York Academy of Sciences. 2013;**1280**:30-34. DOI: 10.1111/nyas.12059

[35] Alghasham A, Rasheed Z. Therapeutic targets for rheumatoid arthritis: Progress and promises. Autoimmunity. 2014;**47**:77-94. DOI: 10.3109/08916934.2013.873413

[36] Malemud CJ. The PI3K/Akt/PTEN/mTOR pathway: A fruitful target for inducing cell death in rheumatoid arthritis? Future Medicinal Chemistry. 2015;**7**:1137-1147. DOI: 10.4155/fmc.15.55

[37] Tristano AG. Tyrosine kinases as targets in rheumatoid arthritis. International Immunopharmacology. 2009;**9**:1-9. DOI: 10.1016/j.intimp.2008.09.010

[38] Malemud CJ. The discovery of novel experimental therapies for inflammatory arthritis. Mediators of Inflammation. 2009;**2009**:698769. DOI: 10.1155/2009/698769

[39] Tan SL, Liao C, Lucas MC, et al. Targeting the SyK-BTK axis for the treatment of immunological and hematological disorders: Recent progress and therapeutic perspectives. Pharmacologic Therapy. 2013;**138**:294-309. DOI: 10.1016/j.pharmthera.2013.02.001

[40] Malemud CJ. Investigative drugs for rheumatoid arthritis: Novel targets. Journal of Autoimmune Disorders. 2016;**2**:12

[41] Wu L, Huang X, Li L, et al. Insights on the biology and pathology of HIF-1α/-2α, TGFβ/BMP. Wnt/β-catenin, and NF-κB pathways in osteoarthritis. Current Pharmaceutical Design. 2012;**18**:3293-3312. PMID: 22646092

[42] Husa M, Petursson F, Lotz M, et al. C/EBP homologous protein drives pro-catabolic responses in chondrocytes. Arthritis Research & Therapy. 2013;**15**:R218. DOI: 10.1186/ar4415

[43] Wang X, Xu Z, Wang J, et al. DUSP19, a downstream effector of leptin, inhibits chondrocyte apoptosis via dephosphorylating JNK during osteoarthritis pathogenesis. Molecular BioSystems. 2016;**12**:721-728. DOI: 10.1039/c5mb00776c

[44] Huang Y, Huang Q, Su H, et al. TAR DNA-binding protein 43 inhibits inflammatory responses and protects chondrocyte function by modulating RACK1 expression in osteoarthritis. Biomedicine & Pharmacotherapy. 2017;**85**:362-371. DOI: 10.1016/j.biopha.2016.11.037

[45] Yu C, Chen WP, Wang XH. MicroRNA and osteoarthritis. Journal of International Medical Research. 2011;**39**:1-9. DOI: 10.1177/147323001103900101

[46] Diaz-Prado S, Cicione C, Mulños-López E, et al. Characterization of microRNA expression in normal and osteoarthritic human chondrocytes. BMC Musculoskeletal Disorders. 2012;**13**:144. DOI: 10.1186/1471-2474-13-144

[47] Genemaras AA, Ennis H, Kaplan L. Inflammatory cytokines induce specific time- and concentration-dependent MicroRNA release by chondrocytes, synoviocytes and meniscus cells. Journal of Orthopaedic Research. 2016;**34**:779-790. DOI: 10.1002/jor.23086

[48] Cong L, Zhu Y, Tu G. A bioinformatics analysis of microRNAs in osteoarthritis. Osteoarthritis and Cartilage. 2017;**25**:1362-1371. DOI: 10.1016/j.joca.2017.03.012

[49] Zamli Z, Adams MA, Tarlton JF, et al. Increased chondrocyte apoptosis is associated with the progression of osteoarthritis in spontaneous Guinea pig models of the disease. International Journal of Molecular Sciences. 2013;**14**:17729-17743. DOI: 10.3390/ijms140917729

[50] Karouzakis E, Neidhart M, Gay RE, et al. Molecular and cellular basis of rheumatoid joint destruction. Immunology Letters. 2006;**106**:8-13. DOI: 10.1016/j.imlet.2006.04.011

[51] Huber LC, Distler O, Tarner I, et al. Synovial fibroblasts: Key player in rheumatoid arthritis. Rheumatology (Oxford, England). 2006;**45**:669-675. DOI: 10.1093/rheumatology/kel065

[52] Johnson EQ, Charchandi A, Babis GC, et al. Apoptosis in osteoarthritis: Morphology, mechanisms, and potential means for therapeutic intervention. Journal of Surgery Orthopedic Advances. 2008;**17**:147-152. PMID: 18851798

[53] Thomas CM, Fuller CJ, Whittles CE, et al. Chondrocyte death by apoptosis is associated with the initiation and severity of articular cartilage degradation. International Journal of Rheumatic Diseases. 2011;**14**:191-198. DOI: 10.1111/j.1756-185X.2010.01578.x

[54] Dowthwaite GP, Bishop JC, Redman SN, et al. The surface of articular cartilage contains a progenitor cell population. Journal of Cell Science. 2004;**117**:889-897. DOI: 10.1242/jcs.00912

[55] Alsalameh S, Amin R, Gemba T, et al. Identification of mesenchymal progenitor cells in normal and osteoarthritic human articular cartilage. Arthritis and Rheumatism. 2004;**50**:1522-1532. DOI: 10.1002/art.20269

[56] Koeling S, Kruegel J, Imer M, et al. Migratory chondrogenic progenitor cells from repair tissue during the later stages of human osteoarthritis. Cell Stem Cell. 2009;**4**:324-335. DOI: 10.1016/j.stem.2009.01.015

[57] Schimke B, Trautman S, Mai B, et al. Interleukin 17 inhibits progenitor cells in rheumatoid arthritis cartilage. European Journal of Immunology. 2016;**46**:440-445. DOI: 10.1002/eji.201545910

[58] Malemud CJ. Apoptosis resistance in rheumatoid arthritis synovial tissue. Journal of Clinical and Cellular Immunology. 2011;**S3**:006

[59] Malemud CJ, Mobasheri A, editors. International Journal of Medical Sciences. Special Issue: Apoptotic Chondrocytes and Osteoarthritis

[60] Liu-Bryan R, Terkeltaub R. Emerging regulators of the inflammatory process in osteoarthritis. Nature Reviews. Rheumatology. 2015;**11**:35-44. DOI: 10.1038/nrrheum.2014.162

[61] Malemud CJ. Biologic basis of osteoarthritis: State of the evidence. Current Opinion in Rheumatology. 2015;**27**:289-294. DOI: 10.1097/BOR.0000000000000162

[62] Miossec P. An update on the cytokine network in rheumatoid arthritis. Current Opinion in Rheumatology. 2004;**16**:218-222. DOI: 10.1097/BOR.0000000000000162

[63] Brennan F, Beech J. Update on cytokines in rheumatoid arthritis. Current Opinion in Rheumatology. 2007;**19**:296-301. DOI: 10.1097/BOR.0b013e32805e87f1

[64] Malemud CJ, Reddy SK. Targeting cytokines, chemokines and adhesion molecules in rheumatoid arthritis. Current Rheumatology Reviews. 2008;**4**:219-234

[65] Houard X, Goldring MB, Berenbaum F. Homeostatic mechanisms in articular cartilage and role of inflammation in osteoarthritis. Current Rheumatology Reports. 2013;**15**:375. DOI: 10.1007/s11926-013-0375-6

[66] Malemud CJ. Growth hormone, VEGF and FGF: Involvement in rheumatoid arthritis. Clinica Chimica Acta. 2007;**375**:10-19. DOI: 10.1016/j.cca.2006.06.033

[67] Stannus O, Jones G, Cicuttini F, et al. Circulating levels of IL-6 and TNF-α are associated with knee radiographic osteoarthritis and knee cartilage loss in older adults. Osteoarthritis and Cartilage. 2010;**18**:1441-1447. DOI: 10.1016/j.joca.2010.08.016

[68] Abe H, Sakai T, Ando W, et al. Synovial fluid cytokine levels in hip disease. Rheumatology (Oxford, England). 2014;**53**:165-172. DOI: 10.1093/rheumatology/ket334

[69] Zan PF, Yao J, Wu Z, et al. Cyclin D1 gene silencing promotes IL-1β-induced apoptosis in rat chondrocytes. Journal of Cellular Biochemistry. 2018;**119**:290-299. DOI: 10.1002/jcb.26172

[70] Islam N, Haqqi TM, Jepsen KJ, et al. Hydrostatic pressure induces apoptosis in human chondrocytes from osteoarthritic cartilage through up-regulation of tumor necrosis factor-α, inducible nitric oxide synthase, p53, c-myc and bax-α and suppression of bcl-2. Journal of Cellular Biochemistry. 2002;**87**:266-278. DOI: 10.1002/jcb.10317

[71] Caramés B, López-Armada MJ, Cillero-Pastor B, et al. Differential effects of tumor necrosis factor-α and interleukin-1-β on cell death in human articular chondrocytes. Osteoarthritis and Cartilage. 2008;**16**:715-722. DOI: 10.1016/j.joca.2007.10.006

[72] Malemud CJ, Sun Y, Pearlman E, et al. Monosodium urate and tumor necrosis factor-α increase apoptosis in human chondrocyte cultures. Rheumatology (Sunnyvale). 2012;**2**:113. DOI: 10.4172/2161-1149.1000113

[73] Wang Y, Li de L, Zhang XB, et al. Increase of TNFα-stimulated osteoarthritic chondrocytes apoptosis and decrease of matrix metalloproteinase-9 by NF-κB inhibition. Biomedical and Environmental Sciences. 2013;**26**:277-283. DOI: 10.3967/0895-3988.2013.04.006

[74] Cheleschi S, Cantarini L, Pascarelli NA, et al. Possible chondroprotective of canakinumab: An in vitro study of human osteoarthritic chondrocytes. Cytokine. 2015;**71**:165-172. DOI: 10.1016/j.cyto.2014.10.023

[75] Lu H, Zeng C, Chen M, et al. Lentiviral vector-mediated over-expression of Sox9 protected chondrocytes from IL-1β induced degeneration and apoptosis. International Journal of Clinical and Experimental Pathology. 2015;**8**:10038-10049. PMCID: PMC4637526

[76] Shi X, Ye H, Yao X, et al. The involvement and possible mechanism of NR4A1 in chondrocyte apoptosis during osteoarthritis. American Journal of Translational Research. 2017;**9**:746-754. PMCID: PMC5340710

[77] Malemud CJ, Lewis AC, Wylie MA, et al. U0126, an inhibitor of MEK1/2, increases tumor necrosis factor-α-induced apoptosis, but not interleukin-6-induced apoptosis in C-28/I2 human chondrocytes. Journal of Autoimmune Disorders. 2015;**1**:4. PMCID: PMC4739803

[78] Malemud CJ. Anticytokine therapy for osteoarthritis. Evidence to date. Drugs & Aging. 2010;**27**:95-115. DOI: 10.2165/11319950-000000000-00000

[79] Malemud CJ. Suppression of pro-inflammatory cytokines via targeting of STAT-responsive genes. In: El-Shemy H, editor. Drug Discovery. Rijeka: InTech Publishing; 2013. pp. 373-411

[80] Meszaros EC, Malemud CJ. Phosphorylation of STAT proteins by recombinant human IL-6 in immortalized human chondrocyte cell lines, T/C28a2 and C28/I2. Journal of Inflammation Research. 2017;**10**:1-8. DOI: 10.2147.JIR.593797

[81] Arora V, Cheung HH, Plenchette S, et al. Degradation of survivin by the X-linked inhibitor of apoptosis (XIAP)-XAF1 complex. The Journal of Biological Chemistry. 2007;**282**:26202-26209. DOI: 10.1074/jbc.M700776200

[82] Lewis AC, Malemud CJ. Correction of dysfunctional apoptosis in arthritis by pharmacologic interventions: Focus on altering the activity of inhibitor of apoptosis protein. In: Pandalai SG, editor. Recent Research Developments in Pharmacology. Kerala: Research Signpost; 2011. pp. 69-84

[83] Smolewski P, Robak T. Inhibitors of apoptosis proteins (IAPs) as potential molecular targets for therapy of hematological disorders. Current Molecular Medicine. 2011;**11**:633-649. PMID: 21902653

[84] Saleem M, Qadir MI, Perveen N, et al. Inhibitors of apoptosis proteins: New targets for anticancer therapy. Chemical Biology & Drug Design. 2013;**82**:243-251. DOI: 10.1111/cbdd. 12176

[85] Malemud CJ. Suppressor of cytokine signaling and rheumatoid arthritis. Integrative Molecular Medicine. 2016;**3**:17-20

[86] He Q, Sun C, Lei W, et al. SOCS1 regulates apoptosis and inflammation by inhibiting IL-4 signaling in IL-1β-stimulated human osteoarthritic chondrocytes. BioMed Research International. 2017;**2017**:4601959. DOI: 10.1055/2017/4601959

[87] Blanco FJ, Rego I, Ruiz-Romero C. The role of mitochondria in osteoarthritis. Nature Reviews Rheumatology. 2011;**7**:161-169. DOI: 10.1038/nrrheum.2010.213

[88] Takada K, Hirose J, Yamabe S, et al. Endoplasmic reticulum stress mediates nitric-oxide-induced chondrocyte apoptosis. Biomedical Reports. 2013;**1**:315-319. DOI: 10.3892/br.2013.52

[89] Uehara Y, Hirose J, Yamabe S, et al. Endoplasmic reticulum-stress-induced apoptosis contributes to articular cartilage degeneration via C/EBP homologous protein. Osteoarthritis and Cartilage. 2014;**22**:1007-1017. DOI: 10.1016/j.joca.2014.04.025

[90] Hughes A, Oxford AE, Tawara K, et al. Endoplasmic reticulum stress and unfolded protein response in cartilage pathophysiology: Contributing factors to apoptosis and osteoarthritis. International Journal of Molecular Sciences. 2017;**18**. pii: E665. DOI: 10.3390/ijms18030665

[91] Li XF, Zhang Z, Chen ZK, et al. Piezo protein induces the apoptosis of human osteoarthritis-derived chondrocytes by activating caspase-12, the signaling marker of ER stress. International Journal of Molecular Medicine. 2017;**40**:845-853. DOI: 10.3892/ijmm.2017.3075

[92] Li D, Xie G, Wang W. Reactive oxygen species: The 2-edged sword of osteoarthritis. The American Journal of Medical Sciences. 2012;**344**:486-490. DOI: 10.1097/MAJ.0b013e3182579dc6

[93] Wu Q, Zhong ZM, Zhu SY, et al. Advanced oxidation protein products induce chondrocyte apoptosis via receptor for advanced glycation end products-mediated, redox-dependent intrinsic apoptosis pathway. Apoptosis. 2016;**21**:36-50. DOI: 10.1007/s10495-015-1191-4

[94] Angelotti F, Parma A, Cafaro G, et al. One year in review 2017: Pathogenesis of rheumatoid arthritis. Clinical and Experimental Rheumatology. 2017;**35**:368-378. PMID: 28631608

[95] Battistelli M, Salucci S, Olivotto E, et al. Cell death in human articular chondrocytes. A morpho-functional study in micromass model. Apoptosis. 2014;**19**:1471-1483. DOI: 10.1007/s10495-014-1017-9

[96] Gu YY, Chen J, Meng ZL, et al. Research progress on osteoarthritis mechanisms. Biomedical Pharmacotherapy. 2017;**93**:1246-1252. DOI: 10.1016/j.biopha.2017.07.034

[97] Hwang HS, Kim HA. Chondrocyte apoptosis in the pathogenesis of osteoarthritis. International Journal of Molecular Sciences. 2015;**16**:26035-26054. DOI: 10.3390/ijms161125943

[98] Roach HI, Aigner T, Kouri JB. Chondropotosis: A variant of apoptotic cell death in osteoarthritis. Apoptosis. 2004;**9**:265-277 15258458

[99] Lin NY, Beyer C, Giessl A, et al. Autophagy regulates TNFα-mediated joint destruction in experimental arthritis. Annals of the Rheumatic Diseases. 2013;**72**:761-768. DOI: 10.1136/annrheumdis-2012-201671

[100] Dai Y, Hu S. Recent insights into the role of autophagy in the pathogenesis of rheumatoid arthritis. Rheumatology (Oxford, England). 2016;**55**:403-410. DOI: 10.1093/rheumatology/kev337

[101] Speziali A, Delcogliano M, Tei M, et al. Chondropenia: Current concept review. Musculoskeletal Surgery. 2015;**99**:189-200. DOI: 10.1007/s12306-015-0377-9

[102] Chang J, Wang W, Zhang H, et al. The dual role of autophagy in chondrocyte responses in the pathogenesis of articular cartilage degeneration in osteoarthritis. International Journal of Molecular Medicine. 2013;**32**:1311-1318. DOI: 10.3892/ijmm.2013.1520

[103] Musumeci G, Castrogiovanni P, Trovato FM, et al. Biomarkers of chondrocyte apoptosis and autophagy in osteoarthritis. International Journal of Molecular Sciences. 2015;**16**:20560-20575. DOI: 10.3390/ijms160920560

[104] Jeon H, Im GI. Autophagy in osteoarthritis. Connective Tissue Research. 2017;**58**:497-508. DOI: 10.1080/03008207.2016.1240790

[105] Li YS, Zhang FJ, Zeng C, et al. Autophagy in osteoarthritis. Joint, Bone, Spine. 2016;**83**: 143-148. DOI: 10.1016/j.jbspin.2015.06.009

[106] Wylie MA, Malemud CJ. Perspective: Deregulation of apoptosis in arthritis by altered signal transduction. International Journal of Clinical Rheumatology. 2013;**8**:483-490. DOI: 10.2217/IJR.13.31

[107] Musumeci G, Loreto C, Carnazza M, et al. Characterization of apoptosis in articular cartilage derived from the knee joints of patients with osteoarthritis. Knee Surgery, Sports Traumatology, Arthroscopy. 2011;**19**:307-313. DOI: 10.1007/s00167-010-1215-0

[108] Huang ZM, Du SH, Huang LG, et al. Leptin promotes apoptosis and inhibits autophagy of chondrocytes through upregulating lysyl oxidase-like 3 during osteoarthritis pathogenesis. Osteoarthritis and Cartilage. 2016;**24**:1246-1253. DOI: 10.1016/j.joca.2016.02.009

[109] Zhang Y, Vasheghani F, Li YH, et al. Cartilage-specific deletion of mTOR upregulates autophagy and protects mice from osteoarthritis. Annals of Rheumatic Diseases. 2015;**74**:1432-1440. DOI: 10.1136/annrheumdis-2013-204599

[110] Shen C, Cai GQ, Peng JP, et al. Autophagy protects chondrocytes from glucocorticoid-induced apoptosis via ROS/Akt/FOXO3 signaling. Osteoarthritis and Cartilage. 2015;**23**:2279-2287. DOI: 10.1016/j.joca.2015.06.020

[111] Huang W, Ao P, Li J, et al. Autophagy protects advanced glycation end product-induced apoptosis and expression of MMP-3 and MMP-13 in rat chondrocytes. Biomedical Research International. 2017;**2017**:6341919. DOI: 10.1155/2017/6341919

[112] Sera SR, Zur Nieden NI. microRNA regulation of skeletal development. Current Osteoporosis Reports. 2017;**15**:353-366. DOI: 10.1007/s11914-017-0379-7

[113] Churov AV, Oleinik EK, Knip M. MicroRNAs in rheumatoid arthritis: Altered expression and diagnostic potential. Autoimmune Reviews. 2015;**14**:1029-1037. DOI: 10.1016/j.autrev.2015.07.005

[114] Haftmann C, Stittrich AB, Zimmermann J, et al. miR-148a is upregulated by Twist1 and t-bet and promotes Th1-survival by regulating the proapoptotic gene Bim. European Journal of Immunology. 2015;**45**:1192-1205. DOI: 10.1002/eji.201444633

[115] D'Adamo S, Cetrullo S, Minguzzi M, et al. MicroRNAs and autophagy: Fine players in the control of chondrocyte homeostatic activities in osteoarthritis. Oxidative Medicine and Cellular Longevity. 2017;**2017**:3720128. DOI: 10.1155/2017/3720128

[116] Malemud CJ. Chondrocyte apoptosis in rheumatoid arthritis: Is preventive therapy possible? Immunotherapy (Los Angel). 2015;**1**. pii: 102. PMID: 26878072

[117] Jin L, Zhao J, Jing W, et al. Role of miR-146a in human chondrocyte apoptosis in response to mechanical pressure injury in vitro. International Journal of Molecular Medicine. 2014;**34**:451-463. DOI: 10.3892/ijmm.2014.1808

[118] Zhong JH, Li J, Liu CF, et al. Effects of microRNA-146a on the proliferation and apoptosis of human osteoarthritis chondrocytes by targeting TRAF6 through the NF-κB signaling pathway. BioScience Reports. 2017;**37**. pii: BSR20160578. DOI: 10.1042/BSR20160578

[119] West C, McDermott MF. Effects of microRNA-146a on the proliferation and apoptosis of human osteochondrocytes by targeting TRAF6 through the NF-κB signalling pathway. BioScience Reports. 2017;**37**:BSR20170180. DOI: 10.1042/BSR20170180

[120] Li J, Huang J, Dai L, et al. miR-146a, an IL-1β responsive miRNA, induces vascular endothelial growth factor and chondrocyte apoptosis by targeting Smad4. Arthritis Research & Therapy. 2012;**14**:R75. DOI: 10.1187/ar3798

[121] Abouheif MM, Nakasa T, Shibuya H, et al. Silencing microRNA-34a inhibits chondrocyte apoptosis in a rat osteoarthritis model in vitro. Rheumatology (Oxford, England). 2010;**49**:2054-2060. DOI: 10.1093/rheumatology/keg247

[122] Yan S, Wang M, Zhao J, et al. Micro-RNA-34a affects chondrocyte apoptosis and proliferation by targeting the SIRT1/p53 signaling pathway during the pathogenesis of osteoarthritis. International Journal of Molecular Medicine. 2016;**38**:201-209. DOI: 10.3892/ijmm.2016.2618

[123] Chen H, Wang J, Hu B, et al. MiR-34a promotes Fas-mediated cartilage endplate chondrocyte apoptosis by targeting Bcl-2. Molecular and Cellular Biochemistry. 2015;**406**:21-30. DOI: 10.1007/s11010-015-2420-4

[124] Zhai X, Meng R, Li H, et al. miR-181a modulates chondrocyte apoptosis by targeting glycerol-3-phosphate dehydrogenase 1-like protein (GPD1L) in osteoarthritis. Medical Science Monitor. 2017;**23**:1224-1231. PMCID: PMC5360418

[125] Wu XF, Zhou ZH, Zou J. MicroRNA-181 inhibits proliferation and promotes apoptosis of chondrocytes in osteoarthritis by targeting PTEN. Biochemistry and Cell Biology. 2017;**95**:437-444. DOI: 10.1139/bcb-2016-0078

[126] Malemud CJ. Matrix metalloproteases and synovial joint pathology. In: Khalil RA, editor. Progress in Molecular Biology and Translational Science. Vol. 148. Burlington: Academic Press; 2017. pp. 306-325

[127] Wang GL, Wu YB, Liu JT, et al. Upregulation of miR-98 inhibits apoptosis in cartilage cells in osteoarthritis. Genetic Testing and Molecular Biomarkers. 2016;**20**:645-653. DOI: 10.1089/gtmb/2016.0011

[128] Wang J, Chen L, Jin S, et al. MiR-98 promotes chondrocyte apoptosis by decreasing Bcl-2 expression in a rat model of osteoarthritis. Acta Biochimica Biophysica Sin (Shanghai). 2016;**48**:923-929. DOI: 10.1093/abbs/gmw084

[129] Wang J, Chen L, Jin S, et al. Altered expression of microRNA-98 in IL-1β-induced cartilage degradation and its role in chondrocyte apoptosis. Molecular Medicine Reports. 2017;**16**:3208-3216. DOI: 10.3892/mmr.2017.7028

[130] Song J, Kim D, Chun CH, et al. MicroRNA-9 regulates survival of chondroblasts and cartilage integrity by targeting protogenin. Cell Communication and Signaling. 2013; **11**:66. DOI: 10.1186/1478-811X-11-66

[131] Chen H, Tian Y. MiR-15a-5p regulates viability and matrix degradation of human osteoarthritis chondrocytes via targeting VEGFA. Bioscience Trends. 2017;**10**:482-488. DOI: 10.5582/bst.2016.01187

[132] Wang X, Guo Y, Wang C, et al. MicroRNA-142-3p inhibits chondrocyte apoptosis and inflammation in osteoarthritis by targeting HMGB1. Inflammation. 2016;**39**:1718-1728. DOI: 10.1007/s10753-016-0406-3

[133] Zhang G, Sun Y, Wang Y, et al. MiR-502-5p inhibits IL-1β-induced chondrocyte injury by targeting TRAF2. Cellular Immunology. 2016;**302**:50-57. DOI: 10.1016/j.cellimm.2016.01.007

[134] Bai R, Zhao AQ, Zhao ZQ, et al. MicroRNA-195 induced apoptosis in hypoxic chondrocytes by targeting hypoxia-inducible factor 1 alpha. European Review for Medical and Pharmacological Sciences. 2015;**19**:545-551. PMID: 25753868

[135] Makki MS, Haqqi TM. miR-139 modulates MCPIP1/IL-6 expression and induces apoptosis in human chondrocytes. Experimental & Molecular Medicine. 2015;**47**:e189. DOI: 10.1038/emm.2015.66

[136] Chen L, Li Q, Wang J, et al. MiR-29b-3p promotes chondrocyte apoptosis and facilitates the occurrence and development of osteoarthritis by targeting PRGN. Journal of Cellular and Molecular Medicine. 2017;**21**:3347-3359. DOI: 10.1111/jcmm.13237

[137] Li Y, Li S, Luo Y, et al. LncRNA PVT1 regulates chondrocyte apoptosis in osteoarthritis by acting as a sponge for miR-488-3p. DNA Cell Biology. 2017;**36**:571-580. DOI: 10.1089/dna.2017.3678

[138] Zhao C, Wang Y, Jin H, et al. Knockdown of microRNA-203 alleviates LPS-induced injury by targeting MCL-1 in C28/I2 chondrocytes. Experimental Cell Research. 2017;**359**:171-178. DOI: 10.1016/j.yexcr.2017.07.034

[139] Winsauer G, Resch U, Hofer-Warbinek R, et al. XIAP regulates bi-phasic NF-κB induction involving physical interaction and ubiquitination of MEKK2. Cell Signaling. 2008;**11**:2107-2112. DOI: 10.1016/j.cellsig.2008.08.004

[140] Rajalingam K, Dikic I. Inhibitors of apoptosis catch ubiquitin. Biochemical Journal. 2009; **417**:e1-e3. DOI: 10.1042/BJ20082215

[141] Chen Q, Gao Y, Kao X, et al. SNP-induced apoptosis may be mediated with caspase inhibitor by JNK signaling pathways in rabbit articular chondrocytes. The Journal of Toxicological Sciences. 2012;**37**:157-167. PMID: 22293420

[142] Ye Z, Chen Y, Zhang R, et al. C-Jun N-terminal kinase—C-Jun pathway transactivates Bim to promote osteoarthritis. Canadian Journal of Physiology and Pharmacology. 2014; **92**:132-139. DOI: 10.1139/cjpp-2013-0228

[143] Xu L, Zhai L, Ge Q, et al. Vacuolar protein sorting 4B (VPS4B) regulates apoptosis of chondrocytes via p38 mitogen-activated protein kinases (MAPK) in osteoarthritis. Inflammation. DOI: 10.1007/s10753-017-0633-2

[144] Sun HY, Hu KZ, Yin ZS. Inhibition of p38-MAPK signaling pathway suppresses the apoptosis and expression of proinflammatory cytokines in human osteoarthritis chondrocytes. Cytokine. 2017;**90**:135-143. DOI: 10.1016/j.cyto.2016.11.002

[145] Shi J, Zhang C, Yi Z, et al. Explore the variation of MMP3, JNK, p38 MAPKs, and autophagy at the early stages of osteoarthritis. IUBMB. 2016;**68**:293-302. DOI: 10.1002/iub.1482

[146] Zhang ZM, Shen C, Li H, et al. Leptin induces the apoptosis of chondrocytes in an in vitro model of osteoarthritis via the JAK2-STAT3 signaling pathway. Molecular Medicine Reports. 2016;**13**:3684-3690. DOI: 10.3892/mmr.2016.4970

[147] Li D, Wu Z, Duan Y, et al. TNFα-mediated apoptosis in human osteoarthritic chondrocytes sensitized by PI3K-NFκB inhibitor, not mTOR inhibitor. Rheumatology International. 2012;**32**:2017-2022. DOI: 10.1007/s00296-011-1929-4

[148] Yin MH, Wang YT, Li Q, et al. Oligomeric proanthocyanidins inhibit apoptosis of chondrocytes induced by interleukin-1β. Molecular Medicine Reports. . DOI: 10.3892/mmr.2017.7124

[149] Rao Z, Wang S, Wang J. Peroxiredoxin 4 inhibits IL-1β-induced chondrocyte apoptosis via PI3K/AKT signaling. Biomedicine & Pharmacotherapy. 2017;**90**:414-420. DOI: 10.1016/j.biopha.2017.03.075

[150] Fu D, Shang X, Ni Z, et al. Shikonin inhibits inflammation and chondrocyte apoptosis by regulation of the PI3K/Akt signaling pathway in a rat model of osteoarthritis. Experimental and Therapeutic Medicine. 2016;**12**:2735-2740. DOI: 10.3892/etm.2016.3642

[151] Wu Z, Li M, Zheng W, et al. Silencing of both ATF4 and PERK inhibits cell cycle progression and promotes the apoptosis of differentiating chondrocytes. International Journal of Molecular Medicine. 2017;**40**:101-111. DOI: 10.3892/ijmm.2017.2985

[152] Zhang FJ, Luo W, Lei GH. Role of HIF-1α and HIF-2α in osteoarthritis. Joint, Bone, Spine. 2015;**82**:144-147. DOI: 10.1016/j.ibspin.2014.10.003

[153] Zhang LO, Zhao GZ, Xu XY, et al. Integrin-β1 regulates chondrocyte proliferation and apoptosis through the upregulation of G1T1 expression. International Journal of Molecular Medicine. 2015;**35**:1074-1080. DOI: 10.3892/ijmm.2015.2114

[154] Wei Z, Li HH. IGFBP-1 may trigger osteoarthritis by inducing apoptosis of chondrocytes through Nur77 translocation. International Journal of Clinical and Experimental Pathology. 2015;**8**:15599-15610. PMCID: PMC4730042

[155] Bao G, Xu L, Xu X, et al. SGBT promotes the caspase-dependent apoptosis in chondrocytes of osteoarthritis. Inflammation. 2016;**39**:601-610. DOI: 10.1007/s10753-015-0285-z

[156] Huang Z, Li J, Du S, et al. Effects of UCP4 on the proliferation and apoptosis of chondrocytes: Its possible involvement and regulation in osteoarthritis. PLoS One. 2016;**11**:e0150684. DOI: 10.1371/journal.pone.0150684

[157] Wang Z, Tran C, Bhatia NJ, et al. Del1 knockout mice developed more severe osteoarthritis associated with increased susceptibility of chondrocytes to apoptosis. PLoS One. 2016;**11**:e0160684. DOI: 10.1371/journal.pone.0160684

[158] Kobayashi H, Chang SH, Mori D, et al. Biphasic regulation of chondrocytes by Rela through induction of anti-apoptotic and catabolic target genes. Nature Communications. 2016;**7**:13336. DOI: 10.1038/ncomms13336

[159] Song B, Song H, Wang W, et al. Beclin 1 overexpression inhibits chondrocyte apoptosis and downregulates extracellular matrix metabolism in osteoarthritis. Molecular Medicine Reports. 2017;**16**:3958-3964. DOI: 10.3892/mmr.2017.7064

[160] Liu J, Meng Q, Jing H, et al. Astragaloside IV protects against apoptosis in human degenerative chondrocytes through autophagy activation. Molecular Medicine Reports. 2017;**16**:3269-3275. DOI: 10.3892/mmr.2017.6980

[161] Gao H, Gui J, Wang L, et al. Aquaporin 1 contributes to chondrocyte apoptosis in a rat model of osteoarthritis. International Journal of Molecular Medicine. 2016;**38**:1752-1758. DOI: 10.3892/ijmm.2016.2785

[162] Won Y, Shin Y, Chun CH, et al. Pleiotropic roles of metallothioneins as regulators of chondrocyte apoptosis and catabolic and anabolic pathways during osteoarthritis pathogenesis. Annals of the Rheumatic Diseases. 2016;**75**:2045-2052. DOI: 10.1136/annrheumdis-2015-208406

[163] He Ds HXJ, Yan YQ, et al. Underlying mechanism of Sirt1 on apoptosis and extracellular matrix degradation of osteoarthritis chondrocytes. Molecular Medicine Reports. 2017;**16**:845-850. DOI: 10.3892/mmr.2017.6659

[164] Berenbaum F, Griffin TM, Liu-Bryan R. 2017; review: Metabolic regulation of inflammation in osteoarthritis. Arthritis & Rheumatology. 2017;**69**:9-21. DOI: 10.1002/art.39842

[165] Sorice M, Iannuccelli C, Manganelli V, et al. Autophagy generates citrullinated peptides in human synoviocytes: A possible trigger for anti-citrullinated peptide antibodies. Rheumatology (Oxford, England). 2016;**55**:1374-1385. DOI: 10.1093/rheumatology/kew178

[166] Ireland JM, Unanue ER. Autophagy in antigen-presenting cells results in presentation of citrullinated peptides to CD4 T cells. Journal of Experimental Medicine. 2011;**208**:2625-2632. DOI: 10.1084/jem.20110640

[167] Van Loosdregt J, Rossetti M, Spreafico R, et al. Increased autophagy in $CD4^+$ T cells of rheumatoid arthritis patients results in T-cell hyperactivation and apoptosis resistance. European Journal of Immunology. 2016;**46**:2862-2870. DOI: 10.1002/eji.201646375

[168] Dalbeth N, Smith T, Gray S, Doyle A, Antill P, Lobo M, et al. Cellular characterisation of magnetic resonance imaging bone oedema in rheumatoid arthritis; implications for pathogenesis of erosive disease. Annals of the Rheumatic Diseases. 2009;**68**:279-282. DOI: 10.1136/ard.2008.096024

[169] Yang J, Zhao S, Yang X, et al. Inhibition of B-cell apoptosis is mediated through increased expression of Bcl-2 in patients with rheumatoid arthritis. International Journal of Rheumatic Diseases. 2016;**19**:134-140. DOI: 10.1111/1756-185X.12706

[170] Störch H, Zimmerman B, Resch B, et al. Activated human B cells induce inflammatory fibroblasts with cartilage-destructive properties and become functionally suppressed in return. Annals of the Rheumatic Diseases. 2016;**75**:924-932. DOI: 10.1136/annrheumdis-2014-206965

[171] Meednu N, Zhang H, Owen T, et al. Production of RANKL by memory B cells: A link between B cells and bone erosion and rheumatoid arthritis. Arthritis & Rheumatology. 2016;**68**:805-816. DOI: 10.1002/art.39489

[172] Taherian E, Rao A, Malemud CJ, et al. The biological and clinical activity of anti-malarial drugs in autoimmune disorders. Current Rheumatology Reviews. 2013;**9**:45-62. PMID: 25198367

[173] Lee WK, Kang JS. Modulation of apoptosis and differentiation by the treatment of sulfasalazine in rabbit articular chondrocytes. Toxicology Research. 2016;**32**:115-121. DOI: 10.5487/TR.2016/32.2.115

[174] Nasi S, Ea HK, So A, et al. Revisiting the role of interleukin-1 pathway in osteoarthritis: Interleukin-1α and -1β and NALP3 inflammasome are not involved in pathological features of the murine meniscectomy model of osteoarthritis. Frontiers in Pharmacology. 2017;**8**:282. DOI: 10.3389/fphar.2017.00282

[175] Campbell L, Raheem I, Malemud CJ, et al. The relationship between NALP3 and autoinflammatory syndromes. International Journal of Molecular Sciences. 2016;**17**:725. DOI: 10.3390/ijms17050725

[176] Siegelin MD, Gaiser T, Siegelin Y. The XIAP inhibitor Embelin enhances TRAIL-mediated apoptosis in malignant glioma cells by down-regulation of the short isoform of FLIP. Neurochemistry International. 2009;**55**:423-430. DOI: 10.1016/j.neuint.2009.04.011

[177] Malemud CJ. The small molecular weight inhibitor of protein kinase revolution for the treatment of rheumatoid arthritis. In: Vallisuta O, Olimat S, editors. Drug Discovery and Development—From Molecules to Medicine. Rijeka: InTech Publishing; 2015. p. 163-179. DOI: http://dx.doi.org/10.5772/59639

3

Going Small: Using Biophysical Screening to Implement Fragment Based Drug Discovery

John J. Bowling, William R. Shadrick,
Elizabeth C. Griffith and Richard E. Lee

Abstract

Screening against biochemical targets with compact chemical fragments has developed a reputation as a successful early-stage drug discovery approach, thanks to recent drug approvals. Having weak initial target affinities, fragments require the use of sensitive biophysical technologies (NMR, SPR, thermal shift, ITC, and X-ray crystallography) to accommodate the practical limits of going smaller. Application of optimized fragment biophysical screening approaches now routinely allows for the rapid identification of fragments with high binding efficiencies. The aim of this chapter is to provide an introduction to fragment library selection and to discuss the suitability of screening approaches adapted for lower-throughput biophysical techniques. A general description of metrics that are being used in the progression of fragment hits, the need for orthogonal assay testing, and guidance on potential pitfalls are included to assist scientists, considering initiating their own fragment discovery program.

Keywords: fragment-based drug discovery, biophysical screening, efficiency metrics, nuclear magnetic resonance spectroscopy, surface plasmon resonance, thermal shift assay, isothermal titration calorimetry, fluorescence polarization, X-ray crystallography

1. Introduction

"Going small" with fragment-based drug discovery (FBDD) denotes using low molecular weight compounds to probe a therapeutic target. This also includes using smaller tailored libraries and lower screening throughput in more carefully measured assays. This is a consequence of being reliant on biophysical technologies, as compared to classical high-throughput screening (HTS) approaches performed in 384-well plates that detect product formation. FBDD at its core is target-based drug discovery, but the initial approach of fragment screening differs from standard lead-like screening, which utilizes much larger higher molecular weight screening libraries.

In theory, modern target-based drug discovery screening libraries are designed to maximize coverage of chemical space. This is especially important for groups that use high-throughput technologies (HTS) and screen against diverse targets. These target-based programs tend to rely on screening the highest practical number of chemical entities from their screening libraries, sometimes accumulating millions of compounds [1]. However, with over 166 billion possible synthetically accessible organic molecules containing up to 17 heavy atoms (nonhydrogen) [2], even the biggest screening libraries cannot possibly statistically represent this vast chemical space [3].

From modeling described in a 2001 article, Hann and colleagues showed how higher molecular complexity (i.e., ligand size) significantly decreased the probability of protein-site molecular recognition [4]. The authors outlined this as a primary shortcoming of the combinatorial chemistry/HTS approach to drug discovery and promoted the idea that screening smaller libraries with reduced complexity could be a complementary approach. Thus, by reducing compound complexity, FBDD evades the pitfall of scaffold bias which develops in large lead-like screening libraries.

In this chapter, the reader should come to appreciate how going small is an intrinsically orthogonal screening platform that is easily integrated with established biophysical techniques. The methods, examples, and citations discussed are intended to guide a newcomer to FBDD, specifically scientists who have some prior experience with drug screening principles.

2. The rise of fragments as a screening ideology

Fragment-based drug discovery started as a concept published in 1981 [5] by biochemist William P. Jencks, who characterized the binding affinities of molecules to proteins as being built from components. Citing several examples, he described how the balance of Gibbs-free energy for a two-component molecule binding to a protein could also be described through the equation $\Delta G^0_{AB} = \Delta G^i_A + \Delta G^i_B + \Delta G^s$, where ΔG^i values are the "intrinsic binding energies" of the components and ΔG^s is their "connection Gibbs energy." A key aspect of the concept is that the component's contribution to the balance of the observed binding energy (ΔG^0_{AB}) would be relatively significant but weak, thus creating a challenge for detection. Jencks' concept was obscured at the time due to the excitement around combi-chem/HTS drug discovery approaches. In 1996, the conceptual observations of Jencks were experimentally validated by the team of Fesik. His team successfully produced a drug lead by linking fragment hits detected by a sensitive two-dimensional nuclear magnetic resonance (NMR) spectroscopy binding assay (often referred to as SAR-by-NMR) [6]. Since then, fragment-based drug discovery has energized the pharmaceutical industry. In 2011, a drug for BRAF-mutated metastatic melanoma became the first FDA-approved drug discovered via FBDD [7]. A second, for chronic lymphocytic leukemia, was approved in 2016 [8], with several related candidates currently making their way through the pipeline [9].

3. Fragment primary screening

At present, NMR, surface plasmon resonance (SPR), thermal shift assay (TSA), isothermal titration calorimetry (ITC), and X-ray crystallography (Sections 3.2–3.4, 4.1 and 4.2) are the most widely used techniques in FDBB. Given their respective throughput capacities NMR, SPR, and TSA are often used as the primary screening technology with ITC and X-ray crystallography reserved as secondary screening. **Figure 1** shows the effective ligand affinity coverage of each technique which partly demonstrates their utility with FBDD. All biophysical screening techniques work best in combination and individual hits need careful orthogonal validation. Crystallography is the gold standard as the information gained allows for rapid ligand advancement. However, its application as a primary screen is often impractical due to resource and time limitations. High concentration inhibitor biochemical or fluorescence polarization (FP) assays can be used in some cases for orthogonal validation of primary screening hits where crystallography is not an option.

The workflow represented in **Figure 2** shows how these techniques might be organized into a traditional screening paradigm. It is common to use some of these techniques in parallel, particularly at the secondary screening stage since there are always fewer compounds to evaluate. Pragmatically, scientists should obtain structural insights at this secondary stage to validate primary screening results. Structural information is preferred when deciding to progress a fragment to the hit generation stage (discussed further in Section 5.2).

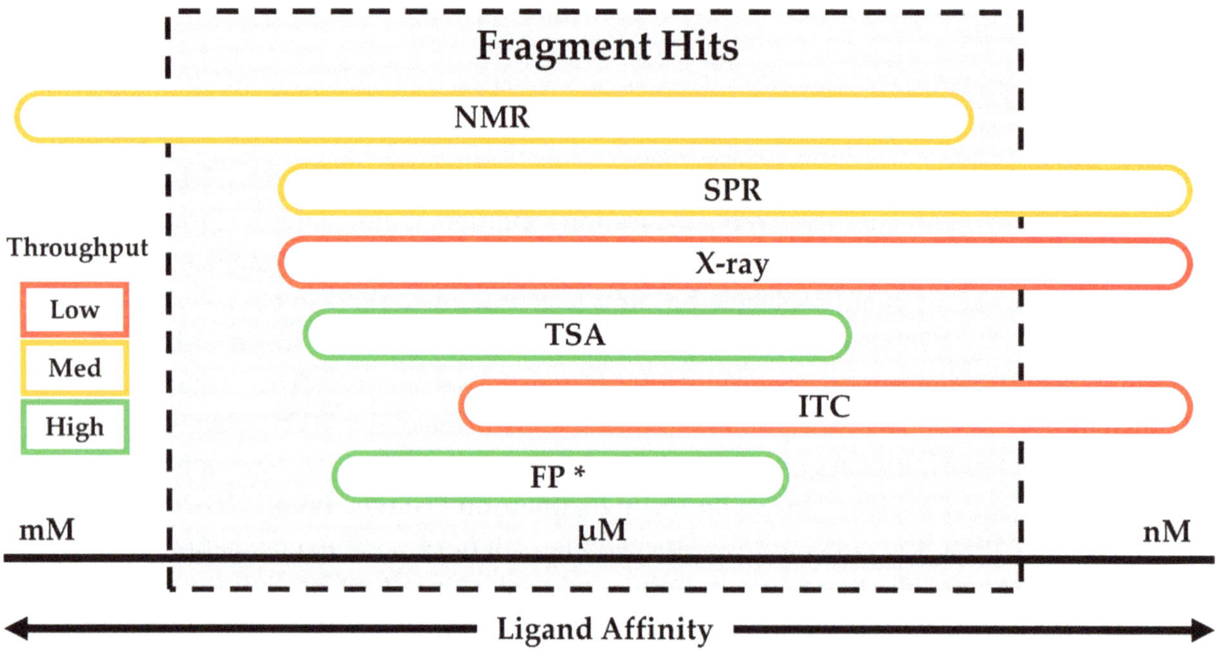

Figure 1. The range of fragment affinities covered by the biophysical techniques described in this chapter. The techniques are ranked from the top downwards in order of their typical frequency of use in FBDD programs (SPR being a close second). NMR (yellow outline) is represented as a medium-throughput method but can be low-throughput based on the availability of protein and whether recycling is required. *Fluorescence polarization, technically a biochemical technique and highly dependent on probe affinity, is included for comparison but can be applied to fragment screening.

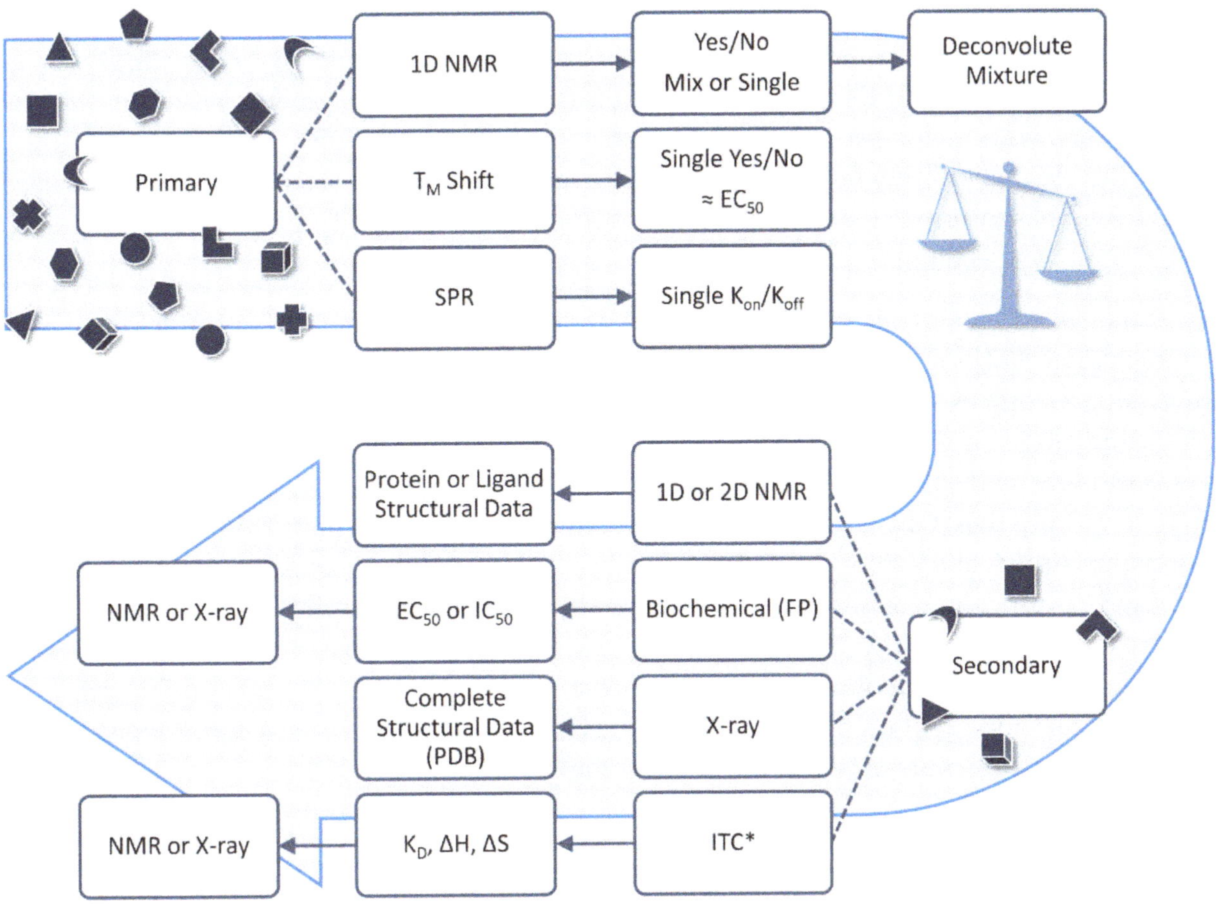

Figure 2. An example of the typical FBDD screening workflow. The workflow assumes structural information by X-ray or NMR. The hierarchy will not accurately depict the resources of all drug discovery programs. Dashed connections represent screening options at the primary and secondary screening stages. Arrows point to the results from each screen to be ranked or compared to those of other techniques. Fragments promoted to secondary screening will eventually require structural information to be progressed to hit generation. *The ITC technique is typically used for ranking fragment hits after secondary screening.

3.1. Fragment library design

An obvious first step for any primary fragment screening is to resource compounds for the screen. However, wielding a proper fragment library as a tool for hit generation conflicts with traditional lead-like screening methods. Central to the conflict is the regular use of high concentrations of compounds to accommodate expected low binding affinities. Practical pitfalls, such as compound aggregation, compound precipitation, dramatic pH changes, detector saturation, and nonspecific interactions, are a minor concern when nanomolar concentrations are used during screening of larger molecular weight molecules, but can become major issues when millimolar concentrations are used in fragment screening.

In 2003, scientists at Astex Pharmaceuticals published a synopsis of their emerging fragment drug-discovery program and noted that the average physical properties of their fragment hits fell conveniently within different orders of 3 (molecular weight <300, hydrogen bond donors ≤3, hydrogen bond acceptors ≤3, and ClogP ≤3) [10]. As a compliment to Lipinski's rule of 5 (RO5), the fragment rule of 3 (RO3) was a convenient target toward which chemical suppliers built fragment libraries from their existing stores. Ten years later, Astex Pharmaceuticals revised their position [11], stating that similar to the RO5 described by Lipinski, RO3 was more of a guideline and that their refined library consisted of fragments with less than 17 heteroatoms with molecular mass <230 Daltons. This exemplifies how well-constructed fragment libraries should rely heavily on practicality to be effective tools and speaks to the need for additional scrutiny of (in order of importance) solubility, stability, and reactivity for effective fragment screening.

Commercial and nonprofit access to fragment libraries exists, and several examples have been characterized [12, 13]. A custom library allows for existing libraries to be used in addition to catalog resources with some tailoring based on specific cheminformatics principles, such as optimization of the representative chemical space, avoidance of nuisance compounds, and guidance with pharmacophore models. One early-stage example of note is the Global Fragment Initiative (GFI) by Pfizer [14], wherein the library was built from compounds on hand, purchased, and synthesized. Each member of the GFI library was rigorously characterized and empirically tested for aqueous solubility up to 1 mM, with the intent of using the library for multiple biophysical techniques. How a fragment library is procured will depend on an acceptable balance of convenience and cost, but it is highly recommended that the end user have methods in place to reliably assess each compound for practical use at high concentrations. For an example of this workflow, see **Figure 3**.

Fragment hits can have limited traction toward chemical expansion or linking as a consequence of their size. As a safeguard, Merck strategically redesigned its general FBDD library to accommodate more structure-activity relationships and to fill structural gaps by visual inspection [15]. The purposeful move away from diversity in its general library was a concerted effort of cheminformatics and crowdsourcing of medicinal chemists to gain pipeline traction. The strategy leads to larger general screening libraries and effectively restricts widespread application to appropriately equipped programs. Regardless, any FBDD program

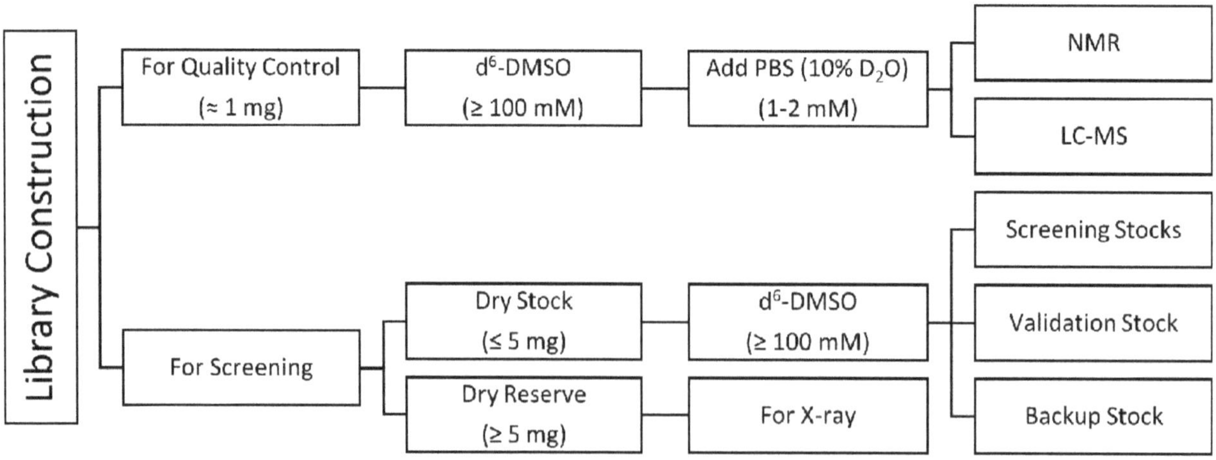

Figure 3. A suggested library construction workflow for FBDD. Once compounds are obtained as dry stocks, the workflow proceeds left to right. Having redundancy built into the screening stocks helps rule out contamination or mishandling. It is presumed that fragments will eventually be used in NMR studies, therefore dissolved using deuterated solvents (d6-DMSO and D_2O). Rigid quality control is recommended to eliminate spoiled or misidentified compounds and repeated on hits or on the event of significant additions of fragments to the library.

design must account for this pitfall and ensure the potential to develop fragment hits through chemistry or catalogs.

Finally, Pan-Assay Interference Compounds (PAINS) are a well-known classification of chemical entities to activity across multiple assays and proteins, and they have been thoroughly reviewed in regards to their practical impacts on FBDD [16], and related cheminformatics filters are available via the Internet [17]. The reduced chemical complexity of fragments does inherently diminish the number of "worst offenders" in its library and often bad fragments are quickly identified and triaged from screening libraries.

In conclusion, for FBDD, it is prudent to prioritize highly soluble fragment libraries with a diversity of ring shapes that can match a broad range of hydrogen bonding interactions from the protein target. A minimalistic approach would be to only eliminate mostly predictable fragment "show stoppers," containing toxicophores subject to xenobiotic metabolism, since it is often easy to scaffold hop in the early stages of FBDD to remove unwanted motifs.

3.2. Nuclear magnetic resonance

Modern NMR spectroscopy is best known for enabling the three-dimensional characterization of ordered molecular structures in solution and was the first technique to be used for fragment screening [6]. It is also one of the few biophysical techniques that can easily be switched between perspectives of the small molecule and the protein at run time. A growing list of NMR experiments used in fragment screening can help validate hits without using additional biophysical techniques.

Samples are prepared *in situ* by using automation (such as the Gilson GX-271 in **Figure 4**) or by pipetting manually. One immediate benefit of the manual method is the ease with which a scientist can eliminate precipitated or turbid samples by optical analytics. Individual inspection of samples is time-consuming but a must for any successful FBDD program, providing important feedback about the fragment library. Fragments must be dissolved in deuterated solvent (e.g., 99.9% d6-DMSO, Cambridge Isotope Laboratories, Inc., USA) for programs using NMR at any stage (see **Figure 3**). Typical concentration ratios for test samples are 10:1 up to 30:1 fragment to protein in the chosen buffer (phosphate buffers being the most common). Prior knowledge of the K_d and stoichiometry is not required but can be used to tune concentrations to avoid unintended site saturation by an individual fragment, which is a general concern when screening fragment mixtures or performing competition experiments. Finally, the issue of whether or not to use surfactants (e.g., 0.05% Triton X100) to help eliminate false positives is best left to a case by case basis, but if used, the conditions should be consistent with orthogonal techniques, with the exception of crystallography.

Spectroscopy experiments that indicate binding from the fragment's perspective are structurally less informative but have a higher dynamic range than do protein-detected experiments. Because significant cost savings can be made by using unlabeled protein, early-stage, budget-conscious programs may focus on using the ligand-detected suite of experiments shown in **Figure 4**, often acquiring them in parallel for each sample. The saturation transfer difference (STD) experiment can provide a binding-epitope map, as magnetization can only travel

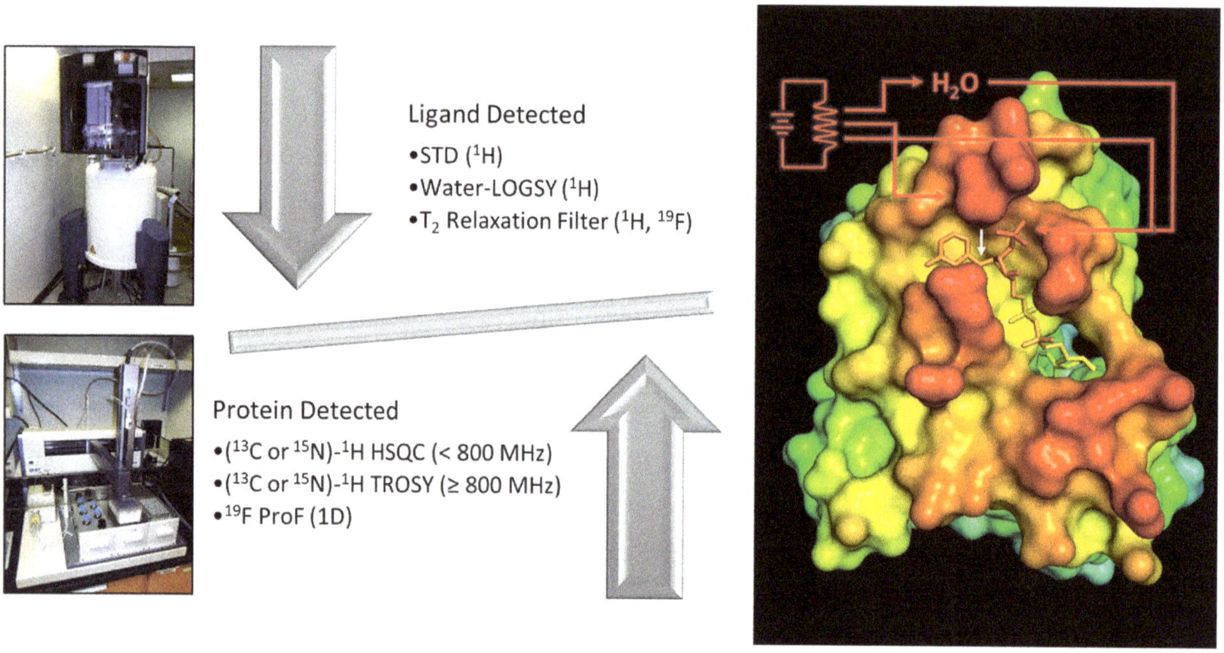

Figure 4. Screening fragments by NMR may include the use of automated sample preparation and handling. Common NMR experiments used in FBDD programs are listed, categorized according to their use of the magnetization pathways indicated. For ligand-detected experiments, additional pathways to the unbound ligand also exist. The white arrow indicates magnetization transfer from the protein to its bound ligand and is specific to the saturation transfer difference (STD) experiment.

through the protein to the bound fragment [18]. The epitope map enables a scientist using unlabeled protein to identify the portions of the fragment in closest proximity to the protein and, conversely, the portions available for expansion or linking for hit generation. Specialized experiments, such as the interligand nuclear Overhauser effect and target immobilized NMR screening (ILOE [19] and TINS [20], respectively), are best reserved for the study of difficult proteins or competition experiments. From the protein perspective, several variants of the two-dimensional HSQC experiment (typically ^1H nuclei measured directly and X nuclei, indirectly) that helps to disperse the numerous signals in a protein target and depend on the protein isotopic enrichment strategy. TROSY (another HSQC variant) can be used for large, usually perdeuterated proteins but requires a high-field instrument (i.e., 800 MHz and up); the discovery of methods to selectively label methyls [21] has simplified the resulting spectra and enabled screening on lower-field instruments (e.g., 500 MHz) [22].

To reduce protein consumption, NMR FBDD relies on the screening of equimolar fragment mixtures. This step is immediately followed by mixture dereplication, usually involving manual interpretation of spectra, although with careful sample preparation and a well-curated fragment spectral database, hits can be identified by software (e.g., *Mnova Suite*, Mestrelab Research S.L.; *ACD/Spectrus Suite*, Advanced Chemistry Development, Inc.; *Topspin*, Bruker Inc.). Individual reference spectra are acquired during the quality control steps of the fragment library design, and mixtures are then designed to avoid spectral overlap and reactivity. The number of fragments used per mixture is not standardized; but, basic statistical principles support using as few fragments as possible while avoiding mixing acids with bases or nucleophiles with electrophiles. For ^{1}H-observed experiments, 5–7 compounds per mixture is a reasonable starting point. Validation of hits is accomplished by a second round of screening individual fragments. At the validation stage, the use of spectroscopy experiments that provide binding site information (e.g., HSQC, STD mapping, ILOE) is highly recommended if crystallography is not readily available. Any resulting structural information is crucial for promoting the fragment into the downstream processes of medicinal chemistry and hit generation.

With the exception of WaterLOGSY, titration and analysis of the resulting signal of these NMR experiments can provide binding affinity scores for fragments with reasonable accuracy. In addition to the previously described STD experiment, ^{19}F NMR screening by filtered transverse relaxation (T_2), a filter also referred to as a Carr-Purcell-Meiboom-Gill (CPMG) scheme, can be a powerful option if used in competition with a known fluorinated ligand having a K_d measured carefully by using more rigorous techniques (e.g., SPR, ITC, FP). The potential benefit is that one sample can be analyzed for fragments in competition with or, perhaps, having an allosteric contribution to binding, and binding affinity is back-calculated relative to an internal nonbinding control or electric reference signal [23].

There are relatively few drawbacks to using available NMR facilities in a FBDD program considering the method's ability to contribute to every aspect of the workflow, such as library quality control and hit generation. The two drawbacks that are most often cited are the speed of the screen from sample preparation to data analysis and the demands on protein production for screening by NMR.

3.3. Surface plasmon resonance

Surface plasmon resonance shares the spotlight with NMR as a major screening technique for FBDD programs. The hurdles that come with using an immobilized protein for screening are counterbalanced by increased sensitivity and immediate access to kinetics data. Although absolute binding kinetics are not assured when dealing with weak affinities, for well-optimized experiments, obtaining k_a (binding), k_d (dissociation) rates, and the K_D (binding constant) value is certainly possible. Consequently, interpreting the resulting sensorgram can be challenging; but thankfully, the biosensor community has over 25 years of experiments to help set standards—hundreds just in 2009 [24]. With improvements in software to include experiment wizards, relatively new users can screen numerous fragments.

These experiments generally have long lead in times, as protein immobilization chemistry and buffer conditions need to be carefully perfected prior to screening experiments. Setting aside the routine instrument maintenance and screen validation using appropriate controls, the traditional stages of each experiment have been buffer and compound preparation, target immobilization, start-up samples (i.e., buffer match, blanks, and positive controls), fragment primary screen, data reduction and analysis, hit selection, and secondary dose response of hits.

Successful FBDD programs focus most practical attention on the preparation of the chip immobilization surface, ensuring stability between experiments. This focus on stability assumes that the loading conditions for the protein have been standardized and validated across multiple coupling methods, such as a covalent amine coupling [25] (to amine termini or lysine) or the less-amenable (regarding FBDD) coupling by protein tags (e.g., biotinylation or poly-histidine).

Once the target is loaded, screening samples should be prepared as single-point concentrations, for example 100 μM. The concentrations can be variable, but the expectation is that they are carefully prepared to avoid common problems such as precipitation and aggregate formation that may produce nonstoichiometric binding to the target. The use of detergents is allowable for the sake of the target but further complicates buffer matching in the reference channel. Troublesome fragments identified by their atypical sensorgrams are usually triaged from screening collections.

Once the data have been collected, data reduction and normalization follows and requires some practice to prosecute these steps efficiently. An experienced scientist can perform a first pass of the entire data set to quickly exclude sensorgrams for which a reasonable curve fit is unlikely due to compound incompatibilities or systemic problems with the instrument (**Figure 5**). Next, data reduction can seem like a tedious process to simply "clean" the sensorgrams; but in addition to aligning the injection time points, it checks the soundness of the blank injections, which yield important problem-solving data. Finally, the configuration of most instruments requires multiple runs to cover entire fragment libraries, so run-to-run variation naturally exists. Normalization seeks to enable the comparison of experimental responses, regardless of target density, binding activity, molecular weight, and buffer mismatch. The most expedient way to achieve this is by using the known concentration and bind-

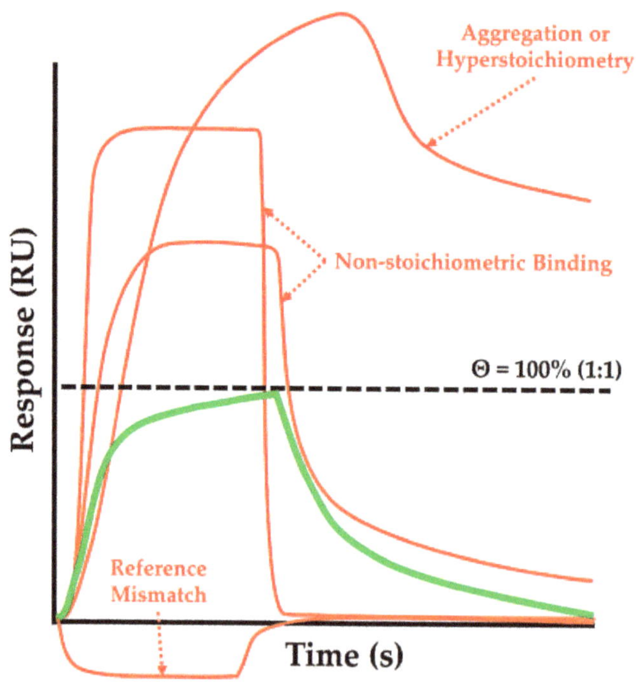

Figure 5. Ideal (green) and unfortunate (red) sensorgrams simulate binding and nonbinding events during the SPR experiment. Aggregation is typically concentration-dependent, whereas incorrect stoichiometry will not fit simple binding models. Relative occupancy (θ) of 100%, with a 1:1 stoichiometry indicated at the dashed line, represents how using high concentrations of fragments that appear to bind do so nonspecifically, binding weakly to multiple sites on the protein, chip surface, or nothing at all.

ing affinities of the control compound injections to convert the response unit (RU) to a relative occupancy (θ), wherein 100% would be saturated binding (i.e., R_{eq}/R_{max}).

Recently developed methods have increased the throughput of dose response studies, providing kinetic information earlier in the screening workflow and practically eliminating the need for a secondary set of experiments for hits. For example, a nonbinding diluent (i.e., 20%, w/v sucrose) can be used to create a range of compound concentrations from the same sample [26], or individually prepared sample concentrations can be sequentially injected (e.g., "single cycle kinetics" or kinetic titration) [27]. Both methods save time by avoiding multiple regeneration steps. Further gains have been realized by using Taylor dispersion injections [28] in a longer flow path (e.g., OneStep™, SensiQ Technologies Inc.) to deliberately produce a gradient of analyte concentration flowing across the chip surface: by modeling [29] this dispersion from a known initial concentration, the same kinetic data can be obtained during the injection phase of the experiment.

3.4. Thermal shift assay

Protein exists in a thermodynamic equilibrium between the folded and unfolded state. As the temperature of the system increases, the ratio of folded to unfolded protein shifts toward the unfolded state, making it possible to determine the temperature at which half of the protein is in the unfolded state. This point is referred to as the melting temperature of the protein (T_m). The thermal shift assay relies on ligand-induced conformational stabilization, which is based on the energetic coupling of ligand binding and protein denaturation. In short, fragment binding alters the ratio of folded to unfolded protein by stabilizing the folded state (**Figure 6**). Adding a stabilizing fragment will shift the T_m, allowing for the calculation of ΔT_m

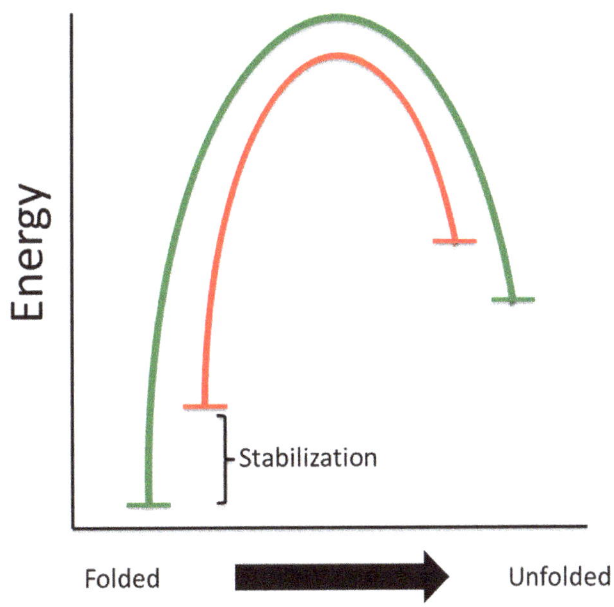

Figure 6. This figure demonstrates the theory associated with thermal shift interactions. Ligand binding causes stabilization of the protein in the more ordered folded state (represented in green). Thus, more thermal energy is required to move ligand stabilized protein from the folded to the unfolded state. Protein in the absence of ligand is represented in red. This protein requires less thermal energy to shift to the disordered state.

as an indicator of fragment binding [30–32]. Several methods available to measure the ratio of folded to unfolded protein in a given condition are: circular dichroism, infrared spectroscopy, differential scanning calorimetry, measurement of the intrinsic fluorescence of exposed tryptophan residues, and TSA, which is the most commonly applied technique. These methods were first adapted for use in TSA as a simple and inexpensive biophysical method for drug discovery in 2001 [30]. This work determined that ligand-induced protein stabilization could be tracked with environmentally sensitive dyes over a range of experimental temperatures. In an aqueous environment, the dye is quenched, giving minimal quantum yield. As the protein is denatured in the increasing temperature, its hydrophobic core is exposed to react with the dye. This interaction measurably increases the quantum yield of the dye.

Thermal shift has since been revised and optimized for use as an economical fragment screening method. A typical TSA has minimal requirements for the quantity of the target protein. A pilot assay should be completed wherein the concentration of protein is altered over a given range, as running TSA with an excess of protein can saturate the detector. Alternatively, too little protein will give a flat curve and negatively affect the signal-to-noise ratio in the resulting data (**Figure 7**). Thermal shift assays are commonly completed with 1–10 μM target protein, which should be as pure as possible. Gross impurities within the sample protein could lead to multiple curves, reducing the accuracy of the resulting data.

In addition to protein, TSA requires an environmentally sensitive dye. Historically napthylamine sulfonic acid dyes (such as 1,8-ANS, 2,6-ANS, or 2,6-TNS) were used for this purpose. Currently, SYPRO Orange is used more commonly as its fluorescence (Ex/Em of 300, 550/630 nm) is better adapted to rtPCR instruments. This dye is supplied from the vendor as a 5000X concentrate in DMSO. A pilot assay should be conducted to determine the appropriate concentration of SYPRO Orange for a given assay, as is done for protein concentration. In practice, many assays can be effectively run at a 5X concentration of SYPRO Orange. After the appropriate dye concentration has been established, a master mix of dye and buffer can be applied to the assay plate. At this point the plate is ready for the application of a fragment library.

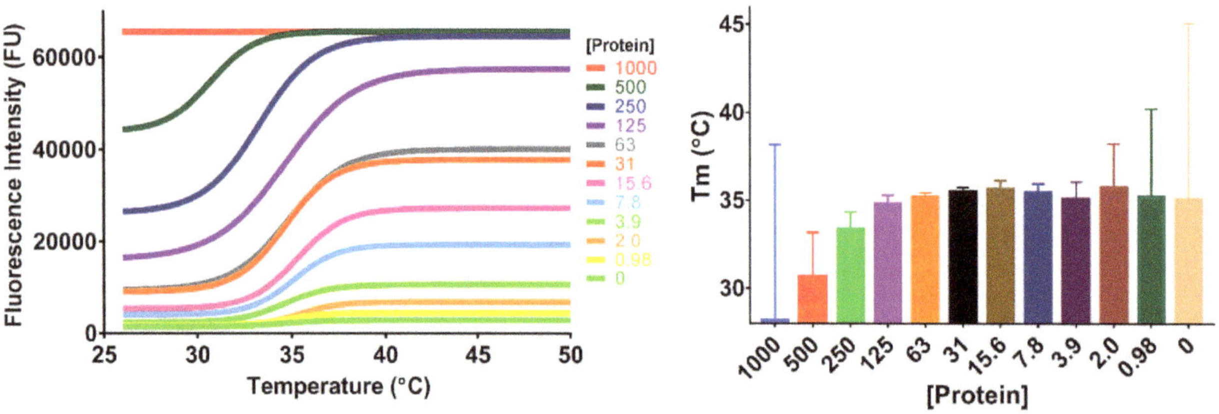

Figure 7. The importance of protein concentration in TSA. As protein concentration moves above or below the optimal range for the assay the curves fail to accurately represent the system and will increase the error of melting temperature calculation.

As in many fragment-screening assays, the quality of the library is paramount. In the assay development stage, a pilot assay should be run in which the concentration of solubilizing agent is varied over a range to define any effects that the agent might have on the stability of the protein. If time and availability of fragments allow, then a screen of fragment alone should be performed to check for fluorescence in the absence of ligand; this additional screen could yield data that is useful for removing problem compounds within the library. With an appropriate fragment library, it is possible to apply fragment to the screening plates. This is typically accomplished by using a pin tool or similar device capable of accurately delivering small volumes. After the plate has been exposed to the fragment library, it should be sealed with a fluorescently inert plate seal to avoid sample evaporation during the course of the assay. The assay plate should then be centrifuged to remove any air pockets from the samples, as these might reduce the quality of the data.

It has been established that TSA can be completed in a standard qPCR instrument [33]. The minimal requirement is the ability to evenly heat the samples over a suitable range of temperatures and record fluorescence. Deconvolution of resulting data output is variable based on instrumentation. This step can be time consuming and automation in data processing is helpful if large-scale projects are planned. Results should be recorded as fluorescent units recorded at each temperature in each well. This information can then be moved into data analysis software (e.g., *Graphpad Prism*, Graphpad Software, Inc.). Plotting fluorescence units against temperature should result in a sigmoidal curve reflecting the folded and unfolded states of the protein over a range of temperatures (**Figure 8a** and **b**). The signal commonly drops after it has reached a plateau. This drop is the result of aggregation in the protein-dye complex after denaturation [33]. Failure to remove data points resulting from this drop in signal can detrimentally affect subsequent curve fitting (**Figure 8a** and **b**). The Boltzmann equation can be adapted to calculate the exact T_m for each protein. Alternatively, it is possible to plot the derivative of the signal against temperature, recording the maximum of this derivative as the melting temperature (**Figure 8c**). The appropriate method for calculating the T_m can vary by target. Different methods should be tested to determine which calculation most accurately reflects the T_m of the experimental protein [32]. The thermal stability of a protein is increased to varying degrees when ligand is bound. The extent of this shift can vary greatly. In the case of fragment binding, thermal stabilization can be as little as 0.5 °C, making it crucial to establish the baseline stability of the protein within the experimental environment. It is then possible to establish the threshold of ΔT_m for a positive result in fragment stabilization of the ligand. As a rule of thumb, the standard deviation should not be greater than 10% of the ΔT_m [34].

There are many benefits to using TSA for the initial biophysical screening of a fragment library. First, the assay does not rely on the biochemical activity of the target and can be performed with limited knowledge of the target's function, which is beneficial for FBLD because fragment binding often does not yield a measurable biochemical result. Additionally, TSA requires only a small amount of minimally stable protein whose thermal stability can be tracked in the presence and absence of the ligand [30]. Thermal shift assays can be completed by using widely available RT-PCR instruments [33] and is relatively simple to perform with

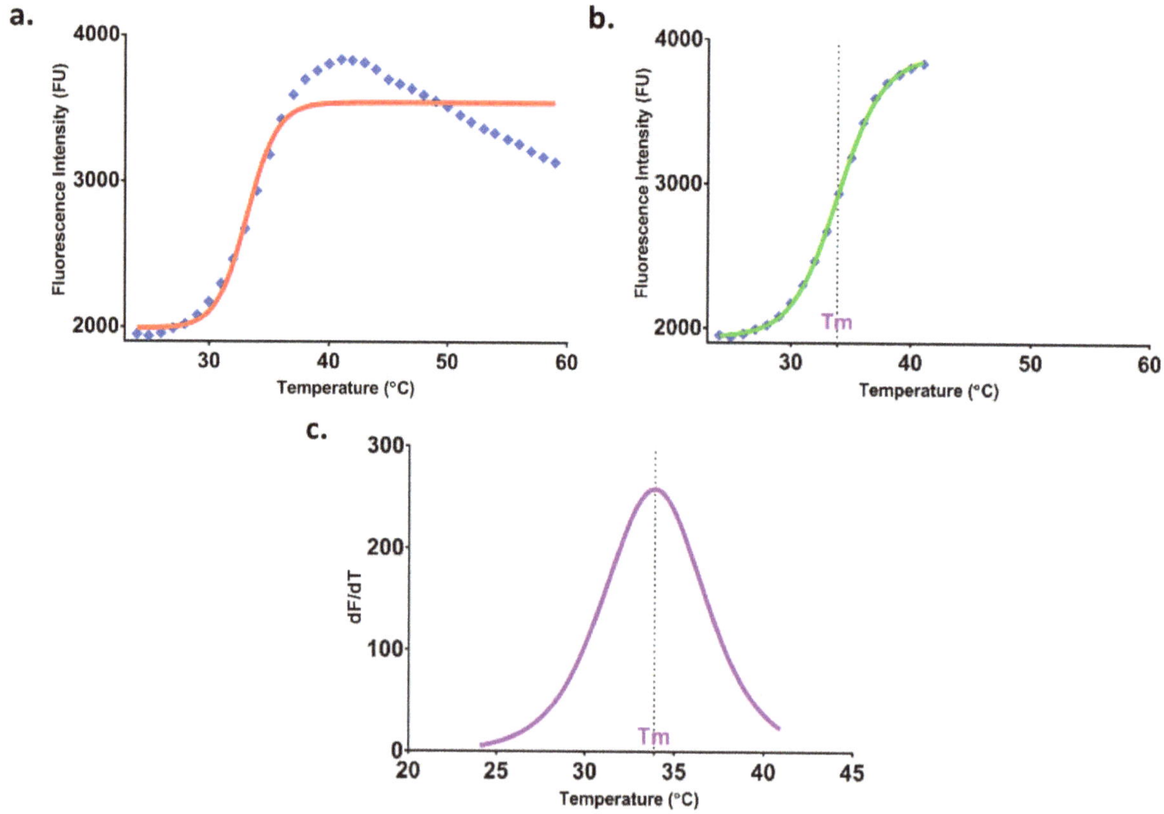

Figure 8. Curve fitting. (a) In this figure fluorescence intensity is plotted against temperature in blue. Above 41°C the dye begins to denature causing a decrease in signal. Fitting the full curve with the Boltzman equation (shown in red) would give an inaccurate estimation of T_m. (b) In this figure fluorescence intensity is plotted against temperature in blue. The data here is trimmed as signal begins to decrease improving the curve fitting (shown in green). (c) In this figure the change in fluorescence intensity over the change in temperature is plotted against temperature in purple.

limited training, reducing the up-front cost of implementing. This medium- to high-throughput assay typically enables the testing of up to 384 compounds in only 30–40 min.

Thermal shift assay is not a silver bullet *per se* and has some limitations and drawbacks. Traditional methods of assaying thermal shift will not work if a protein does not contain a hydrophobic core, as there will be nothing for the dye to differentially interact with when the target unfolds. Similarly, this assay will not produce valuable data if the surface of the protein is hydrophobic because the dye will fluoresce before the protein unfolds. Changing the dye used in the assay can mitigate these issues. The fluorescent readout of this assay also creates limitations. Some fragments commonly found in screening libraries fluoresce and interfere with the signal from SYPRO Orange. This phenomenon is readily evident upon inspection of the resulting data but requires a deconvolution step to avoid false-positive or false-negative results. Additionally, TSA does not provide accurate affinity data. However, a concentration versus ΔT_m curve can be fit to generate an EC_{50} value that can estimate the range in which subsequent biochemical or biophysical assays can be more effective [34, 35]. With these limitations in mind, TSA can be a powerful tool for detecting fragment binding.

3.5. Fragment validation

For the purposes of validation, a "good" fragment hit should be spatially described within a known target site via crystal structure, two-dimensional NMR studies, or at least, a ligand epitope map. The structural information enables the chemical expansion or linking of fragments during hit generation.

Hit rates in fragment-based screening are typically high, frequently at least an order of magnitude higher than those of ligand-based screening. Hits in the primary screen can be narrowed by using an orthogonal technique of comparable throughput for validation. Considering the numerous techniques available at the primary screening stage, the path to validation can be variable. Using an orthogonal approach to primary screening assumes that fragments that are hit by both techniques will translate successfully in secondary screening.

Using multiple techniques for fragment primary screening may yield a diminishing return. For example, after solving 71 crystal structures from soaking 361 fragments and statistically comparing the results of other fragment screening techniques [36], one group found that nearly half of the 71 "good" fragment hits were missed by other techniques. When used in combination, hit validation was statistically worse, but this fact was heightened by the inclusion of hits that were originally missed by crystallography. Therefore, orthogonal primary screening with at least two techniques still achieves the goal of fragment hit validation. However, if the primary fragment screening techniques do not provide meaningful structure characterization, then NMR or crystallography is required in a secondary screening capacity.

4. Fragment secondary screening

4.1. X-ray crystallography

Several companies, including Astex Pharmaceuticals, SGX Pharmaceuticals, Plexxikon, and Abbott, have effectively used structural biology in their fragment-based lead discovery efforts. This valuable tool avoids the pitfalls of false-positive results and nonspecific binding that may result from other fragment-screening methods. Any fragment hit discovered via crystallography is inherently validated for the given target. Crystallography gives a clear picture of the fragment binding posture within the active site. This information can greatly facilitate the design of libraries based on the initial hit.

Using crystallography as a method of fragment-based lead discovery has some limitations. It has long been associated with slow throughput. Additionally, some targets, such as membrane-associated proteins, do not readily lend themselves to crystallization. Crystallography often requires extensive and time-consuming efforts to arrive at crystallization conditions suitable for fragment soaking experiments. Even if these conditions have been determined, ready access to a suitable beam line and expertise in crystallography and data reduction can be hurdles in the rest of the lead discovery process. Protein in crystallization conditions is in a crystal lattice, which does not completely reflect a physiological environment. This artificial environment can lead to artifacts in the data and an inaccurate picture of fragment binding.

Although a crystal structure is rich in information, it does not reflect the potency or the biochemical activity of the bound fragment. With a wealth of structural information, it will not be possible to rank hits based on these criteria; orthogonal assays are critical for these purposes, and crystallography alone will not suffice.

The process of generating a fragment structure typically follows a set path. First, protein must be purified. Then, crystallization conditions for the purified protein are determined. Crystals can then either be grown in the presence of a fragment or soaked into a preexisting crystal. The resulting crystals are flash frozen and used for data collection either in house or at a larger beam line. The data is analyzed to generate a three-dimensional model of the fragment binding site within the target protein. This model can be used in iterative design efforts to grow the fragment into the binding site or link it to other fragments in neighboring sites.

Perhaps one of the most critical hurdles to successfully implementing structural biology into the FBLD process is having a suitable supply of the target protein. In most cases, protein used for X-ray crystallography must be pure and in high yields. A typical screen for crystallization conditions is completed by using as much as 20 mg/ml of protein. If initial crystal screening efforts using native protein are not effective, then it may be necessary to modify the target via removal of mobile loop regions or trimming the terminal ends. Creating multiple variants is commonly a valuable step in generating robust high-resolution structural data.

Once protein is available with sufficient yield and purity, screening for crystallization conditions begins. This is typically performed as a high-throughput screen with as many as 1000 set conditions in a single experiment. Many commercially available sparse matrix and additive crystallization screens use conditions that have historically yielded crystals. When these experiments yield a hit, the conditions can then be optimized to yield larger, highly reproducible crystals. Suitable crystals for fragment soaking should have fairly high resolution (<2 Å). Starting with a higher resolution structure improves resulting maps and increases the chances of producing an accurate model of fragment binding. If multiple crystallization conditions are available, it is best to choose the one that more closely represents physiological conditions, even at a slight cost to resolution. This trade-off will result in fragments with best chance of advancement to be prioritized.

Fragments suitable for X-ray crystallography benefit from good solubility, as insoluble fragments have a low probability of yielding a structure with suitable occupancy of the ligand. Compounds are soaked at high concentrations to improve the chances of high occupancy within the structure. Given this fact, a fragment should have a solubility of at least 1 mM [37]. SGX pharmaceuticals benefited from generating a brominated fragment library, which enabled detection of anomalous scatter as an indication of successful soaking, streamlining the data collection process. To further increase throughput, fragments were soaked in mixtures composed of fragments with diverse shapes. Resulting structures could then be deconvoluted based on the shape of the ligand in the active site [36]. Fragment mixtures do run the risk of decreasing the effective concentration of individual fragments in the mixture because high fragment concentration contributes to high-occupancy crystal structures, which can be detrimental to an experiment. In addition, these mixtures increase the chances of damaging the crystal in the soaking process, and fragments within the mix can interact with one another, skewing the results of the experiment. In one report, fragment mixtures resulted in 11 structures, whereas 20 structures resulted from individual soaking experiments [37]. These data suggest that if time and resources permit, soaking individual fragments is preferable to using mixtures.

If all other factors fall into place, a data set is collected. Improper treatment of this data set can result in an inaccurate and misleading model of fragment binding. Methods of data reduction and refinement are highly variable, and model building is a continuously evolving process. Certain steps in model building are especially pertinent when dealing with fragments. When searching for ligand density in a map, it is tempting to perform a quick refinement, and presume the location of a ligand. This approach is especially hazardous when modeling small fragments. If the map is not of high enough quality when the search for ligands begins, it is possible that water, a poorly resolved side chain, or even highly conserved buffers could masquerade as bound fragments [38]. It is best to perform several rounds of refinement before the ligand hunt begins. Model in any waters and then refine a few more times [37]. If the fragment is bound, a convincing map should take shape, and the creation of an accurate model of the target protein bound to fragments should be possible.

As technology progresses, many of the limitations of structural biology are being addressed. Most notably, throughput is being increased by incorporating automation. As this occurs, obtaining structural data is no longer the rate-limiting step in lead development. In several cases, automation of this process has improved to the extent that structural studies are successfully being used as a primary screen. Although this approach might not yet be a feasible option in laboratories with limited resources and limited access to beam lines, it holds promise for an improved fragment screening process in the future.

4.2. Isothermal titration calorimetry

Calorimetry measures the thermodynamics of a molecular interaction via observations of heat change in a reaction occurring in an adiabatic (thermodynamically closed) system [39]. In the context of drug discovery, the molecular interaction most commonly measured is the heat of binding of a small molecule to a protein target, although reaction kinetics can be measured under specific circumstances [40]. Measuring the heat associated with a molecular interaction allows direct measurement of the extent of breakage and formation of noncovalent interactions upon complex formation [39]. Using other methods, such as coupled reactions (e.g., product release) and fluorescent binding techniques, the change in enthalpy can only be inferred via the Van't Hoff relationship [41].

Classically, calorimetry has been applied to measurement of a binding interaction in two different ways: isothermal titration calorimetry, which measures heat release upon binding; and differential scanning calorimetry (DSC), which measures thermal stabilization of a protein due to binding of a small molecule. These methods offer a very detailed look at the thermodynamics of binding and have been used successfully in optimization after initial fragment hits have been identified. For the purposes of this chapter, discussion will be limited to ITC, as it is more directly applicable to FBDD. As a direct measurement of the heat of binding, ITC allows the researcher to remove the effects of fluorescent tags, antibody relationships, or coupling chemistry from the investigation of a binding relationship. Because ITC is a solution-based method, surface physical effects that interfere with binding (often seen with SPR) are not an issue.

Directly determining the thermodynamic components of overall binding allows a researcher to optimize a lead compound for a chosen target through specific binding interactions while minimizing off-target effects that often derail drug discovery programs. When combined with X-ray-based binding information or applied to analysis of structure-activity relationships, ITC can be a powerful tool in drug discovery. Overall binding of a small molecule to a target (as expressed by K_D) can be broken down into enthalpic (specific interactions such as H-bonding and π-stacking) and entropic (nonspecific events such as bound water release and increases in conformational flexibility) components.

The normal range of dissociation constants that can be measured by ITC is from 10 nM to 100 μM [41]. This range can be extended below 1 nM or above 1 mM by using displacement methods [42, 43], although a suitable displacement ligand (independently characterized) must be identified beforehand. Displacement ITC has not yet gained wide acceptance in drug discovery as of this writing, with most researchers reporting results of direct binding studies. Most fragments have binding affinities in the millimolar range, limiting the applicability of ITC as a screening method. In addition, large amounts of protein are typically required (usually 0.1–0.3 mg of protein per experiment, this moderate amount adds up for multiple samples and repeats). Each titration requires a moderate amount of time (45 min–1 h), but for a large number of samples, experiment time becomes a hurdle to using ITC as a screening method.

For these reasons, ITC is usually brought in to the drug discovery process after screening, as part of hit validation and lead optimization [44]. Fewer compounds are involved, allowing more focus on the large amount of information provided by ITC [44–46]. After a compound of interest is identified, a small set of structurally similar compounds can be purchased or synthesized to gain insight into the nature of binding to a target [47, 48]. At this stage, ITC offers the most benefit, as small molecules can be identified that maximize enthalpic interactions and minimize entropic interactions with the target.

Recent research into high-throughput calorimetry offer solutions to researchers wanting to incorporate calorimetry into an earlier stage in their screening cascade. Research into technologies in pursuit of the so-called "lab on a chip" has led to the development of both microfluidic [49] and droplet-based systems [50–52]. The droplet-based system has been applied to both binding and kinetics.

4.3. Fluorescence polarization

Biochemical screening is not a typical choice for the primary screening of fragments but can be used to verify an inhibition of function, and inhibition by a known mechanism which may help discriminate fragments binding to alternative target sites.

Fluorescence polarization-based assays are an option in FBDD when preliminary information about a target, such as small molecules that bind, is known. FP assays are competition assays in that they indirectly measure the effect of a compound on binding of an enzyme to a fluorescent probe. A fluorescent probe ideally starts out as a small molecule that binds tightly to an enzyme with known stoichiometry. This small molecule is chemically modified by the addition of a fluorescent label via an aliphatic or polyol linker to generate a fluorescent probe. Signal readout, represented in millipolarization units (mP), is calculated by measuring the amount of plane-polarized light passing through two filters (perpendicular and parallel to the plane of incident light) that remains after interaction with a solution containing probe and calculating the ratio of parallel to perpendicular light [53, 54]. In an FP assay, a plate reader measures the difference in relative tumbling between a free probe (high amount of tumbling, leading to more scattered emission, and thus low FP signal) and probe bound to a protein (low amount of tumbling, with more ordered emission relative to incident light, leading to high FP signal).

Depending on assay design, FP can be applied to either binding or activity assays, with ready-to-use kits available from BellBrook Labs [55] or Cayman Chemical [56]. Activity assays using FP rely on endpoint detection of binding to a probe, thus, are modified binding assays. For applications for which no kit is available, a small amount of synthesis can combine a small molecule of interest with a wide variety of synthetic fluorophores available from major vendors. When designing a probe for FP, resources such as the Molecular Probes Handbook [57] can be valuable.

FP is less commonly used in fragment screening than perhaps it should be. The range of binding affinities normally found in fragment libraries is in the high-μM to low-millimolar range, previously considered to be out of the range of FP when tight binding probes are used [58]. Although still somewhat limited in application by the need for a well-characterized probe, FP offers an inexpensive way to screen large numbers of compounds and has been used for many years in conventional drug discovery programs. With the advent of fragment-based techniques, FP is finding use both as a site directed primary [59, 60] and secondary [61–64] screening method, and has been used to validate new methods [65].

5. Fragment hit progression

For fragments, it is important to see activity in more than one assay, but equivalent potency in assays is not so important, and is not the best way to determine which molecules to promote. Various combinations of advanced metrics (i.e., efficiencies) with empirically driven evaluations (e.g., PAINS, metabolic stability) can help scientists make informed decisions on hit progression. An outside example of the successful application of metrics is sabermetrics. Today widely used in baseball, but also heavily scrutinized and evolving, sabermetrics uses advanced statistics to define in-game performance and improve decision-making by managers. Just like a game manager, scientists have to be aware of the limitations and effects of following a metric's indication, being consistent about hit progression occasionally in the light of conflicting results. Some experts [66] suggest using ligand efficiencies that can be easily determined without a calculator to facilitate discussions. Several metric-focused reviews are available to consult; one in particular covers a large number of reported hit-lead programs [67] for a wider perspective.

5.1. Empirically based fragment evaluations

Fragment screening methods virtually ensure that most screens will produce multiple hits for any target. Thus, the challenge to the researcher is not identifying compounds that interfere with a specific enzyme but determining which of many is the best to carry forward. Several metrics have emerged to guide the selection of fragment lead molecules through the drug discovery process: these metrics combine physical properties (e.g., molecular weight, cLogP, polar surface area, number of H-bond donors and acceptors) with potency data. The earliest of these was simply termed ligand efficiency (LE) and involved dividing the free energy (ΔG) of binding by the total number of nonhydrogen atoms in the molecule [68]. With the introduction of LE, researchers now havea relatively simple way to keep focused on the specificity of binding to the target, potentially avoiding downstream problems due to nonspecific binding [69].

Another metric in wide use in FBDD is lipophilic ligand efficiency (LLE) [70], which takes into account the total lipophilicity and potency of a molecule (IC_{50}, K_D, K_i). A useful modification of LLE (LLE_{Astex}) also controls for molecule size [71]. These statistical means of grading performance can support the early and late stages of the FBDD workflow and can be extended into progression analyses used during lead development (**Figure 9**). Which metric to use is up to the individual researcher and is based on the specific goals of the research program. Further reading to find an appropriate metric to use is recommended.

5.2. Hit generation

Fragments that progress to the hit-generation stage typically do so with structural insight that either describes the fragment bound to its protein target or the binding epitope mapped

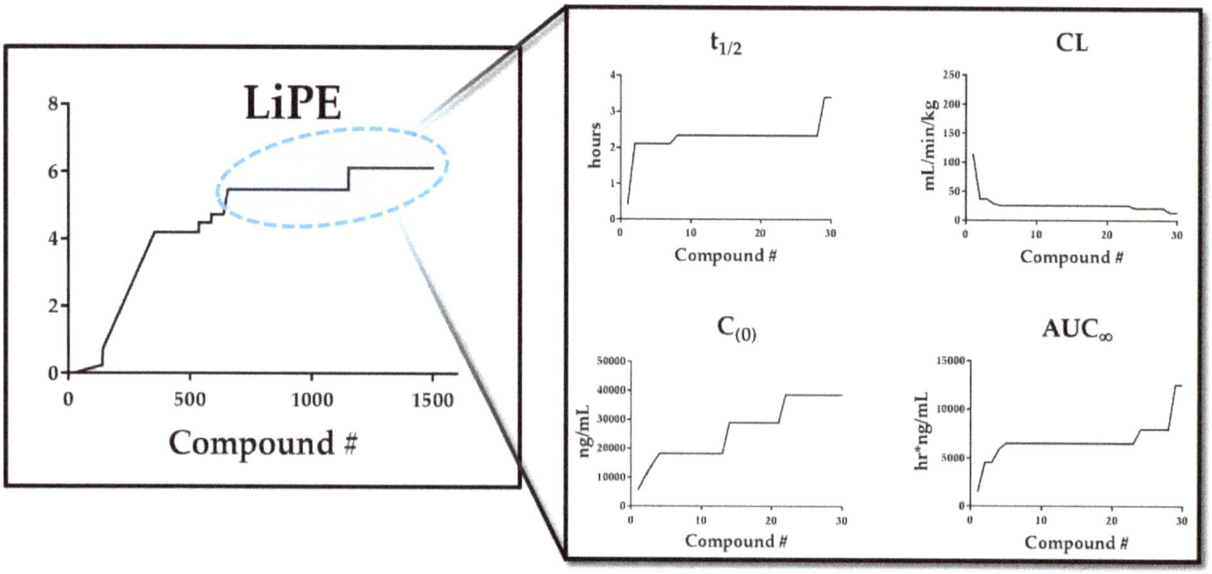

Figure 9. A typical progression analysis found in lead development can also include ligand efficiency metrics in a seamless fashion.

onto the fragment. A typical downstream workflow for hit generation includes a path that is structure blind, but this is essentially a diversion from traditional target-based discovery and may lead to an SAR bottleneck. The hit-generation stage refers to acquisition and screening of larger nonfragment ligands, which are obtained by catalog or synthetically prepared. This workflow includes either a chemical elaboration of individual fragments or the linking of at least two fragments, which then requires some optimization of the linker between them.

The hit generation phase is a practical place for virtual screening to be used to assist in fragment development. Method comparisons [72, 73] suggest that the currently available force fields and docking procedures based on lead-like molecules will provide adequate results for fragments (i.e., better than randomized screening). However, the careful consideration of a scoring function to reliably discern weak interactions cannot be overemphasized. Scientists have recognized this distinction within FBDD and have sought to improve the scoring functions for fragments [74]. One notable viewpoint is that fragment elaboration or linking may be facilitated when binding poses are expressed as Gibbs energy [75].

6. Conclusions

Considering that FBDD has been attributed to at least two FDA drug approvals, and that the platform is relatively easy to integrate into existing technologies, many companies and academic groups have started their own fragment-based discovery programs. The biophysical techniques each group uses will be dictated by the target, available facilities, and individual preferences of the investigators. Generally speaking, as long as the protein target has been successfully used with a technique in lead-like screening and structural information is available, there are virtually no other major obstacles to generating new chemical matter for a given target-based screening program. What remains are practical challenges, two of which bear repeating for those who are in the beginning stages of FBDD.

First, the key practical difference between lead-like screening and fragment screening is the use of high concentrations of the fragments. The increased concentration impacts the compound library that is used and the clarity at which hits are delineated. Some suggestions have been made as to the optimal concentrations to use for a given technique. These are only suggestions and will likely change based on the system and techniques employed. With some practice, these procedures can be suitably optimized and need less attention going forward.

Second, is the challenge of directing fragment build out and/or fragment linking chemistry which can be resource intensive. As such, medicinal chemists are aided by the use of a preferred ligand efficiency metric early in the FBDD process to assist the ranking of fragment hits. Certainly other empirical and nonempirical factors will influence the progression of fragments, but metrics will help organize the structure-activity relationship which is a key driver of the expansion or linking of fragments during hit generation.

Acknowledgments

The authors would like to acknowledge the funding support from the National Institutes of Health grant R01AI110578, and the American Lebanese Syrian Associated Charities (ALSAC), St Jude Children's Research Hospital. We thank Cherise Guess, PhD, ELS, of the SJCRH Department of Scientific Editing for her assistance with editing.

Author details

John J. Bowling[1], William R. Shadrick[1], Elizabeth C. Griffith[1] and Richard E. Lee[1, 2*]

*Address all correspondence to: Richard.Lee@stjude.org

1 Department of Chemical Biology and Therapeutics, St. Jude Children's Research Hospital, Memphis, TN, United States

2 Department of Pharmaceutical Sciences, University of Tennessee Health Science Center, Memphis, TN, United States

References

[1] Macarron R, Banks MN, Bojanic D, Burns DJ, Cirovic DA, Garyantes T, Green DVS, Hertzberg RP, Janzen WP, Paslay JW, Schopfer U, Sittampalam GS. Impact of high-throughput screening in biomedical research. Nat Rev Drug Discov. 2011; 10(3): 188–95. DOI: 10.1038/nrd3368

[2] Reymond J-L. The chemical space project. Acc Chem Res. 2015; 48(3): 722–30. DOI: 10.1021/ar500432k

[3] Hert J, Irwin JJ, Laggner C, Keiser MJ, Shoichet BK. Quantifying biogenic bias in screening libraries. Nat Chem Biol. 2009; 5(7): 479–83. DOI: 10.1038/nchembio.180

[4] Hann MM, Leach AR, Harper G. Molecular complexity and its impact on the probability of finding leads for drug discovery. J Chem Inf Comp Sci. 2001; 41(3): 856–64. DOI: 10.1021/ci000403i

[5] Jencks WP. On the attribution and additivity of binding energies. Proc Natl Acad Sci USA. 1981; 78(7): 4046–50. DOI: N/A

[6] Shuker SB, Hajduk PJ, Meadows RP, Fesik SW. Discovering high-affinity ligands for proteins: SAR by NMR. Science. 1996; 274(5292): 1531–4. DOI: 10.1126/science.274.5292.1531

[7] Bollag G, Tsai J, Zhang J, Zhang C, Ibrahim P, Nolop K, Hirth P. Vemurafenib: the first drug approved for BRAF-mutant cancer. Nat Rev Drug Discov. 2012; 11(11): 873–86. DOI: 10.1038/nrd3847

[8] Deeks ED. Venetoclax: first global approval. Drugs. 2016; 76(9): 979–87. DOI: 10.1007/s40265-016-0596-x

[9] Erlanson DA, Fesik SW, Hubbard RE, Jahnke W, Jhoti H. Twenty years on: the impact of fragments on drug discovery. Nat Rev Drug Discov. 2016; 15(9): 605–19. DOI: 10.1038/nrd.2016.109

[10] Congreve M, Carr R, Murray C, Jhoti H. A 'Rule of Three' for fragment-based lead discovery? Drug Discov Today. 2003; 8(19): 876–7. DOI: 10.1016/S1359-6446(03)02831-9

[11] Jhoti H, Williams G, Rees DC, Murray CW. The 'rule of three' for fragment-based drug discovery: where are we now? Nat Rev Drug Discov. 2013; 12(8): 644. DOI: 10.1038/nrd3926-c1

[12] Keseru GM, Erlanson DA, Ferenczy GG, Hann MM, Murray CW, Pickett SD. Design principles for fragment libraries: maximizing the value of learnings from pharma fragment-based drug discovery (FBDD) programs for use in academia. J Med Chem. 2016; 59(18): 8189–206. DOI: 10.1021/acs.jmedchem.6b00197

[13] Swain C. Fragment Collections [Internet]. 2016. Available from: http://www.cambridgemedchemconsulting.com/resources/hit_identification/fragment_collections.html [Accessed: 2016-09-09]

[14] Lau WF, Withka JM, Hepworth D, Magee TV, Du YJ, Bakken GA, Miller MD, Hendsch ZS, Thanabal V, Kolodziej SA, Xing L, Hu Q, Narasimhan LS, Love R, Charlton ME, Hughes S, van Hoorn WP, Mills JE. Design of a multi-purpose fragment screening library using molecular complexity and orthogonal diversity metrics. J Comput Aid Mol Des. 2011; 25(7): 621–36. DOI: 10.1007/s10822-011-9434-0

[15] Kutchukian PS, So S-S, Fischer C, Waller CL. Fragment library design: using cheminformatics and expert chemists to fill gaps in existing fragment libraries. In: Klon EA, editor. Fragment-Based Methods in Drug Discovery. New York, NY: Springer New York; 2015. pp. 43–53. DOI: 10.1007/978-1-4939-2486-8_5

[16] Davis BJ, Erlanson DA. Learning from our mistakes: the 'unknown knowns' in fragment screening. Bioorg Med Chem Lett. 2013; 23(10): 2844–52. DOI: 10.1016/j.bmcl.2013.03.028

[17] Lagorce D, Sperandio O, Baell JB, Miteva MA, Villoutreix BO. FAF-Drugs3: a web server for compound property calculation and chemical library design. Nucleic Acid Res. 2015; 43(W1): W200–W7. DOI: 10.1093/nar/gkv353

[18] Mayer M, Meyer B. Group epitope mapping by saturation transfer difference NMR to identify segments of a ligand in direct contact with a protein receptor. J Am Chem Soc. 2001; 123(25): 6108–17. DOI: 10.1021/ja0100120

[19] Sledz P, Silvestre HL, Hung AW, Ciulli A, Blundell TL, Abell C. Optimization of the interligand Overhauser effect for fragment linking: application to inhibitor discovery against mycobacterium tuberculosis pantothenate synthetase. J Am Chem Soc. 2010; 132(13): 4544–5. DOI: 10.1021/ja100595u

[20] Vanwetswinkel S, Heetebrij RJ, van Duynhoven J, Hollander JG, Filippov DV, Hajduk PJ, Siegal G. TINS, Target immobilized NMR screening: an efficient and sensitive method for ligand discovery. Chem Biol. 2005; 12(2): 207–16. DOI: 10.1016/j.chembiol.2004.12.004

[21] Gardner KH, Kay LE. Production and incorporation of 15N, 13C, 2H (1H-δ1 methyl) isoleucine into proteins for multidimensional NMR studies. J Am Chem Soc. 1997; 119(32): 7599–600. DOI: 10.1021/ja9706514

[22] Hajduk PJ, Augeri DJ, Mack J, Mendoza R, Yang J, Betz SF, Fesik SW. NMR-Based screening of proteins containing 13C-labeled methyl groups. J Am Chem Soc. 2000; 122(33): 7898–904. DOI: 10.1021/ja000350l

[23] Dalvit C. Ligand- and substrate-based 19F NMR screening: principles and applications to drug discovery. Prog Nucl Mag Res Sp. 2007; 51(4): 243–71. DOI: 10.1016/j.pnmrs.2007.07.002

[24] Rich RL, Myszka DG. Survey of the 2009 commercial optical biosensor literature. J Mol Recognit. 2011; 24(6): 892–914. DOI: 10.1002/jmr.1138

[25] Johnsson B, Löfås S, Lindquist G. Immobilization of proteins to a carboxymethyldextran-modified gold surface for biospecific interaction analysis in surface plasmon resonance sensors. Anal Biochem. 1991; 198(2): 268–77. DOI: 10.1016/0003-2697(91)90424-R

[26] Rich RL, Quinn JG, Morton T, Stepp JD, Myszka DG. Biosensor-based fragment screening using FastStep injections. Anal Biochem. 2010; 407(2): 270–7. DOI: 10.1016/j.ab.2010.08.024

[27] Karlsson R, Katsamba PS, Nordin H, Pol E, Myszka DG. Analyzing a kinetic titration series using affinity biosensors. Anal Biochem. 2006; 349(1): 136–47. DOI: 10.1016/j.ab.2005.09.034

[28] Quinn JG. Evaluation of Taylor dispersion injections: determining kinetic/affinity interaction constants and diffusion coefficients in label-free biosensing. Anal Biochem. 2012; 421(2): 401–10. DOI: 10.1016/j.ab.2011.11.023

[29] Quinn JG. Modeling Taylor dispersion injections: determination of kinetic/affinity interaction constants and diffusion coefficients in label-free biosensing. Anal Biochem. 2012; 421(2): 391–400. DOI: 10.1016/j.ab.2011.11.024

[30] Pantoliano MW, Petrella EC, Kwasnoski JD, Lobanov VS, Myslik J, Graf E, Carver T, Asel E, Springer BA, Lane P, Salemme FR. High-density miniaturized thermal shift assays as a general strategy for drug discovery. J Biomol Screen. 2001; 6(6): 429–40. DOI: 10.1089/108705701753364922

[31] Ciulli A. Biophysical screening for the discovery of small-molecule ligands. In: Williams M, Daviter T, editors. Methods in Molecular Biology. 2nd ed. New York: Springer; 2013. pp. 357–88. DOI: 10.1007/978-1-62703-398-5_13

[32] Schiebel J, Radeva N, Koster H, Metz A, Krotzky T, Kuhnert M, Diederich WE, Heine A, Neumann L, Atmanene C, Roecklin D, Vivat-Hannah V, Renaud JP, Meinecke R, Schlinck

N, Sitte A, Popp F, Zeeb M, Klebe G. One question, multiple answers: biochemical and biophysical screening methods retrieve deviating fragment hit lists. Chemmedchem. 2015; 10(9): 1511–21. DOI: 10.1002/cmdc.201500267

[33] Lo MC, Aulabaugh A, Jin G, Cowling R, Bard J, Malamas M, Ellestad G. Evaluation of fluorescence-based thermal shift assays for hit identification in drug discovery. Anal Biochem. 2004; 332(1): 153–9. DOI: 10.1016/j.ab.2004.04.031

[34] Vivoli M, Novak HR, Littlechild JA, Harmer NJ. Determination of protein-ligand interactions using differential scanning fluorimetry. J Vis Exp. 2014; 91: 51809. DOI: 10.3791/51809

[35] Groftehauge MK, Hajizadeh NR, Swann MJ, Pohl E. Protein-ligand interactions investigated by thermal shift assays (TSA) and dual polarization interferometry (DPI). Acta Crystallogr D. 2015; 71(Pt 1): 36–44. DOI: 10.1107/S1399004714016617

[36] Schiebel J, Radeva N, Krimmer SG, Wang X, Stieler M, Ehrmann FR, Fu K, Metz A, Huschmann FU, Weiss MS, Mueller U, Heine A, Klebe G. Six biophysical screening methods miss a large proportion of crystallographically discovered fragment hits: a case study. ACS Chem Biol. 2016; 11(6): 1693–701. DOI: 10.1021/acschembio.5b01034

[37] Schiebel J, Krimmer SG, Rower K, Knorlein A, Wang X, Park AY, Stieler M, Ehrmann FR, Fu K, Radeva N, Krug M, Huschmann FU, Glockner S, Weiss MS, Mueller U, Klebe G, Heine A. High-throughput crystallography: reliable and efficient identification of fragment hits. Structure. 2016; 24(8): 1398–409. DOI: 10.1016/j.str.2016.06.010

[38] Kleywegt GJ. Crystallographic refinement of ligand complexes. Acta Crystallogr D. 2007; 63(Pt 1): 94–100. DOI: 10.1107/S0907444906022657

[39] Ladbury JE, Klebe G, Freire E. Adding calorimetric data to decision making in lead discovery: a hot tip. Nat Rev Drug Discov. 2010; 9(1): 23–7. DOI: 10.1038/nrd3054

[40] Hansen LD, Transtrum MK, Quinn C, Demarse N. Enzyme-catalyzed and binding reaction kinetics determined by titration calorimetry. Biochim Biophys Acta. 2016; 1860(5): 957–66. DOI: 10.1016/j.bbagen.2015.12.018

[41] Ladbury JE. Calorimetry as a tool for understanding biomolecular interactions and an aid to drug design. Biochem Soc T. 2010; 38(4): 888–93. DOI: 10.1042/bst0380888

[42] Velazquez-Campoy A, Freire E. Isothermal titration calorimetry to determine association constants for high-affinity ligands. Nat Protoc. 2006; 1(1): 186–91. DOI: 10.1038/nprot.2006.28

[43] Ruhmann E, Betz M, Fricke M, Heine A, Schafer M, Klebe G. Thermodynamic signatures of fragment binding: validation of direct versus displacement ITC titrations. Biochim Biophys Acta. 2015; 1850(4): 647–56. DOI: 10.1016/j.bbagen.2014.12.007

[44] Mashalidis EH, Sledz P, Lang S, Abell C. A three-stage biophysical screening cascade for fragment-based drug discovery. Nat Protoc. 2013; 8(11): 2309–24. DOI: 10.1038/nprot.2013.130

[45] Ladbury JE. Isothermal titration calorimetry: application to structure-based drug design. Thermochim Acta. 2001; 380(2): 209–15. DOI: 10.1016/S0040-6031(01)00674-8

[46] Scott DE, Ehebauer MT, Pukala T, Marsh M, Blundell TL, Venkitaraman AR, Abell C, Hyvonen M. Using a fragment-based approach to target protein-protein interactions. Chembiochem. 2013; 14(3): 332–42. DOI: 10.1002/cbic.201200521

[47] Banerjee DR, Dutta D, Saha B, Bhattacharyya S, Senapati K, Das AK, Basak A. Design, synthesis and characterization of novel inhibitors against mycobacterial beta-ketoacyl CoA reductase FabG4. Org Biomol Chem. 2014; 12(1): 73–85. DOI: 10.1039/c3ob41676c

[48] Kišonaite M, Zubriene A, Čapkauskaite E, Smirnov A, Smirnoviene J, Kairys V, Michailoviene V, Manakova E, Gražulis S, Matulis D. Intrinsic thermodynamics and structure correlation of benzenesulfonamides with a pyrimidine moiety binding to carbonic anhydrases I, II, VII, XII, and XIII. Plos One. 2014; 9(12): e114106. DOI: 10.1371/journal.pone.0114106

[49] Wolf A, Hartmann T, Bertolini M, Schemberg J, Grodrian A, Lemke K, Förster T, Kessler E, Hänschke F, Mertens F, Paus R, Lerchner J. Toward high-throughput chip calorimetry by use of segmented-flow technology. Thermochim Acta. 2015; 603: 172–83. DOI: 10.1016/j.tca.2014.10.021

[50] Recht MI, Nienaber V, Torres FE. Fragment-based screening for enzyme inhibitors using calorimetry. Method Enzymol. 2016; 567: 47–69. DOI: 10.1016/bs.mie.2015.07.023

[51] Recht MI, Sridhar V, Badger J, Bounaud PY, Logan C, Chie-Leon B, Nienaber V, Torres FE. Identification and optimization of PDE10A inhibitors using fragment-based screening by nanocalorimetry and X-ray crystallography. J Biomol Screen. 2014; 19(4): 497–507. DOI: 10.1177/1087057113516493

[52] Torres FE, Kuhn P, De Bruyker D, Bell AG, Wolkin MV, Peeters E, Williamson JR, Anderson GB, Schmitz GP, Recht MI, Schweizer S, Scott LG, Ho JH, Elrod SA, Schultz PG, Lerner RA, Bruce RH. Enthalpy arrays. Proc Natl Acad Sci U S A. 2004; 101(26): 9517–22. DOI: 10.1073/pnas.0403573101

[53] Lea WA, Simeonov A. Fluorescence polarization assays in small molecule screening. Expert Opin Drug Discov. 2011; 6(1): 17–32. DOI: 10.1517/17460441.2011.537322

[54] Rossi AM, Taylor CW. Analysis of protein-ligand interactions by fluorescence polarization. Nat Protoc. 2011; 6(3): 365–87. DOI: 10.1038/nprot.2011.305

[55] BellBrook Labs. Transcreener® HTS Assays [Internet]. 2016. Available from: https://www.bellbrooklabs.com/products-services/transcreener-hts-assays/[Accessed: 2016-09-23]

[56] Cayman Chemical. Assay Kits [Internet]. 2016. Available from: https://www.caymanchem.com/Products/kits [Accessed: 2016-09-23]

[57] Thermo Fisher Scientific. The Molecular Probes Handbook [Internet]. 2016. Available from: http://www.thermofisher.com/us/en/home/references/molecular-probes-the-handbook.html [Accessed: 2016-09-23]

[58] Xinyi H. Fluorescence polarization competition assay: the range of resolvable inhibitor potency is limited by the affinity of the fluorescent ligand. J Biomol Screen. 2003; 8(1): 34–8. DOI: 10.1177/1087057102239666

[59] Baughman BM, Jake Slavish P, DuBois RM, Boyd VA, White SW, Webb TR. Identification of influenza endonuclease inhibitors using a novel fluorescence polarization assay. ACS Chem Biol. 2012; 7(3): 526–34. DOI: 10.1021/cb200439z

[60] Carson MW, Zhang J, Chalmers MJ, Bocchinfuso WP, Holifield KD, Masquelin T, Stites RE, Stayrook KR, Griffin PR, Dodge JA. HDX reveals unique fragment ligands for the vitamin D receptor. Bioorg Med Chem Lett. 2014; 24(15): 3459–63. DOI: 10.1016/j.bmcl.2014.05.070

[61] Davies NGM, Browne H, Davis B, Drysdale MJ, Foloppe N, Geoffrey S, Gibbons B, Hart T, Hubbard R, Jensen MR, Mansell H, Massey A, Matassova N, Moore JD, Murray J, Pratt R, Ray S, Robertson A, Roughley SD, Schoepfer J, Scriven K, Simmonite H, Stokes S, Surgenor A, Webb P, Wood M, Wright L, Brough P. Targeting conserved water molecules: design of 4-aryl-5-cyanopyrrolo[2,3-d]pyrimidine Hsp90 inhibitors using fragment-based screening and structure-based optimization. Bioorg Med Chem. 2012; 20(22): 6770–89. DOI: 10.1016/j.bmc.2012.08.050

[62] Yin Z, Whittell LR, Wang Y, Jergic S, Liu M, Harry EJ, Dixon NE, Beck JL, Kelso MJ, Oakley AJ. Discovery of lead compounds targeting the bacterial sliding clamp using a fragment-based approach. J Med Chem. 2014; 57(6): 2799–806. DOI: 10.1021/jm500122r

[63] Yu W, Xiao H, Lin J, Li C. Discovery of novel STAT3 small molecule inhibitors via in silico site-directed fragment-based drug design. J Med Chem. 2013; 56(11): 4402–12. DOI: 10.1021/jm400080c

[64] Zhao L, Cao D, Chen T, Wang Y, Miao Z, Xu Y, Chen W, Wang X, Li Y, Du Z, Xiong B, Li J, Xu C, Zhang N, He J, Shen J. Fragment-based drug discovery of 2-thiazolidinones as inhibitors of the histone reader BRD4 bromodomain. J Med Chem. 2013; 56(10): 3833–51. DOI: 10.1021/jm301793a

[65] Meiby E, Simmonite H, le Strat L, Davis B, Matassova N, Moore JD, Mrosek M, Murray J, Hubbard RE, Ohlson S. Fragment screening by weak affinity chromatography: comparison with established techniques for screening against HSP90. Anal Chem. 2013; 85(14): 6756–66. DOI: 10.1021/ac400715t

[66] Zartler E. Practical Fragments [Internet]. Erlanson D, editor. Blogger: Google Inc. 2015. [2016/08/01]. Available from: http://practicalfragments.blogspot.com/2015/09/is-this-still-thing-and-why.html

[67] Ferenczy GG, Keseru GM. How are fragments optimized? A retrospective analysis of 145 fragment optimizations. J Med Chem. 2013; 56(6): 2478–86. DOI: 10.1021/jm301851v

[68] Hopkins AL, Groom CR, Alex A. Ligand efficiency: a useful metric for lead selection. Drug Discov Today. 2004; 9(10): 430–1. DOI: 10.1016/s1359-6446(04)03069-7

[69] Hughes JP, Rees S, Kalindjian SB, Philpott KL. Principles of early drug discovery. Brit J Pharmacol. 2011; 162(6): 1239–49. DOI: 10.1111/j.1476-5381.2010.01127.x

[70] Leeson PD, Springthorpe B. The influence of drug-like concepts on decision-making in medicinal chemistry. Nat Rev Drug Discov. 2007; 6(11): 881–90. DOI: 10.1038/nrd2445

[71] Mortenson PN, Murray CW. Assessing the lipophilicity of fragments and early hits. J Comput Aid Mol Des. 2011; 25(7): 663–7. DOI: 10.1007/s10822-011-9435-z

[72] Kawatkar S, Wang H, Czerminski R, Joseph-McCarthy D. Virtual fragment screening: an exploration of various docking and scoring protocols for fragments using Glide. J Comput Aid Mol Des. 2009; 23(8): 527–39. DOI: 10.1007/s10822-009-9281-4

[73] Sándor M, Kiss R, Keseru GM. Virtual fragment docking by glide: a validation study on 190 protein-fragment complexes. J Chem Inf Model. 2010; 50(6): 1165–72. DOI: 10.1021/ci1000407

[74] Wang J-C, Lin J-H. Scoring functions for prediction of protein-ligand interactions. Curr Pharm Design. 2013; 19(12): 2174–82. DOI: 10.2174/1381612811319120005

[75] Kozakov D, Hall DR, Jehle S, Luo L, Ochiana SO, Jones EV, Pollastri M, Allen KN, Whitty A, Vajda S. Ligand deconstruction: why some fragment binding positions are conserved and others are not. Proc Nat Acad Sci. 2015; 112(20): E2585–E94. DOI: 10.1073/pnas.1501567112

4

Biomedical and Pharmaceutical Applications of Inductively Coupled Plasma-Mass Spectrometry (ICP-MS)

Desam Nagarjuna Reddy,
Abdul Jabbar Al-Rajab and
Gowkanapalli Ramachandra Reddy

Abstract

Medical science is a field of study that is relevant to all people, but the development of pharmaceutical, biomedical and life science is of particular importance. In these fields, further studies are being established to determine with incredible accuracy the quantities and concentration of inorganic elements and organic compounds, such as nucleotides, sulphur and phosphorous containing peptides and proteins, to be used in all kinds of drugs. Since 1980, inductively coupled plasma-mass spectrometry (ICP-MS) has emerged as a new and powerful technique for elemental and isotopic analysis. It provides a means for the analysis of an extremely wide range of elements and the co-analysis of most elements in the periodic table. It can also be used for qualitative, quantitative and semi-quantitative analysis and for the measurement of isotopic ratios through mass-to-charge ratios. In recent years, ICP-MS has emerged as the best technique for the quantification of inorganic impurities in pharmaceutical and biomedical applications. This chapter focuses on introducing the applications of ICP-MS in the pharmaceutical and biomedical fields. Some problems facing ICP-MS are also presented at the end of this chapter.

Keywords: pharmaceutical analysis, biomedical analysis, inductively coupled plasma-mass spectrometry (ICP-MS)

1. Introduction

Within the field of pharmaceuticals, two fundamental issues are necessary for drug therapy: safety and efficiency. The impact of elemental impurities in drugs must be investigated using pharmacological and toxicological profiles so that the safety requirements and dosage forms of bulk drug scan be determined. This is vital because unwanted pharmacological and toxicological effects may result from elemental impurities and improper drug dosage forms. As such, all products intended for human consumption must be characterised as completely as possible to ensure quality and safety and to ensure that elemental impurities are being monitored and controlled. Thus, pharmaceutical analysis is one of the most important activities related to ensuring the safety of drugs [1].

1.1. Heavy metals in drugs

During the synthesis of pharmaceuticals, inorganic impurities can result from several different sources and phases, including solvents, raw materials, reagents, catalysts, electrodes, reaction vessels, plumbing and other equipment used. These impurities are often a result of the manufacturing process. Routinely monitored as impurities in several drugs are cadmium, copper, chromium, mercury, iridium, molybdenum, nickel, osmium, lead, tungsten, palladium, platinum, rhodium, and ruthenium and vanadium and their derivatives [2]. For the synthesis of many pharmaceuticals, tungsten-containing catalysts are used in the intermediate reaction process. In the pharmaceutical industry, monitoring heavy metals is an important activity for both reaction intermediates and final drug substances, not only because of their ability to catalyse decomposition but also because of their potential for toxicity. Even at very low doses, heavy metals such as lead, cadmium, mercury and chromium pose a serious health risk when used for pharmaceutical purposes [3]. Long exposures can cause physiological and behavioural issues. For instance, daily exposure to 0.06 mg of lead for a period of 1 month is sufficient to cause long-term problems such as kidney impairment, demineralization and obstructive lung disease. In pharmaceutical and biomedical substances, the presence of heavy metals is monitored and limited by regulatory authorities. Tests are performed to ensure that no inorganic-based reagents or contaminates are introduced into the drugs at any step during the manufacturing process. The determination of residues of metal catalysts and reagents has moved increasingly into the focus of regulatory guidance within the last 5 years [4]. The European medicines agency has published guidelines on the specification requirements for inorganic metal catalysts and reagents [5]. The United States Pharmacopoeia (USP), British Pharmacopoeia (BP), European Pharmacopoeia (EP) and Japanese Pharmacopoeia (JP) have proposed the collective monitoring of the total metal content in pharmaceutical products. For example, the EP has proposed a limit of 20 μ.g/g of platinum in calcium folinate. In aqueous solutions, metal sulphide precipitation results in a clear visual difference of colour, but this are not the case for similarly treated standard metal solutions. In both cases, determining the exact presence of heavy metals is a process that is time consuming and not selective, specific or accurate. Thus, there is a great need to develop a highly sensitive and more selective technique to determine the presence of heavy metals in pharmaceutical substances and, accordingly, to ensure the safety and efficacy of drugs intended for human consumption.

1.2. Atomic spectrometric techniques used in pharmaceutical and biomedical analysis

Spectrophotometric techniques are widely used for trace elemental analysis, including atomic absorption spectrophotometer (AAS), inductively coupled plasma-atomic emission

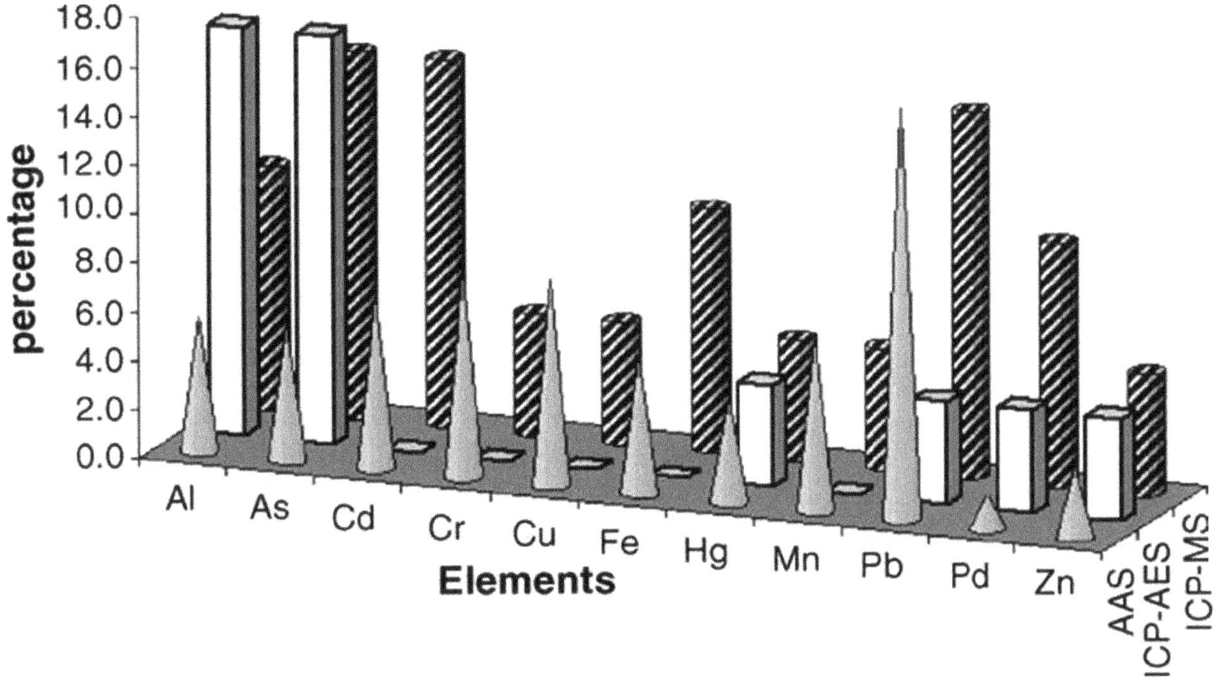

Figure 1. Usage pattern of different spectrophotometric techniques in detection of trace metals in drugs and pharmaceutical industry.

spectrophotometer (ICP-AES) and inductively coupled plasma-mass spectrometry (ICP-MS) [3, 6]. AAS is used extensively, often for analysing different samples. Flame-AAS (F-AAS) or low graphite furnace (GF-AAS) is used for samples with a high concentration of metals. Because of its high detection limit, the application of this technique to the analysis of impurities is limited. However, each metal present can be individually analysed to a high level of specificity because of the hollow-cathode lamp used.

ICP-AES is an important technique for the trace elemental analysis of pharmaceutical samples [7, 8]. While it is a powerful technique for multielemental analysis, it does suffer from spectral interferences and low levels of accuracy. At present, ICP-MS has emerged as the most powerful, sensitive and selective technique for the determination of elemental impurities in trace and ultra-trace concentrations in pharmaceutical and bulk drug substances. Hence, ICP-MS provides a major service to the pharmaceutical and bulk drug industries in allowing them to identify and quantify elemental impurities. However, there are limitations to ICP-MS in that it is very expensive and lacks certified reference standards for most drugs and pharmaceutical products. The pattern of the various spectrometric techniques used recently is shown in **Figure 1**.

2. Principle and instrumentation of ICP-MS

The hyphenated ICP-MS principle and construction are essentially identical. Plasma employs the ionisation source for the ICP, and positively charged ions detect the mass analyser in the mass spectrometer (MS). Generally, argon gas is used to generate plasma at a high frequency (30 MHz), with energy in the range of 1000–2000 W, since in the periodic table most elements excite and ionise at plasma temperatures in the range of 6000–10,000 K. The torch is made with quartz and consists of three concentric tubes through which the argon flows. The periodic table shown in the **Figure 2** makes multielemental analysis possible. A schematic diagram of the ICP-MS instrumentation is shown in **Figure 3**.

When a sample is introduced into the plasma, it goes through desolvation, vaporisation, atomisation and ionisation before entering the mass analyser. There are many methods for introducing the samples, which can be solid, liquid or gas, into the plasma. Most commonly, liquid samples are introduced using pneumatic nebulization.

From ICP, the MS extracts the ions at a low pressure, via sampling and skimmer cones. Later, ions travel towards the quadrupole mass analyser through a series of ion lenses. Positively charged ions are then separated according to the mass-to-charge ratio. Ions can then be detected by an electron multiplier and amplified. The quadrupole mass analyser is widely used ICP-MS, and the double-focusing field mass analyser is used to achieve more separation and to decrease isobaric interference (such as ^{40}Ar, $^{35}Cl^{+}$ interference with $^{75}As^{+}$). A speciation analysis can also be performed using time-of-flight mass spectrometry (TOFMS). Another possible separation technique, the introduction of samples into the source of ICP at atmospheric pressure makes its possible of coupling separation techniques to ICP-MS. This decreases the isobaric overlap of the high-resolution mass analyser and interests ions with different mass-to-charge ratios differently via chemical reaction. The percentages of the different elements analysed by ICP-MS in pharmaceutical substances and bulk drugs are shown in **Figure 4**.

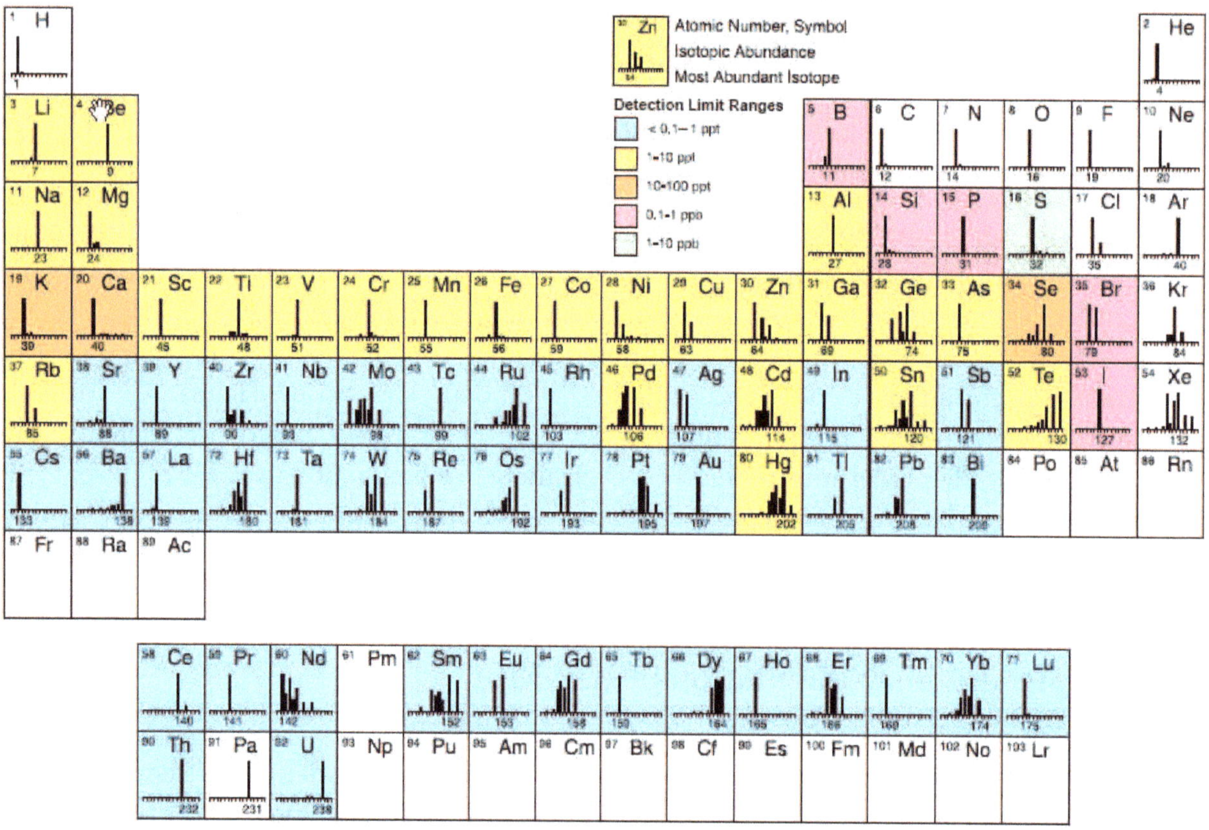

Figure 2. Elements detectable by ICP-MS analysis.

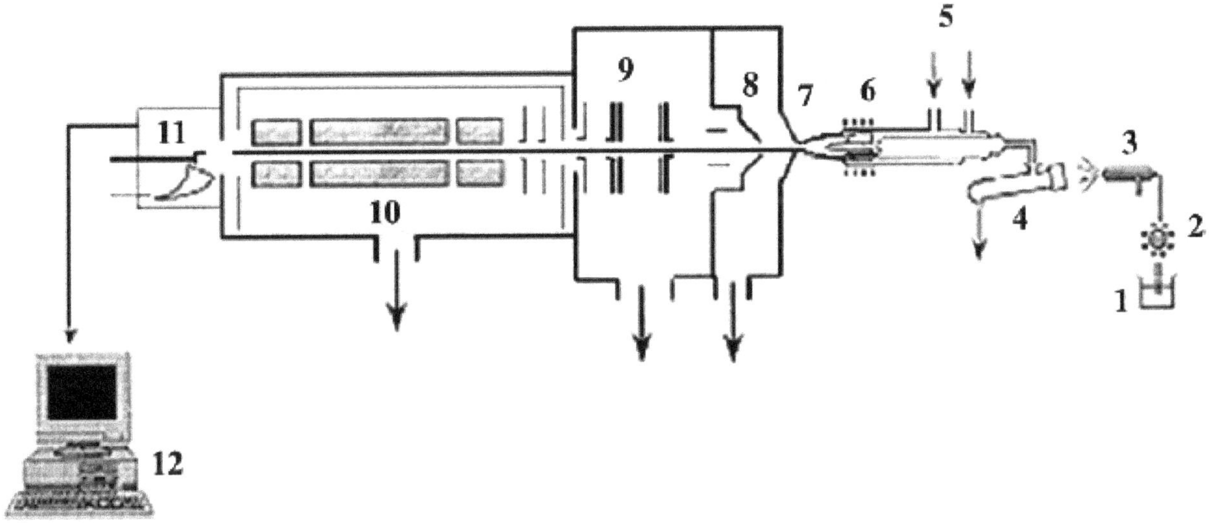

Figure 3. Schematic diagram of inductively coupled plasma-mass spectrometer: 1. Liquid sample, 2. Pump, 3. Nebuliser, 4. Spray chamber, 5. Argon gas torch inlets, 6. Torch, 7. Sampler cone, 8. Skimmer cone, 9. Ion lenses, 10. Quadrupole mass analyser, 11. Electron multiplier detector, and 12. Data collection.

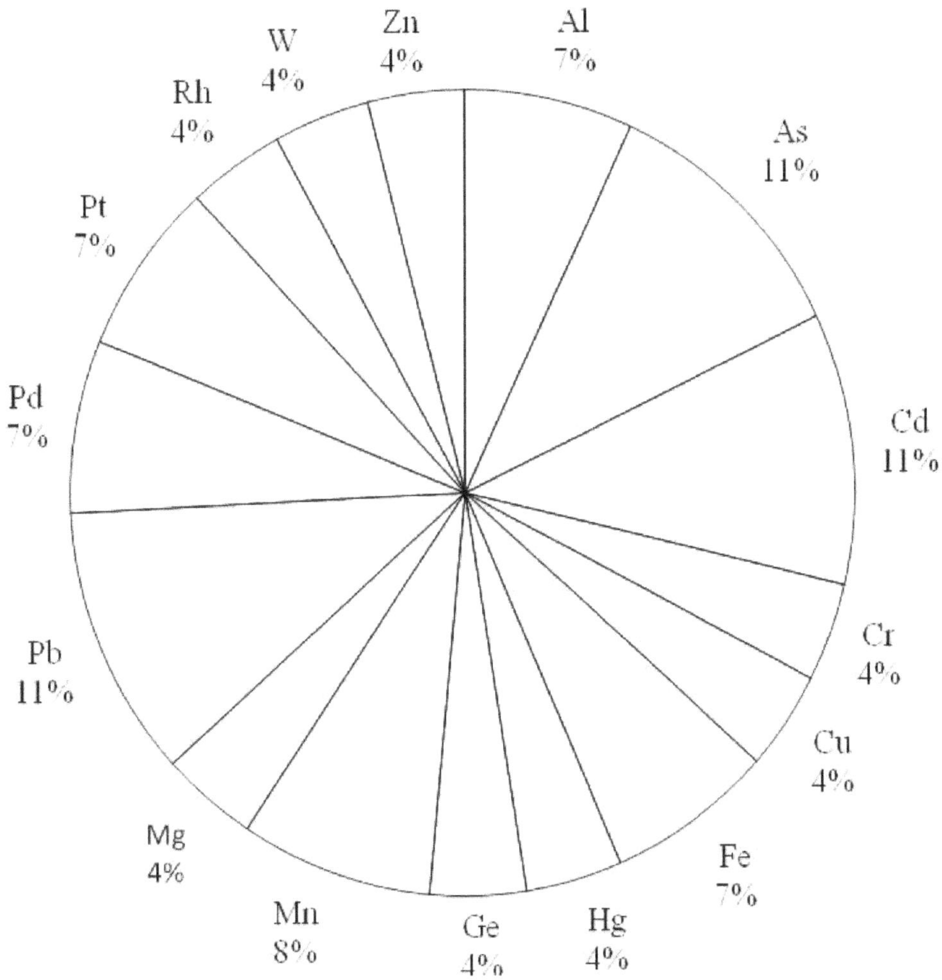

Figure 4. Individual elements analysed by ICP-MS in pharmaceutical substances and bulk drugs.

3. Sample preparations

Samples are normally prepared using dissolution or digestion with a low concentration of mineral acids [9, 10]. For the reproducibility of volatile, low-concentration and low-volume elements, microwave digestion is better than acid digestion. However, microwave digestion and acid digestion are both appropriate for pharmaceutical samples due to the volatility of some metals and trace detection limits. The laser ablation technique [11] can be used for solid samples. Some of the sample preparation methods are summarised in **Table 1**.

Element	Bulk drug/ formulation	Procedure	Medium	Calibration[a]	Reference
W	Bulk drugs	Dissolution	80:20 (v/v) HNO_3	EC with ^{209}Bi for IS	[12]
Fe	Methotrexate	Microwave-assisted	$H_2SO_4 + HNO_3$	EC with ^{56}Fe	[13]
Pd, Pt, Rh	Enalapril maleate Calcium folinate Levodopa	Dissolution Dissolution Dissolution	1:1 HNO_3, 0.3 M, 0.2 M HNO_3, 0.2 M HNO_3	EC with In for IS	[14]
Pd	Fosinopril sodium	Dissolution	25% (v/v) 2-butoxy ethanol and water	EC with In for IS	[15]
69 elements	Drug substances, intermediate and raw materials	Dissolution, sonication	80% (v/v) HNO_3	EC	[16]
Cr, Ni, Sn, Pb	Vitamin E	Microwave digestion Emulsion preparation	$HNO_3 + H_2O_2$, Triton X + Tetralin	EC, Y, In and Tl for IS	[17]
Na, Br, Pd, Ba, I	Methamphetamine HCl	Dissolution	H_2O	EC	[18]
As, Se, Mo, Ru, Pd, Cd, In, Sn, Sb, Pt, Hg, Bi, Ag.	API with various functionalities	Dissolution	2-butoxy ethanol/ water (25:75 v/v)	EC with Co, Au and Rh for IS	[19]
Cr, Cu, Mg, Mn, Mo, P, Se, Zn.	Multimineral and multivitamin	Microwave digestion	HNO_3	EC with Co for IS	[20]
Li, B, V, Cr, Mn, Ni, Zn, Cu, Br, Sr, Sn, Ba, Pt, and Pb	Ecstasy tablets	Dissolution	1% (v/v) HNO_3	EC with Rh for IS	[21]
Ti, Cr, Mn, Fe, Co, Ni, Cu, Zn, Cd, Hg, Pb	Dicyclomine HCl, Ethambutol, Pyrazinamide, Furazolidone	Dissolution and digestion	5% (v/v) HNO_3 $HNO_3 + H_2O_2 + H_2O$	EC	[22]
As, Cd, Hg, Pb	Dietary supplements	Microwave digestion	HNO_3	Ec with Rh, IN Lu, Bi for IS	[23]

[a]EC: external calibration; IS: internal standardisation.

Table 1. Sample preparations procedures for analysis of trace elements in pharmaceutical substances and bulk drugs using ICP-MS.

4. Applications

4.1. Applications of ICP-MS in pharmaceutical samples

4.1.1. Determination of multielements in drugs and pharmaceutical substances

Supplements in the form of gluconate contained the lowest concentration of cadmium, which was detected in many zinc supplements, according to ICP-MS [26]. In calcium supplements, cadmium and lead were detected using ICP-MS, F-AAS and electrothermal-atomic absorption spectroscopy (ETAAS) [27]. Using GF-AAS and inductively coupled plasma-optical emission spectroscopy (ICP-OES), iron and palladium were detected in the bulk drug methotrexate; and the results were compared which obtained from ICP-MS [13]. To avoid polyatomic interferences before quadrupole mass analysis (such as ^{40}Ar, ^{16}O with ^{56}Fe), hexapole collision cell was used. Using ICP-MS, lead and its isotope ratio was investigated in antacids and calcium drug supplements using rhenium as an internal standard [28–30].

Tungsten has been identified in bulk drug substances and their intermediates, with bismuth used as an internal standard [31]. With the help of different isotopes, spectral interferences have been monitored in bulk drug substances. In bulk drug samples, ICP-MS was also used to detect up to 2500 ppm of tungsten [31]. The ICP-MS results are in accordance with those of microwave induced plasma-mass spectrometry (MIP-MS). Hence, ICP-MS has been used for the expeditious screening for inorganic impurities such as rhodium, palladium, platinum, beryllium, vanadium, manganese, cobalt, nickel, copper, zinc, molybdenum, cadmium, tin, thorium and lead, using Rh^{103}, Pd^{105}, Pd^{106}, Pt^{195} and In isotopes as an internal standard.

4.1.2. Multielements in synthetic drugs

Sodium, bromine, palladium, barium and indium have been investigated in methamphetamine hydrochloride, which is prepared using catalyst and reagent methods [18]. Barium, palladium, bromine, iodine and sodium were detected by Emeds and Nagais using ICP-MS. The levels of these elements in N-methylamphetamine were measured, and the results were compared with neutron activation analysis (NAA). ICP-MS has been used to detect multielements in synthetic drugs; these elements include arsenic, selenium, cadmium, indium, tin, antimony, lead, bismuth, silver, palladium, platinum, mercury, molybdenum, and ruthenium. Several ICP-MS procedures have been reported for performing single and multielemental analysis in drugs and pharmaceutical substances, as shown in **Table 2**.

4.1.3. Multielements in herbal drugs

In herbal drugs such as dietary supplements, inorganic impurities are a major concern due to their major toxicity and impurities (e.g., As, Cd, Hg and Pb) [23]. Normally, dietary supplements are analysed using high-resolution ICP-MS. Microwave digestion method is also an accepted method according to National Institute of Standards and Technology (NIST) reference materials.

Drug/formulations	Elements	MDL	Detector	Reference
Dicyclomine HCl, Ethambutol, Pyrazinamide, Furazolidone	Ti, Cr, Mn, Fe, Co, Ni, Cu, Zn, Cd, Hg, Pb	Not reported	Varian ultramass 700	[22]
Neusilin	Al, Mg	40 and 6 μg/g	Laser ablation system: CETACLSX-100, Perkin-Elmer SCIEX, ELAN 6000ICP-MS	[23]
Drug substances, intermediate and raw materials	69 Elements	0.004–19 ppm	Elan 6000 ICP-MS, 1300 Wrf, cross flow nebuliser, Scott spray chamber	[16]
Vitamin E	Cr, Ni, Sn and Pb	3.02, 0.22, 2.92, 0.07 ppb (emulsion) 0.13, 0.05, 0.70, 0.08 ppb (15% HNO_3)	Aglient 7500 ICP-MS, 1100 Wrf Meinhard nebuliser	[17]
Methamphetamine HCl	Na, Br, Pd, Ba, I	Not reported	Seiko ICP-MS SPQ-6100, 1.35 kW quadrupole	[18]
Fosinopril sodium (monopril)	Pd	0.1 μg/g	Plasma Quad PQ11 Turbo plus ICP-MS jacketed Scott type spray chamber, cooled to 5°C, platinum sample cone	[15]
Enalapril maleate, calcium folinate, levodopa	Pd, Pt, Rh	15, 2.8, 2.5 ng/g	Plasma Quad II STE peristaltic pump: spray chamber: double pass, water cooled (10°C)	[14]
API	As, Se, Mo, Ru, Pd, Cd, In, Sn, Sb, Pt, Hg, Bi, Ag.	0.37, 0.42, 0.08, 0.2, 0.18, 0.03, 0.17, 0.35, 0.16, 0.03, 1.82, 1.51, 0.15 μg/g	VG Plasma Quad PQII TURBO plus, ICP-MS and Micro mass platform ICP-MS	[19]
Multimineral and multivitamin	Cr, Cu, Mg, Mn, Mo, P, Se, Zn	48.3, 47.1, 24.3, 9.0, 43.2, 750, 24, 109 ng/l	VG Plasma Quad 3 ICP-MS, 1380 W	[20]
Methotrexate	Fe	0.2 μg/g	Thermo elemental ICP-MS with collision cell technology	[13]
Bulk drug substances	W	0.04 ppm	Perkin-Elmer Elan 6000 ICP-MS, AS-91 auto sampler 1300rf	[12]
Ecstasy tablets	Li, B, V, Cr, Mn, Ni, Zn, Cu, Br, Sr., Sn, Ba, Pt, and Pb	Not reported	Perkin-Elmer SCIEX Elan 6000 ICP-MS, Gibson peristaltic pump, rf1000W, nebuliser ryton cross flow with gem tips	[21]
Dietary supplements	As, Cd, Hg, Pb	8.2, 18, 140, 25 ng/l	Micro mass Plasma Trace-2 HR ICP-MS, rf1350W	[23]
Chinese medicinal material	As, Hg	0.19, 0.32 μg/l	ELAN 6000 ICP-MS rf 1000 W, HP 4500 ICP-MS rf 1200 W, Babington type cross flow nebuliser, peristaltic pump, double pass spray chamber	[24]
Dietary supplements	Pb, Hg, Cd, As, U, Cr, V, Cu, Zn, Mo, Pd, Sn, Sb, Tl, W	Not recorded	Micro mass platform ICP-MS Meinhard concentric nebuliser	[25]

Table 2. Determination of single and multielements in drugs and pharmaceuticals using ICP-MS.

An analysis of arsenic and mercury in Chinese Medicinal Materials (CMM) was completed using ICP-MS, with trace amounts of both arsenic and mercury found [24]. This is notable because of the leaching characteristics of these elements. Mercury and arsenic are often used in traditional Chinese medicine (TCM) and have insoluble sulphides due to the low leaching efficiency of the cinnabar or realgar minerals in the drug formulations [24]. ICP-MS has been used to determine elemental impurities in plant and dietary materials, [25] and indium has been used as an internal standard.

In herbal materials, quality and safety is of major importance. Lead, arsenic and cadmium, in particular, are of considerable importance in herbal materials such as mineralised mint, nettle and black-wrack leaves [32]. In herbal materials, arsenic, cadmium and lead have been quantitatively determined to be in the range 0.2–200 ppb, 0.1–20 ppb and 0.1 ppb–10 ppm, respectively. Also, arsenic was investigated in uncoated TCM using ICP-MS with high-pressure microwave digestion [33].

4.2. Application of ICP-MS in biomedical analysis

The continuous improvement of techniques and their applications in the life sciences sphere, including the combining of organic and inorganic MS, has helped to further advance the field. For inorganic MS and life sciences, ICP-MS has emerged as a key technique in biomedical research. In this section, some of the applications of ICP-MS in the biomedical field will be explored.

4.2.1. Analysis of DNA using ICP-MS

The development of cancer cells and modifications in DNA are commonly caused by the chemical modification of nucleobases, such as styrene oxide. The detection of cancer and DNA adducts is essential, and there are various methods based on standard reference materials, such as mass spectrometry, ^{31}P labelling and immunoassays (however, these are not readily available as they have not been made for three decades). The problem is that identification and unknown modification is not possible. Such problems as selectivity, sensitivity, and qualitative and quantitative technique soften arise when using internal standards, regardless of their structure.

For example, ICP-MS quantitatively engages phosphorus signals in modified nucleotides using bis(4-nitropenyl)phosphate (BNNP) as an internal standard [34, 35]. Hence, ICP-MS has independent elemental selectivity, sensitivity and detection capability.

4.2.2. Analysis of proteins using ICP-MS

In recent years, ICP-MS was used extensively in the field of proteomics [36] for the determination of metal concentrations in proteins and biomedical analysis. In these studies, similarly, bromine was detected quantitatively in rats and human plasma metabolism using ICP-MS [36]. In biological systems, and especially in proteins, metals play an important role as cofactors. Without proteins, there will be an absence of essential metals such as manganese, iron, copper, cobalt, molybdenum and zinc and of essential non-metals such as selenium and iodine.

A deficiency in these metals and non-metals cause diseases as well as catalytic cytotoxic reactions. The field of proteomics determines the metals contained in proteins and, therefore, faces the challenging task of identifying metals and their concentrations, which requires a more selective, sensitive and powerful analytical technique. ICP-MS has been used to identify phosphorus, iron, zinc and copper quantitatively within brain proteins and has been used in the study of neurodegenerative diseases [37, 38]. ICP-MS also represents a powerful technique for the detection of copper, iron and zinc in proteins in the study of Alzheimer's disease and has also analysed copper, zinc and iron with respect to $^{54}Fe/^{55}Fe$, $^{65}Cu/^{63}Cu$ and $^{67}Zn/^{64}Zn$.

4.2.3. Analysis of trace elements in human health

Everybody knows that in human health, some of the elements are essential and others are toxic. However, the benefits and risks of each element depend on the quantity of the intake, the accumulation, the mobility of the element, the storage and interaction of the element in metabolites, the oxidation number, the metal-ligand ratio and the complexity of its interaction with different elements. ICP-MS has become one of the most powerful techniques for elemental speciation studies. In HepG2 cell and liver cell lines, copper and its isotope ratio $^{63}Cu/^{65}Cu$ has been measured accurately using ICP-MS [39], and in human blood and livers, iron and its isotopic ratio has been measured. In the liver, iron and its isotopic composition has been found to be higher than that of the blood and muscles [40].

In vivo, many essential and non-essential elements can interact with each other. Because of these interactions, it is important to anticipate deficiency and excess and to know elemental toxicity levels. To use elemental analysis to determine concentrations, ICP-MS has proved to be an advantageous technique. ICP-MS has been used to identify trace elements that are toxic and those that are essential [41–44]. In human blood and serum, many trace elements can be found, including cobalt, copper, zinc, selenium, rubidium, rhodium, palladium, cadmium, tungsten, platinum, mercury, thallium and lead. Both blood and serum selenium correlated with blood can contain the trace elements lead, mercury, copper and zinc.

5. Brief solution to problems in the application of ICP-MS

ICP-MS is a good analytical method when compared to the other analytical methods available. However, it is not without its drawbacks. These include signal fluctuation and the matrix effect, which occurs when elements that are very close in terms of mass number experience an indistinguishable influence [45]. The matrix effect might be a result of the plasma, the deposition of salts in the orifices, ion extraction or the internal standard [46]. The matrix effect can cause severe interference, but it can be eliminated by selecting a matching standard for the matrix of the isotope being diluted or by ensuring a greater dilution of the specimen. It can be of particular concern for double electric charge ions, such as barium and cerium, as these elements have low second ionisation energy levels. Oxides can be controlled by elevating the temperature of the plasma or slowing the rate of flow. Polyatomic ions and isobars can impede the detecting the mass-to-charge ratio via quantitative analysis, making them very important to analysts.

6. Conclusion

ICP-MS has the power required to sensitively analyse the presence of trace elements; the method has low detection limits, allows for more selectivity of elemental mass, provides insight into the isotope ratio and performs ultra-trace elemental detection. It can be used for the elemental analysis of inorganic and organic elements in all kinds of drugs, including nucleotides, sulphur, and phosphorus containing proteins, providing both a qualitative and quantitative determination with accuracy, making it a vital method for trace element analysis in the pharmaceutical and biomedical fields.

Author details

Desam Nagarjuna Reddy[1]*, Abdul Jabbar Al-Rajab[1] and Gowkanapalli Ramachandra Reddy[2]

*Address all correspondence to: dndnrchem@gmail.com

1 Centre for Environmental Research and Studies, Jazan University, Jazan, Saudi Arabia

2 Department of Polymer Science and Technology, College of Science, Sri Krishnadevaraya University, Anatapur, AP, India

References

[1] Nageswara Rao R, Kumar Talluri MVN. An overview of recent applications of inductively coupled plasma-mass spectrometry (ICP-MS) in determination of inorganic impurities in drugs and pharmaceuticals. Journal of Pharmaceutical and Biomedical Analysis. 2007;**43**:1-13

[2] Wang T, Walden S, Egan R. Development and validation of a general non-digestive method for the determination of palladium in bulk pharmaceutical chemicals and their synthetic intermediates by graphite furnace atomic absorption spectroscopy. Journal of Pharmaceutical and Biomedical Analysis. 1997;**15**:593-599

[3] Bings NH, Bogaerts A, Broekaert JAC. Atomic spectroscopy. Analytical Chemistry. 2006;**78**:3917-3946

[4] Wollein U, Bauer B, Habernegg R, Schramek N. Potential metal impurities in active pharmaceutical substances and finished medicinal products - A market surveillance study. European Journal of Pharmaceutical Sciences. 2015;**77**:100-105

[5] Elemental Impurities—Limits (Chapter 232), 2014. Pharm. Forum 40, USP, Elemental Impurities—Procedures (Chapter 233), Pharm. Forum 40, USP; 2014

[6] Beauchemin D. Inductively coupled plasma mass spectrometry. Analytical Chemistry. 2006;**78**:4111-4136

[7] Stoica AL, Peltea M, Baiulescu GE, Ionica M. Determination of cobalt in pharmaceutical products. Journal of Pharmaceutical and Biomedical Analysis. 2004;**36**:653-656

[8] Wang L, Marley M, Jahansouz H, Bahnck C. Determination of content uniformity and distribution characteristics of an investigational drug in its tablets dosage form and granule by ICP-AES. Journal of Pharmaceutical and Biomedical Analysis. 2003;**33**:955-961

[9] Montaser A, editor. Inductively Coupled Plasma Mass Spectrometry. 1st ed. New York: Wiley-VCH; 1998

[10] Jarvis I. Hand Book of Inductively Coupled Plasma Mass Spectrometry. Glasgow and London: Blackie. pp. 172-224

[11] Gunther D, Hattendorf B. Solid samples analysis using laser ablation inductively coupled plasma mass spectrometry. Trends in Analytical Chemistry. 2005;**24**:255-265

[12] Wang T, Ge Z, Wu J, Li B, Liang AS. Determination of tungsten in bulk drug substance and intermediates by ICP-OES and ICP-MS. Journal of Pharmaceutical and Biomedical Analysis. 1999;**19**:937-943

[13] Niemela M, Kola H, Eilola K, Peramaki P. Development of analytical methods for the determination of sub-ppm concentrations of palladium and iron in methotrexate. Journal of Pharmaceutical and Biomedical Analysis. 2004;**35**:433-439

[14] Lasztity A, Kelko-levai A, Varga I, Zih-Perenyi K, Bertalan E. Development of atomic spectrometric methods for trace metal analysis of pharmaceuticals. Microchemical Journal. 2002;**73**:59-63

[15] Lewen N, Schenkenberger M, Larkin T, Conder S, Brittain H. The determination of palladium in fosinopril sodium (momopril) by ICP-MS. Journal of Pharmaceutical and Biomedical Analysis. 1995;**13**:879-883

[16] Wang T, Wu J, Hartman R, Jia X, Egan RS. A multi element ICP-MS survey method as an alternative to the heavy metals limit test for pharmaceutical materials. Journal of Pharmaceutical and Biomedical Analysis. 2000;**23**:867-890

[17] Ponce de Leon CA, Montes-Bayan M, Caruso JA. Trace element determination in vitamin E using ICP-MS. Analytical and Bioanalytical Chemistry. 2002;**374**:230-234

[18] Kishi T. Journal of Research of the National Bureau of Standards (USA). 1988;**93**:469-471

[19] Lewen N, Mathew S, Schenkenberger M, Raglione T. A rapid ICP-MS screen for heavy metals in pharmaceutical compounds. Journal of Pharmaceutical and Biomedical Analysis. 2004;**35**:739-752

[20] Soltyk K, Lozak A, Ostapczuk P, Fijalek Z. Determination of chromium and selected elements in multimineral and multivitamin preparations and in pharmaceutical raw material. Journal of Pharmaceutical and Biomedical Analysis. 2003;**32**:425-432

[21] Suzuki S-I, Tsuchihashi H, Nakajima K, Matsushita A, Nagao T. Analyses of impurities in methamphetamine by inductively coupled plasma mass spectrometry and ion chromatography. Journal of Chromatography. A. 1988;**437**:322-327

[22] Murty ASRK, Kulshresta UC, Rao TN, Talluri MVNK. Determination of heavy metals in selected drug substances by inductively coupled plasma-mass spectrometry. Indian Journal of Chemical Technology. 2005;**12**(2):229-231

[23] Dolan SP, Nortrup DA, Bolger PM, Capar SG. Analysis of Dietary. Supplements for arsenic, cadmium, mercury, and lead using inductively coupled plasma. Mass Spectrometry. Journal of Agricultural and Food Chemistry. 2003;**51**:1307-1312

[24] Wu XH, Sun DH, Zhuang ZX, Wang XR, Gong HF, Hong JX, Lee FSC. Analysis and leaching characteristics of mercury and arsenic in Chinese medicinal material. Analytica Chimica Acta. 2002;**453**:311-323

[25] Raman P, Patino LC, Nair MG. Evaluation of metal and microbial contamination in botanical supplements. Journal of Agricultural and Food Chemistry. 2004;**52**:7822-7827

[26] Krone CA, Wyse EJ, Ely JTA. Cadmium in zinc-containing mineral supplements. International Journal of Food Sciences and Nutrition. 2001;**52**:379-382

[27] Bourgoin BP, Boomer D, Powell MJ, Willie S, Edgar D, Evans D. Instrumental comparison for the determination of cadmium and lead in calcium supplements and other calcium-rich matrices. Analyst. 1992;**117**:19-22

[28] Amarasiriwardena D, Sharma K, Barnes BM. Fresenius. Journal of Analytical Chemistry. 1998;**362**:493-497

[29] Scelfo GM, Flegal AR. Lead in calcium supplements. Environmental Health Perspectives. 2000;**108**:309-313

[30] Wolf RE. Analysis of lead in antacids and calcium supplements. Atomic Spectroscopy. 1997;**18**:169-174

[31] Okoro H, Fatoki O, Adekola F, Ximba B, Snyman R, Opeolu B. Human exposure, biomarkers, and fate of organotins in the environment. Reviews of Environmental Contamination and Toxicology. 2011;**213**:27-54

[32] Soltyk K, Fijalek Z. Inductively-coupled plasma mass spectrometric (ICP-MS) and graphite-furnace atomic absorption spectrometric (GF-AAS) determinations of arsenic, cadmium and lead impurities in medical herbal raw materials. Analytical Chemistry. 2000;**45**:879-886

[33] Ong E-S, Yong Y-L, Woo S-O. Determination of arsenic in traditional Chinese medicine by microwave digestion with flow injection-inductively coupled plasma mass spectrometry (FI-ICP-MS). Journal of AOAC International. 1999;**82**:963-967

[34] Siethoff C, Feldmann I, Jakubowski N, Linscheid MJ. Quantitative determination of DNA adducts using liquid chromatography/electrospray ionization mass spectrometry and liquid chromatography/high resolution inductively coupled plasma mass spectrometry. Journal of Mass Spectrometry. 1999;**34**:421-426

[35] Edler M, Jakubowski N, Linscheid M. Styrene oxide DNA adducts: Quantitative determination using 31P monitoring. Analytical and Bioanalytical Chemistry. 2005;**381**:205-211

[36] Axelsson BO, Jornten-Karlsson M, Michelsen P, Abou-Shakra F. The potential of inductively coupled plasma mass spectrometry detection for high-performance liquid chromatography combined with accurate mass measurement of organic pharmaceutical compounds. Rapid Communications in Mass Spectrometry. 2001;**15**:375-385

[37] Beauchemin D, Kisilevsky R. A method based on ICP-MS for the analysis of Alzheimer's amyloid plaques. Analytical Chemistry. 1998;**70**:1026-1029

[38] Becker JS, Zoriy M, Pickhardt C, Przybylski M, Becker JS. Investigation of Cu-, Zn- and Fe-containing human brain proteins using isotopic-enriched tracers by LA-ICP-MS and MALDI-FT-ICR-MS. International Journal of Mass Spectrometry. 2005;**242**:135-144

[39] Fosset C, McGaw BA, Reid MD, McArdle HJ. A non-radioactive method for measuring Cu uptake in HepG2 cells. Journal of Inorganic Biochemistry. 2005;**99**:1018-1022

[40] Walczyk T, Blanckenburg FV. Deciphering the iron isotope message of the human body. International Journal of Mass Spectrometry. 2005;**242**:117-134

[41] Barany E, Bergdahl IA, Bratteby LE, Lundh T, Samuelson G, Schutz A, Skerfving S, Oskarsson A. Relationships between trace element concentrations in human blood and serum. Toxicology Letters. 2002;**134**:177-184

[42] Muller ALH, Oliveira JSS, Mello PA, Muller EI, Flores EMM. Study and determination of elemental impurities by ICP-MS in active pharmaceutical ingredients using single reaction chamber digestion in compliance with USP requirements. Talanta. 2015;**136**:161-169

[43] Støving C, Jensen H, Gammelgaard B, Stürup S. Development and validation of an ICP-OES method for quantitation of elemental impurities in tablets according to coming US pharmacopeia chapters. Journal of Pharmaceutical and Biomedical Analysis. 2013;**84**:209-214

[44] Li G, Schoneker D, Ulman KL, Sturm JJ, Thackery LM, Kauffman JF. Elemental impurities in pharmaceutical excipients. Journal of Pharmaceutical Sciences. 2015;**104**:4197-4206

[45] Hobbs SE, Olesik JW. Inductively coupled plasma mass spectrometry signal fluctuations due to individual aerosol droplets and vaporizing particles. Analytical Chemistry. 1992;**64**:274-283

[46] Samantha HT, Horlick G. Matrix-effect observations in inductively coupled plasma mass spectrometry. Journal of Analytical Atomic Spectrometry. 1987;**2**:745-763

5

Quantitative Methods in System-Based Drug Discovery

Yu-Chen Lo , Ren Gui , Hiroshi Honda and
Jorge Z. Torres

Abstract

Modern pharmaceutical industries have faced significant challenges to deliver safe and effective medicines because of significant toxicity and severe side effects of discovered drugs. On the other hand, recent developments and advances in system-based pharmacology aim to address these challenges. In this chapter, we provide an overview of quantitative methods for system-based drug discovery. System-based drug discovery integrates chemical, molecular, and systematic information and applies this knowledge to the designing of small molecules with controlled toxicity and minimized side effects. First, we discuss current approaches for drug discovery and outline their advantages and disadvantages. Next, we introduce basic concepts of systems pharmacology with an emphasis on ligand-based drug discovery and target identification. This is followed by a discussion on structure-based drug design and statistical tools for pharmaceutical research. Finally, we provide an overview of future directions in systems pharmacology that will guide further developments.

Keywords: systems pharmacology, drug discovery, chemoinformatics

1. Introduction

The discovery of effective medicines has been a long-term human endeavor aimed at curing illnesses and improving physiological conditions. Early drug discovery methods often relied on serendipitous findings. For example, penicillin, a substance released by mold, was accidentally discovered to inhibit bacterial growth. However, with the advances of molecular cloning techniques, X-ray crystallography, robotics, and computational aided technology, drugs can now be rationally designed. Additionally, the marriage of combinatorial chemistry and robotics has also created a new drug discovery approach called "high-throughput screening." In a high-throughput screening campaign, a library consisting of millions of molecules is tested against a disease-relevant target to identify potential drug candidates.

However, the application of modern drug discovery methods has not directly translated into increases in the output of new drugs. Although many of these "designer" drugs have been optimized for binding and specificity, they are all low-weight molecular ligands and are likely to interact with multiple off-targets, which contribute to severe side effects in patients taking these medicines. Consequently, a system drug discovery approach that simultaneously optimizes drug binding, target promiscuity, and safety profile has been proposed. In particular, "poly-pharmacology" is a new drug discovery paradigm that aims to study the interactions of many drugs to many targets as many body problems. The binding profile of a compound can be used to modify a ligand structure to maximize on-target binding while minimizing off-target interactions. More recently, "structural poly-pharmacology" has also been proposed, which utilizes the structural data of proteins or drugs to gain a mechanistic understanding of drug action and side effects [1, 2].

System-based drug discovery can be classified as ligand-based and structure-based drug discovery approaches. In the ligand-based drug discovery approach, ligand structure information takes center stage, and only ligand information is used to derive its multitude of chemical and biological properties. On the other hand, the structure-based approach utilizes the structure of the receptor to identify shape-complementary ligands with optimal interactions. Given a validated disease target with a known crystal structure, the structure-based approach can be utilized to discover ligands that bind to the receptor of interest. On the other hand, the ligand-based approach is useful when the target structure is unknown or when the crystal structure of the target is difficult to obtain. In some cases, the system-based drug discovery approach combines both ligand-based and structure-based approaches to facilitate the drug design and discovery process [3].

2. Ligand-based approaches to drug design

2.1. Introduction

Ligand-based drug design, also known as "knowledge-based" drug design, extracts essential chemical features from drugs to construct a learning model to predict drug properties. It has been proposed that a ligand structure contains all the necessary information to accurately infer its mechanism of action. Several chemical descriptors such as molecular weight and lipophilicity are predictors of important pharmacodynamic and pharmacokinetic properties of ligands. A well-known example is Lipinski's rule of five, which describes a set of chemical properties and rules that can be used to differentiate drugs from nondrug molecules [4]. Likewise, the chemical similarity principle has been widely applied in similarity-based drug design. The chemical similarity principle assumes that if two molecules share similar structures, then they will likely have similar biological properties [5]. This concept is the underlying principle of modern chemical database search techniques used to identify similar compounds with improved bioactivities.

2.2. Outline of ligand-based drug design

The chemical similarity search is an established approach for ligand-based drug discovery. Given a compound with known biological properties, it is possible for a drug designer to identify similar compounds with improved biological properties. To compare two ligand structures, it is essential to develop appropriate data structure representations for chemical structure comparisons. Mathematically, the chemical structure can be represented by graphs where atoms represent vertices and edges represent chemical bonds [6]. Several chemoinformatics algorithm can be used to extract essential characteristic from the chemical graph such as the number of vertices, the number of bonds, path, connectivity, and others. These properties then become chemical features that can be used in feature engineering using complex machine learning techniques for similarity comparison.

The most direct chemical search approach is the nearest neighbor where the chemical feature of a ligand, also known as a "chemical fingerprint," is used to search a compound database to identify the most similar compounds using a predefined distance measure [7]. The most commonly used chemical fingerprints include path-based and substructure-based fingerprints. Using path-based fingerprints, such as Daylight fingerprints or Obabel FP2 fingerprints, potential paths at different bond lengths in a molecular graph of a molecule are used as features for the similarity comparison. On the other hand, substructure-based fingerprints such as MACCS keys use predefined substructures and characterize each molecule based on the presence or absence of a particular substructure using a binary array. Overall, path-based fingerprints offer higher search specificity due to the unique path dependency of the molecular graph. However, substructure-based fingerprints can be used to identify scaffold hopping ligands since the fingerprints do not impose requirements on the connectivity of the scaffolds and functional groups [8]. To quantify the chemical similarity between two fingerprints, several distance metrics have been proposed. The most commonly used chemical similarity metric is the Tanimoto index, which computes the shared feature bits between two fingerprints in the range of 0–1. Although there is no predefined threshold to define the similarity level, a value of 0.7–0.8 has been commonly adapted in many chemical similarity search programs.

2.3. Ligand-based drug design (LBDD) process

The similarity-based drug design process is as follows (**Figure 1**):

1. The target molecule is used as a query for the chemical search.

2. Similar ligands with similar biological properties are identified.

3. Original ligands are modified to suggest new molecules with improved activities.

The advantages of LBDD are as follows:

1. Does not necessitate receptor structures.

2. Low computational intensity and fast database searching.

3. Allows for large-scale similarity drug design and target prediction.

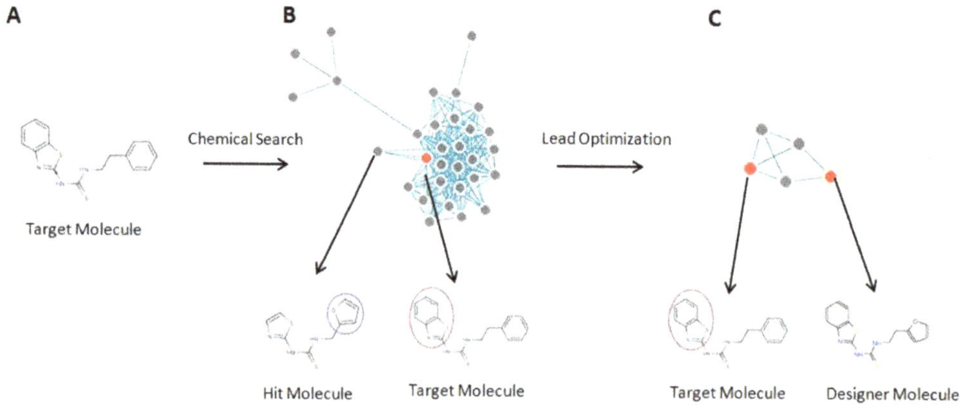

Figure 1. Ligand-based drug design (LBDD) process.

2.4. Target prediction of drugs

While similarity-based methods are prevalently applied in modern drug discovery programs as an efficient way to transition a hit to a lead, the molecular mechanism of the drug is often unknown, and the adverse reaction cannot be predicted. Consequently, drug-target prediction becomes an important follow-up step. Drug-target prediction can be classified as ligand-based or structure-based methods [9]. In ligand-based target prediction, the molecular target of a drug can be inferred from the target-annotated ligand sharing the highest chemical similarity. Chemical bioactivity databases such as ChEMBL, PubChem and DrugBank, and BindingDB have been developed for this application [10]. However, one major limitation of ligand-based target prediction is that there is no natural cutoff for chemical similarity that clearly defines biological similarity, also known as bioactivity cliffs. Approaches such as similarity ensemble approach (SEA) aim to remedy this by calculating similarity values against a random background using an algorithm similar to BLAST [11]. On the other hand, structure-based target prediction methods identify molecular targets based on the structure of the receptor binding sites. For example, panel docking is a common structure-based approach to identify the most probable target based on the docking score. Alternatively, binding site similarity methods that compare the receptor environment of the target ligand to a database of receptor pockets have also proven to be an effective target prediction approach [12].

More recently, network poly-pharmacology has been proposed as a more comprehensive approach to analyze drug-target interactions. Network pharmacology goes beyond the one drug one target hypothesis to multiple drugs multiple targets hypothesis [13]. The goal of this new paradigm is not only to accurately identify on-targets but also other off-targets. One such approach is the drug-target network, which utilizes a bipartite network to analyze complex drug gene interactions. Alternatively, drug-drug networks or chemical similarity networks have also been proposed [8]. The chemical similarity network clusters drugs based on their structure similarity. This approach can be applied for large-scale compound analysis by clustering diverse chemical structures into distinct scaffolds known as chemotypes. Consequently, each chemotype can be correlated with specific molecular targets. Using a consensus statistics scheme similar to that used for functional prediction in protein-protein interaction networks, chemical similarity networks have proven useful for target identification from chemical screening campaigns. In addition, structural poly-pharmacology has also gained substantial attention due to the possibility of correlating structural variations to clinical side effects. One example is CSNAP3D, which uses 3D ligand structure similarity to identify simplified scaffold hopping compounds of complex natural products to suggest new drugs with improved pharmacokinetic properties [1].

2.5. Side effect prediction of drugs

Since severe clinical side effects have contributed to drug failure in the late stages of clinical trials, side effect prediction will need to become an integrated part of the drug design process. Knowing the binding affinity of a drug to an array of proteins makes it possible to predict side effects using several statistical methods such as canonical component analysis (CCA), which identify a set of parameters that optimize the correlation between drug binding features and side effect features [14]. In addition, side effect predictions based on chemoinformatics analysis of the compound structures have also been developed. Many of these approaches provide an accurate prediction of the drug side effects and have been applied in the early stages of clinical drug development.

3. Structure-based approaches to drug design

Modern medicinal chemistry methods and molecular modeling have been employed as powerful tools for the study of structure-activity relationships (SAR) [15]. Structure-based drug design is a drug discovery approach by which synthetic compounds are designed from detailed structural knowledge of the active sites of protein targets associated with particular diseases. This field has involved the integrated application of traditional biology and medicinal chemistry along with advances in biomolecular spectroscopic methods such as X-ray crystallography, nuclear magnetic resonance (NMR), combinatorial chemistry, computer modeling of molecular structure, and protein biophysical chemistry, to focus on the three-dimensional molecular structure and active site characterization of the proteins that control cellular biology. Structure-based drug design is an improvement over traditional drug screening techniques. By identifying the target protein in advance and by discovering the chemical and molecular structure of the protein, it is possible to design a more optimal drug to interact with the protein.

3.1. Basic concept of structure-based drug design

Enzymes are a subset of receptor-like proteins that are directly responsible for catalyzing the biochemical reactions that sustain life. For example, digestive enzymes act to break down the nutrients of our diet. DNA polymerase and related enzymes are crucial for cell division and replication. Enzymes are genetically programmed to be specific for their appropriate molecular targets. Any errors could have grave consequences. Enzymes ensure the specificity of their targets by forming a molecular environment that excludes interactions with inappropriate molecules. The analogy most often mentioned is that of a lock and key. The enzyme is a molecular lock, which contains a keyhole that exhibits a very specific and consistent size and shape. This molecular keyhole is termed the active site of the enzyme and allows interaction with only the appropriate molecular targets. Just as a typical lock is much bigger than the keyhole, the receptor is usually much larger than the active site. The receptor, as specified by our DNA, is a folded protein whose major purpose is to form and maintain the size and shape of the active site.

The most important concept in drug design is to understand the methods by which the active site of the receptor selectivity restricts the binding of inappropriate structures. Any potential molecules that can bind to a receptor are called ligands. In order for a ligand to bind, it must contain a specific combination of atoms that present the correct size, shape, and charge composition needed to bind and interact with the receptor. In brief, the ligand must possess the molecular key that binds the receptor lock.

Computer-aided drug design has played an important role in drug discovery and drug development and has become an indispensable tool in the drug industry. For the purposes of discovering and optimizing biologically active compounds, various types of computer-aided drug design software and resources have been used by computational medicinal chemists. Unsurprisingly, many chemical compounds were discovered and optimized by computer-aided drug design methodologies and have reached the late stages of clinical trials.

3.2. Outline of structure-based drug design

Structure-based drug design is a cyclic process which consists of stepwise procedures (**Figure 2**). It begins with a known target structure, and then, *in silico* studies are conducted in order to identify potential ligands. These molecular modeling procedures are followed by the synthesis of the most promising compounds [16]. Next, using diverse experimental platforms, biological properties such as potency, affinity, and efficacy are evaluated [17]. In the end, given that active compounds are identified, the three-dimensional structure of the ligand-receptor complex can be solved. The available structure allows the visualization of the intermolecular features that support the process of molecular recognition. Structural descriptions of ligand-receptor complexes are useful for the investigation of binding conformations, characterization of key intermolecular interactions, characterization of unknown binding sites, mechanistic studies, and the elucidation of ligand-induced conformational changes [18].

3.3. Process of structure-based drug design (SBDD)

The structure-based drug design process is as follows:

1. An enzyme that is important in a particular pathological condition is chosen.
2. The three-dimensional structure of the active site of the enzyme is determined, often by X-ray crystallography.
3. A chemical is prepared to fit the active site of the enzyme, which can alter the properties of the enzyme, that is, inactivate the enzyme.

The advantages of structure-based drug design are as follows:

1. Useful results are obtained faster than by traditional drug design methods.
2. The process is less expensive than other drug design methods.
3. The compounds are more specific for the active site and potentially less toxic than compounds prepared by other approaches.

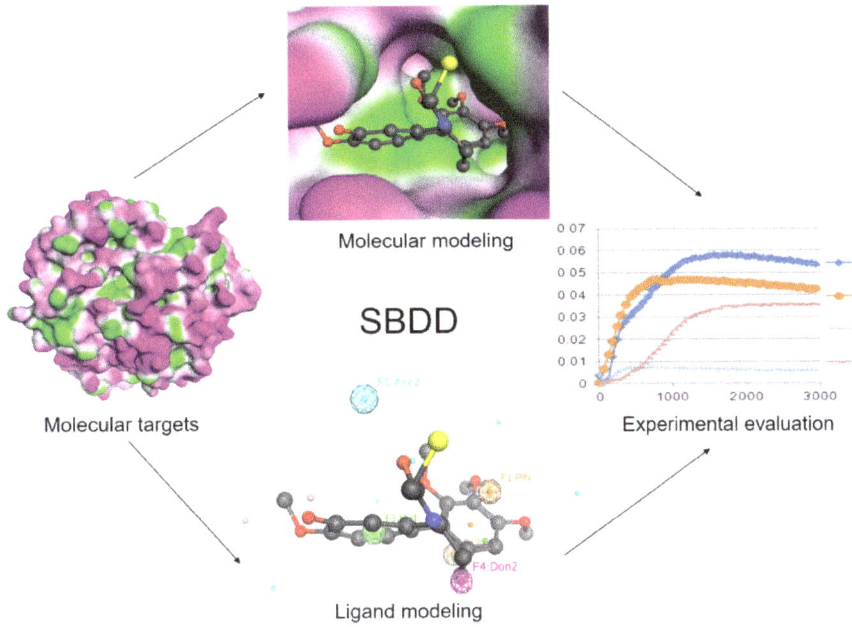

Figure 2. Structure-based drug design (SBDD) process.

3.4. Synthesis of lead compound

The initial drug design phase is followed by the synthesis of the lead compound, quantitative measurements of its ability to interact with the target protein, and X-ray crystallographic analysis of the compound-target complex. This analysis reveals important, empirical information on how the compound actually binds to the target, and the nature and extent of changes induced in the target by the binding. These data, in turn, suggest ways to refine the lead compound to improve its binding to the target protein. The refined lead compound is then synthesized and complexed with the target, and further refined in a reiterative process. If lead compounds are available from other studies, such as screening of combinatorial libraries, these compounds may serve as starting points for this optimization cycle using structure-based drug design.

Once a sufficiently potent compound has been designed and optimized, its activity is evaluated in a biological system to establish the compound's ability to function in a physiological environment. If the compound fails at any stage of the biological evaluation, the design team reviews the structural model and uses crystallography to adjust structural features of the compound to overcome the difficulty. This process continues until a designed compound exhibits the desired properties. The compound is then evaluated in an experimental disease model. If the compound fails, the reasons for failure (e.g., adverse metabolism, plasma binding, distribution, etc.) are determined, and again new modified compounds are designed to overcome the deficiencies without interfering with their ability to interact with the active site of the target protein. The experimental drug is then ready for conventional drug development (e.g., studies in safety assessment, formulation, clinical trials, etc.). This reiterative analysis and compound modification are possible because of the structural data obtained by X-ray crystallographic analysis at each stage. This capability renders structure-based drug design, a powerful tool for rapid and efficient development of drugs that are highly specific for particular protein target sites.

3.5. Docking methodologies

Several docking procedures exist in the literature, from the use of interactive graphics to manipulate the position of the ligand to completely automated procedures, which are becoming increasingly powerful to screen databases of molecules. Many docking algorithms follow a similar pattern. Usually, the first stage is to represent the molecules by their solvent-accessible surfaces. Beginning with a number of different relative orientations, the two molecules can then be brought together. More sophisticated methods carry out their moves by using a Monte Carlo algorithm to direct both rotations and translations. Rapid convergence to a minimum can be achieved by gradually cooling the simulation temperature as the molecule appears to be descending into a potential well.

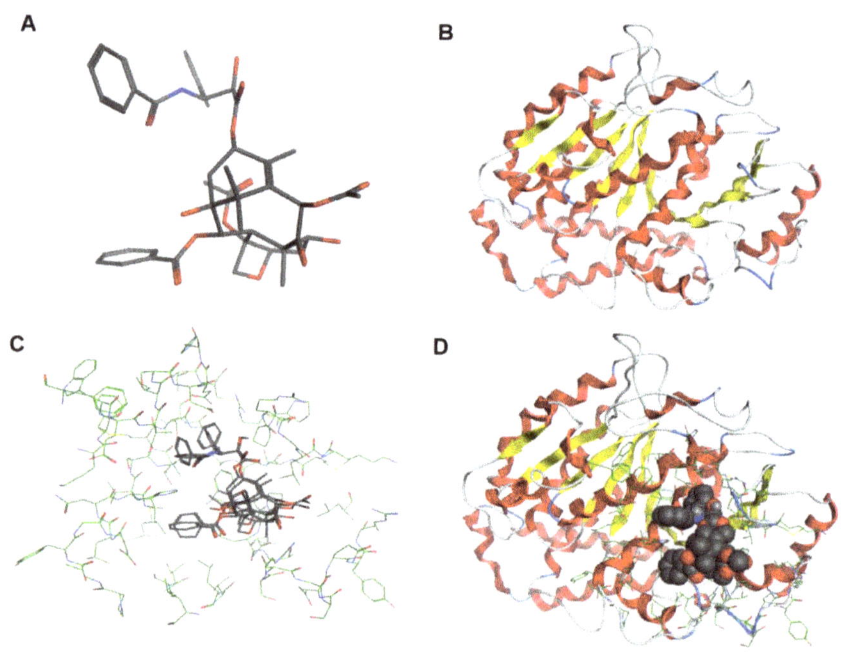

Figure 3. The molecular docking methodology. (A) Prepare the ligand structure, (B) Prepare the receptor structure, (C) Dock the ligand into the receptor surface with multiple potential conformations. (D) The most likely binding mode was identified based on intermolecular interaction between the ligand and the receptor surface. The protein backbone is represented as a cartoon. The ligand and active site residue are shown in stick representation.

Molecular docking is one of the most frequently used methods in structure-based drug design because of its ability to predict, with a substantial degree of accuracy, the conformation of small-molecule ligands within the appropriate target binding site (**Figure 3**) [19]. Following the development of the first algorithms in the 1980s, molecular docking became an essential tool in drug discovery [20]. Highly intensive investigations involving crucial molecular events, including ligand-binding modes and the corresponding intermolecular interactions which stabilize the ligand-receptor complex, could be conveniently performed. Furthermore, molecular docking algorithms execute quantitative predictions of binding energetics, given docked compounds, based on the binding affinity of ligand-receptor complexes [21].

3.6. Computer simulation in drug design

The development of a new drug starts with the design of suitable candidate compounds so-called "ligands" that are selected according to observations about how these compounds are recognized by the target protein and how they bind to it. It is important to know that proteins have dynamic properties: they change their shape in much the way as a machine tool needs to in order to fulfill its function. Now, it is being realized how important it is to have techniques available for studying protein dynamics. Performing experiments is not only expensive but also very time-consuming and, moreover, cannot answer all relevant questions. An alternative is computer-aided simulation of the dynamics of molecules [molecular dynamics (MD) simulations], which is becoming increasingly important to identify the molecular properties that are important and to determine the detailed molecular interactions that are critical for binding.

In some instances, high-performance computing (HPC) is required to cross the threshold where MD simulation becomes a valuable tool for industry. However, in most pharmaceutical companies, HPC is something very new, and supercomputers are simply not available to industrial researchers. With the arrival of affordable high-performance multiprocessor machines and corresponding developments of parallel software, it now becomes possible for industrial researchers to undertake more realistic calculations that were previously out of reach. Scientists at Novo Nordisk, a large Danish pharmaceutical company, are convinced that this new capability will dramatically change the acceptance of MD simulation as a tool in the design of new ligands. During Europort-D, they, for the first time, studied the dynamics of the complex molecular interactions critical for recognition of ligands by their target proteins.

4. Statistical tool for drug design

4.1. Introduction to SPASS for pharmaceutical research

As a sophisticated statistical software, Statistical Package for Social Science (SPSS) can help researchers and users realize their complex statistical tests with result interpretation and the access to data figures, tables, and graphs, which can be quickly and easily displayed in the output view. Even though additional training is usually required before users can maximize its features and the graphing feature is not as simple as an excel spreadsheet, SPSS is still being used by more and more researchers from other fields for applications specific to their research areas, for example, the application of SPSS in clinical trials, with power and sample size calculation functions, comprehensive statistical tests and graphical tools, such as predictive data trends, forecasting and report generation, and the analysis of complex drug assays, etc. [22].

SPSS is being used majorly in pharmaceutical and medical research, where it can provide techniques for the design, implementation, and development of drug campaigns that are important to pharmaceutical research organizations and also provides data mining solutions based on their existing data on quality control and manufacturing, regulatory safety testing, clinical trials, data mining in drug discovery, compliance, and validation [23]. As many pharmaceutical research organizations have experienced that even small improvements in research or processing affect the efficiency and success of the project, SPSS provides a sophisticated analytical platforms to decrease development costs and unnecessary preclinical and clinical trials by integrating with existing data sources.

Overall, the tools in SPSS provide an efficient mechanism to automatically validate the routine analysis reports. In other words, SPSS empowers researchers with tools, which might bring the rapid and solid return on investments in the near future.

4.2. Outlines of the SPASS package

SPSS is a Windows-based program, which can be used to perform data entry and data analysis by tables and graphs (**Figure 4**). Because SPSS is capable of dealing with huge amounts of data with different modules, it is commonly used in the business world and in the Social Sciences [24]. Familiarity with this software will be useful in the field of drug research where big data,

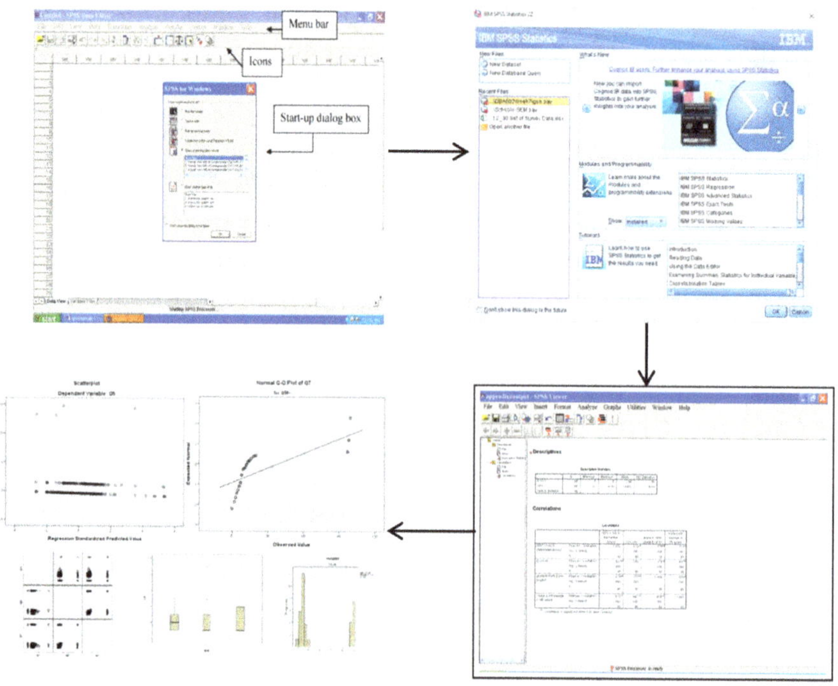

Figure 4. SPSS package in pharmaceutical data analytics application.

such as clinical trials data ranging from simple bioassays and dose-response experiments to long-term survival, and carcinogenicity studies need to be integrated. Unlike Excel, SPSS software can support screen transfers between the data entry view and the output view, which display the results and summarize the data.

4.3. Features of SPSS package

Whether its small and medium enterprises (SME) or large-scale enterprises (LSE), the application of SPSS can provide data accessing in rational data sets, which allows accessing inflexible resources and practices and real-time processing, and mapping of the database [25]. Although other commercial softwares, such as SAS, MATLAB, and others, can also perform such functions, SPSS is a more sophisticated application in statistics analysis. SPSS conducts statistical analysis from basic data, descriptive statistics, such as average and prevalence, and advanced inferential statistics, such as t test, regression model, one-way and factorial analysis of variance (ANOVA), one-way and factorial analysis of covariance (ANCOVA), one-way and factorial multivariate analysis of variance (MANOVA), one-way and factorial multivariate analysis of covariance (MANCOVA), factor analysis, path analysis, and logistic regression [26].

Normally, researchers use SPSS as a tool to collect and analyze data. The data entry screen in SPSS looks like an excel spreadsheet, and users can input variables and quantitative data and save the file as a data file [27]. After data are collected and entered into the data sheet in SPSS, users can also create an output file from the data they used. Then, the users can edit or organize the data in SPSS to check the running results after they choose the module they want. For example, users can check out the frequency distributions of the data to see whether the data set is normally distributed. Furthermore, the researchers can download the tables or graphs directly from the data output view. Because SPSS has the statistical tests built-in to the program, users do not need to do any math calculation or equations to get the results.

5. Conclusion and future direction

Systems pharmacology represents a new paradigm in drug research where ligand and protein information are combined to produce new methods for drug discovery and design. Traditionally, ligand-based approaches utilize information contained within the chemical structure to predict the biological properties of the drug. In particular, chemical similarity database searches can be used to identify molecules with improved activity. However, to be able to design compounds with satisfactory safety profiles, the drug targets will also need to be determined. Target prediction can be performed using ligand or structure data. Both of these approaches require a bioactivity database with pre-characterized activities or functions. If the target structure of the ligand is known, then the structure-based drug discovery approach can be applied. Computer-aided drug design techniques such as molecular docking and molecular dynamic simulation are capable of accurately predicting the binding sites of ligand, docking pose, and binding affinity based on the geometry of the receptor surface. The prediction can then be validated using *in vitro* biochemical assays and X-ray crystallography to validate ligand binding. Thus, a cyclic drug design process is then continued until the strongest binder is found.

Currently, drug discovery has been mainly focused on in vitro optimization. One future direction in system-based drug discovery will necessarily shift to ADMET prediction to assess drug performance *in vivo*. Although several ADMET properties such as drug-likeness can be predicted by simple rules, a more detailed classification of drug properties can be achieved by more advanced machine learning techniques. Likewise, a holistic drug design process that simultaneously optimizes the drug properties based on *in vitro* and *in vivo* data will also hold promise to optimize drug safety and minimize adverse reactions. Consequently, integration of multilevel data from structure, tissue, and the whole organism will be required to achieve a more accurate prediction. In conclusion, we have presented the essential quantitative methods in system-based drug discovery, and the approaches presented here will stimulate further efforts in the progress of drug discovery and design to engineer safer and more effective drugs.

Author details

Yu-Chen Lo[1*], Ren Gui[2], Hiroshi Honda[2] and Jorge Z. Torres[3]

*Address all correspondence to: bennylo@stanford.edu

1 Department of Bioengineering, Stanford University, The United States

2 Department of Bioengineering, Northwestern Polytechnic University, The United States

3 Department of Chemistry and Biochemistry, University of California, Los Angeles, The United States

References

[1] Lo YC, Senese S, Damoiseaux R, Torres JZ. 3D chemical similarity networks for structure-based target prediction and scaffold hopping. ACS Chemical Biology. 2006;11(8):2244–53. doi:10.1021/acschembio.6b00253. PMID: 27285961.

[2] Barelier S, Sterling T, O'Meara MJ, Shoichet BK. The recognition of identical ligands by unrelated proteins. ACS Chemical Biology. 2015;10(12):2772–2784. doi:10.1021/acschembio.5b00683. PMID: 26421501; PMCID: PMCPMC4684825.

[3] Shoichet BK, Walters WP, Jiang H, Bajorath J. Advances in computational medicinal chemistry: A reflection on the evolution of the field and perspective going forward.

Journal of Medicinal Chemistry. 2016;59(9):4033–4034. doi:10.1021/acs.jmedchem.6b00511. PMID: 27054949.

[4] Lipinski CA. Rule of five in 2015 and beyond: Target and ligand structural limitations, ligand chemistry structure and drug discovery project decisions. Advanced Drug Delivery Reviews. 2016;101:34–41. doi:10.1016/j.addr.2016.04.029. PMID: 27154268.

[5] Yan X, Liao C, Liu Z, Hagler AT, Gu Q, Xu J. Chemical structure similarity search for ligand-based virtual screening: Methods and computational resources. Current Drug Targets. 2015:17(14):1580–85. PMID: 26521773.

[6] Le SQ, Ho TB, Phan TT. A novel graph-based similarity measure for 2D chemical structures. Genome Informatics. 2004;15(2):82–91. PMID: 15706494.

[7] Raymond JW, Willett P. Effectiveness of graph-based and fingerprint-based similarity measures for virtual screening of 2D chemical structure databases. Journal of Computer-Aided Molecular Design. 2002;16(1):59–71. PMID: 12197666.

[8] Lo YC, Senese S, Li CM, Hu Q, Huang Y, Damoiseaux R, et al. Large-scale chemical similarity networks for target profiling of compounds identified in cell-based chemical screens. PLoS Computational Biology. 2015;11(3):e1004153. doi:10.1371/journal.pcbi.1004153. PMID: 25826798; PMCID: PMCPMC4380459.

[9] Chen X, Yan CC, Zhang X, Zhang X, Dai F, Yin J, et al. Drug-target interaction prediction: Databases, web servers and computational models. Briefings in Bioinformatics. 2016;17(4):696–712. doi:10.1093/bib/bbv066. PMID: 26283676.

[10] Davies M, Nowotka M, Papadatos G, Dedman N, Gaulton A, Atkinson F, et al. ChEMBL web services: Streamlining access to drug discovery data and utilities. Nucleic Acids Research. 2015;43(W1):W612–W620. doi:10.1093/nar/gkv352. PMID: 25883136; PMCID: PMCPMC4489243.

[11] Keiser MJ, Roth BL, Armbruster BN, Ernsberger P, Irwin JJ, Shoichet BK. Relating protein pharmacology by ligand chemistry. Nature Biotechnology. 2007;25(2):197–206. doi:10.1038/nbt1284. PMID: 17287757.

[12] Liu T, Altman RB. Using multiple microenvironments to find similar ligand-binding sites: Application to kinase inhibitor binding. PLoS Computational Biology. 2011;7(12):e1002326. doi:10.1371/journal.pcbi.1002326. PMID: 22219723; PMCID: PMCPMC3248393.

[13] Westerhoff HV. Network-based pharmacology through systems biology. Drug Discovery Today: Technologies. 2015;15:15–16. doi:10.1016/j.ddtec.2015.05.001. PMID: 26464085.

[14] Liu T, Altman RB. Relating essential proteins to drug side-effects using canonical component analysis: A structure-based approach. Journal of Chemical Information and

Modeling. 2015;55(7):1483–1494. doi:10.1021/acs.jcim.5b00030. PMID: 26121262; PMCID: PMCPMC4875781.

[15] Hughes JP, Rees S, Kalindjian SB, Philpott KL. Principles of early drug discovery. British Journal of Pharmacology. 2011;162(6):1239–1249. doi:10.1111/j.1476-5381.2010.01127.x. PMID: 21091654; PMCID: PMCPMC3058157.

[16] Wilson GL, Lill MA. Integrating structure-based and ligand-based approaches for computational drug design. Future Medicinal Chemistry. 2011;3(6):735–750. doi: 10.4155/fmc.11.18. PMID: 21554079.

[17] Fang Y. Ligand-receptor interaction platforms and their applications for drug discovery. Expert Opinion on Drug Discovery. 2012;7(10):969–988. doi: 10.1517/17460441.2012.715631. PMID: 22860803.

[18] Kahsai AW, Xiao K, Rajagopal S, Ahn S, Shukla AK, Sun J, et al. Multiple ligand-specific conformations of the beta2-adrenergic receptor. Nature Chemical Biology. 2011;7(10): 692–700. doi:10.1038/nchembio.634. PMID: 21857662; PMCID: PMCPMC3404607.

[19] Meng XY, Zhang HX, Mezei M, Cui M. Molecular docking: A powerful approach for structure-based drug discovery. Current Computer-Aided Drug Design. 2011;7(2):146–157. PMID: 21534921; PMCID: PMCPMC3151162.

[20] Lopez-Vallejo F, Caulfield T, Martinez-Mayorga K, Giulianotti MA, Nefzi A, Houghten RA, et al. Integrating virtual screening and combinatorial chemistry for accelerated drug discovery. Combinatorial Chemistry and High Throughput Screening. 2011;14(6): 475–487. PMID: 21521151.

[21] Huang SY, Zou X. Advances and challenges in protein-ligand docking. International Journal of Molecular Sciences. 2010;11(8):3016–3034. doi:10.3390/ijms11083016. PMID: 21152288; PMCID: PMCPMC2996748.

[22] Williams F. Reasoning with Statistics: How to Read Quantitative Research. 4th ed. Fort Worth: Harcourt Brace Jovanovich College Publishers; 1992, Vol. xiii, 220 p.

[23] Sprinthall RC. Basic Statistical Analysis. 6th ed. Boston: Allyn and Bacon; 2000, Vol. xiv, 626 p.

[24] Norusis MJ, SPSS Inc. SPSS 8.0 Guide to Data Analysis. Upper Saddle River, N.J.: Prentice Hall; 1998, Vol. xviii, 563 p.

[25] Harris MB. Basic Statistics for Behavioral Science Research. 2nd ed. Boston: Allyn and Bacon; 1998, Vol. xvi, 576 p.

[26] Asher HB. Causal Modeling. 2nd ed. Beverly Hills: Sage Publications; 1983, 96 p.

[27] George D, Mallery P. SPSS for Windows Step by Step: A Simple Guide and Reference 9.0 Update. 2nd ed. Boston: Allyn and Bacon; 2000, 357 p.

6

Cell-Based Screening to Identify Cytoprotective Compounds

Domokos Gerő

Abstract

Prevention of cellular injury and consequent cell death is expected to provide therapeutic benefit in various diseases, but with the complexity of cell damaging pathways involved, identification and validation of novel potential drug targets is not a trivial task. New drug targets are expected to take part in complex responses with wide-ranging effects on gene expression and cellular function and drug candidates rather modify these effects than act as simple agonists or antagonists to ultimately protect the cells from an injury. Phenotypic screening may help identify cytoprotective compounds in diseases, in which the lack of drug targets makes target-based approaches unfeasible. This chapter gives an overview of the strategy of cell-based assay development, primary screening, hit selection and confirmation. Considerations about the choice of small molecule compound libraries utilized in cell-based models are discussed as well as the use of clinical drugs for drug repurposing or repositioning. The choice of cell types and issues associated with cell culture techniques are overviewed and the most common assays and readouts are briefly described. Finally, the potential pitfalls of data analysis and hit selection are discussed.

Keywords: cell-based screening, high-throughput screening, cytoprotection, drug discovery, chemical genomics, drug target

1. Introduction

The development of small molecule therapeutics for the treatment of diseases has gone through various phases over the last few decades. While the number of approved drugs continuously increased from the 1970s till 1996, when a record number of drugs (53 drugs) was approved by the Center for Drug Evaluation and Research of the U.S. Food and Drug Administration (FDA), a decline has been observed since then with no more than 20–30 new drugs approved each year [1]. In the second half of the twentieth century, drug discovery saw a rise of synthetic organic chemistry that made it economically feasible to produce large combinatorial libraries and biology progressed to provide many novel drug targets with structural details that promoted both high-throughput screening of small molecule libraries and computer-aided drug design as potential methodologies to identify novel therapeutic agents. In 2000, the number of known human drug targets were less than 500 but with the overestimated number of human genes and an expected number of 5–10 drug targets per disease genes, the number of potential drug targets were estimated to lie between 5000 and 10,000 [2–4]. The number of human genes shrank to 19,000 and the identified small molecule drug targets rose to mere 557 (549 for FDA-approved drugs and 8 further targets for drugs approved in the rest of the world) in 2017, while 146 additional human protein targets were curated for biological drugs [5, 6]. In fact, the number of biological drugs and respective targets increased considerably over the last 20 years: in 2000 only 59 biological drugs (recombinant proteins and monoclonal antibodies) were introduced, while 250 unique biological agents were available in 2016 [3, 5]. In 2002, Hopkins and Groom argued that only those disease-modifying genes can be used as drug targets that are druggable (contain domains that small molecules can bind to) and the overlap between the druggable genome and genes linked to diseases may be between 20 and 50% [7]. They predicted that no more than 600–1500 small molecule drug targets existed in humans if we had 30,000 genes. With fewer genes than anticipated, the number of potential drug targets also decreased, which partly explains the lower number of new molecular entities over the last decades. Examining the new first-in-class drugs (compounds that modulate a novel target or biological pathway that was not targeted before their introduction) approved by the FDA during the first decade after 1999, Swinney and Anthony found that 28 of the small molecule drugs were discovered using a phenotypic screening approach compared to 17 drugs discovered by a target-based approach suggesting that phenotypic screening may be more successful because of the unbiased identification of drugs with new molecular mechanisms of action [8–10]. However, the discovery of a first-in-class drug may not be simply attributed to a phenotypic screen or a target-based approach, the two approaches do not mutually exclude each other [11]. The launch of a new chemical entity often roots in a discovery that occurred one or two decades earlier and the development of a drug that reaches the market often involves both approaches [11]. For example, a phenotypic assay may be used for the discovery of a new drug target, while subsequent optimization of drug candidates may occur via a target-based approach, or the two strategies may be combined in multiple cycles during the process. The term of 'phenotypic screening' may be broadly used for all non-target-based approaches or more selectively for testing of compounds in a system-based approach using a target-agnostic assay that monitors phenotypic changes, thus the contribution of phenotypic assays may be differently interpreted in various contexts. Nonetheless, phenotypic screening is making a comeback in drug discovery with large pharmaceutical companies like Novartis AG and GlaxoSmithKline plc admittedly promoting it, but its overall share remains unclear in the efforts of pharmaceutical companies and academics [12].

2. Planning a phenotypic screen

A clear plan is needed for any early drug discovery projects and a phenotypic screen is not an exception [13, 14]. While the steps of the drug discovery project occur in a different order than in a target-based project, it is necessary to establish a clear go/no-go plan for all the steps (**Figure 1**). Since the target is unknown in the beginning of the project and there might be rather wide expectations about the activity of a potential cytoprotective compound, it may not be necessary to define cut-off values in the beginning. However, it is necessary to make

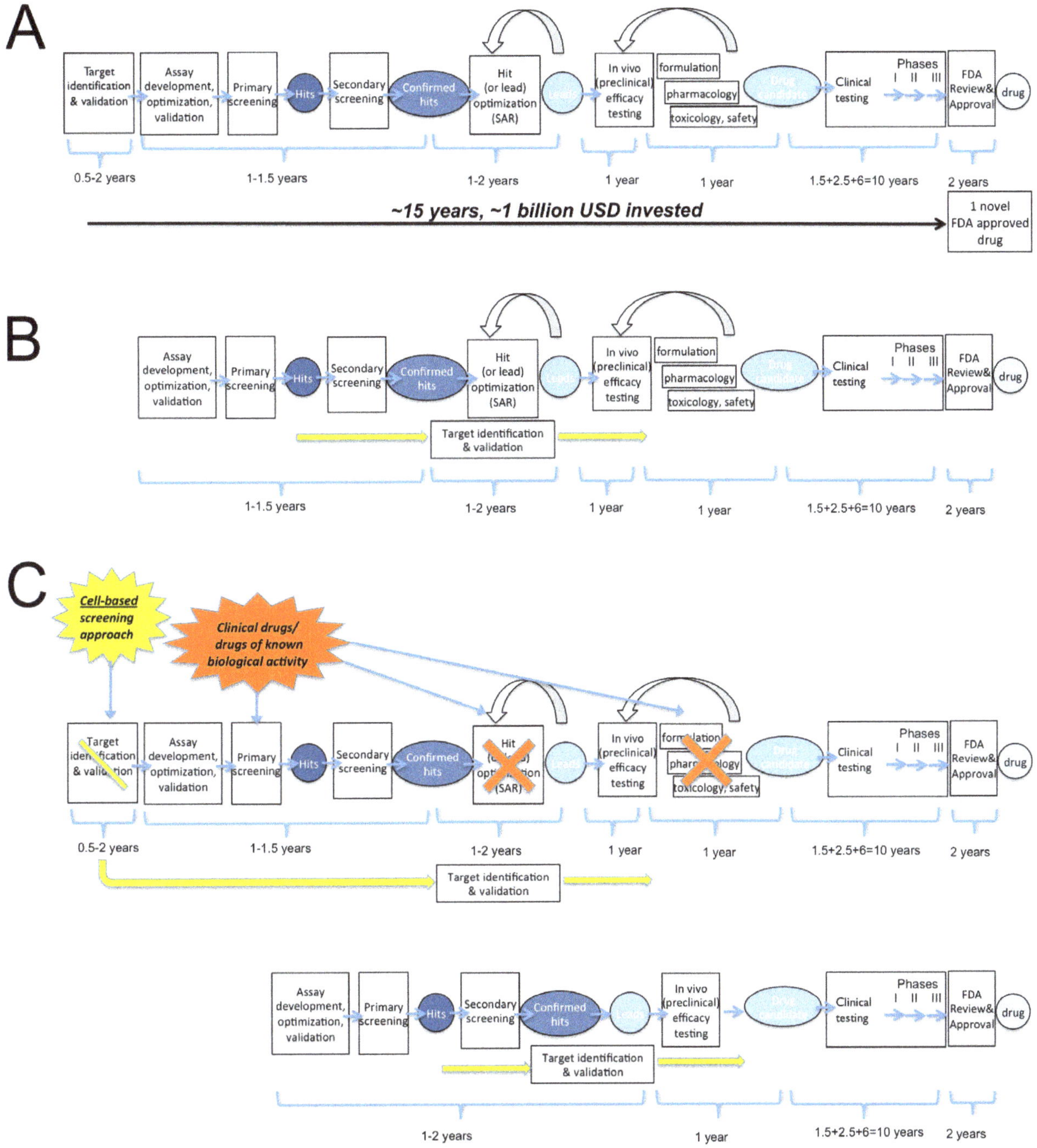

Figure 1. Basic plans of target-based and cell-based drug discovery approaches. (A) Target-based drug discovery represents the standard procedure in drug discovery. (B) Cell-based phenotypic screening skips the target identification step in the beginning of the project. This may lead to considerable time saving, since this step is usually performed simultaneously with the hit optimization. (C) Drug repurposing is possible in cell-based screening projects and it may accelerate the drug discovery process by skipping the hit optimization and toxicology steps. Please note the changes in the order of the respective steps and the expectable savings.

estimations about the market potential of a prospective drug candidate for the disease, so that we can decide on the necessary steps when the costs and potential investments arise. Fortunately, the earliest steps (optimization of the cell-based model and the primary screening) represent relatively low cost, foreseeable expenditures. Actually, the costs of the cell-based screening may not exceed the expenses associated with the identification of a novel target to start up a target-based project. Decisions can be made based on the results of the primary screen whether it is worth proceeding with a hit compound and what kind of secondary tests or models to be used based on the chemical nature of the compound. In general, higher level of flexibility is necessary during a cell-based drug discovery project than in a target-based project due to the unforeseeable nature of the drug target. Still, apart from the cell culture model of the disease it is worth having secondary *in vitro* models and a well-established animal model of the disease planned in the beginning of the project.

Phenotypic assays may be better suited for different disease areas than target-based approaches but there is no clear rule about its applicability. Santos et al. analyzed the therapeutic areas in which new drugs appeared and found that the majority of recent innovation occurred in the areas of cancer and immunology, while very little progress was seen in cardiovascular drugs [5]. On the other hand, the annual direct costs of cardiovascular disease and stroke were double the amounts of cancer-associated costs ($193.1 and $88.7 billion, respectively, in 2011) suggesting that higher progress is expected in this area [15]. When new molecular entities are considered, the lag behind other areas becomes even more apparent over recent years: cancer, infectious diseases and nervous system disorders are the leading areas of drug discovery and they all precede cardiovascular diseases [16–18]. One potential explanation for the disproportional representation of this area is the lack of new druggable targets in cardiovascular diseases, whereas the new cancer drugs and anti-infective agents are new molecular entities, they bind to novel protein targets. The other problem may be related to the nature of the injury: both anti-infective agents and cancer drugs are expected to kill the cells, while in cardiovascular diseases the expectation is to protect the cells from a harmful injury. In most instances, the mechanism of cell killing involves an inhibitory effect on the target, which is easier to attain than a stimulatory effect, just like it is simpler to produce an antagonist than an agonist for a given target since various compounds may block a binding site even if they do not fit perfectly in the active center but only a perfect molecular match can activate the target [19]. Phenotypic screening may provide a solution for the difficulties of cardiovascular drug discovery, since it is possible to find compounds that reduce the cellular injury even in the absence of a known drug target [20].

Orphan diseases represent another potential area of drug discovery using cell-based assays. Orphan diseases are rare disorders that affect small percentage of the population and thus possess a limited market potential, which led to the loss of interest by pharmaceutical companies and the lack of drug treatment in the majority of cases. The definition of orphan diseases are somewhat questionable, since there is no exact prevalence value associated with the term but in most cases if a disease affects less than 1 in 1000 or 2000 people, we call it a low prevalence or orphan disease [21–24]. While the incidence of rare diseases is low, the European Organization for Rare Diseases (EURORDIS) estimates that there are 5000–7000 distinct rare diseases and they affect approximately 6–8% of the population of the European Union [25].

The majority of these disorders are inherited diseases and drug therapy may be necessary throughout the lifetime that increases their market potential. Most governments have recognized the disproportionality of the potential profits and the necessary investments in case of rare diseases and have issued legislations to promote the development of new drug therapies for orphan diseases [26, 27]. As most of these diseases have a disease-linked gene and the mutations are easily reproduced in cellular models, they may represent the most important target diseases for cell-based phenotypic screening. Furthermore, if we accept the prediction about the number of druggable targets by Hopkins and Groom [7], the logical consequence is that many of these diseases will not be cured by an independent molecular entity but will share therapeutic drugs either with other orphan diseases or with more common illnesses. Thus, testing clinically used compounds with a drug repurposing approach may prove successful in many of these disorders, which reduces the overall costs of subsequent steps.

Cellular injury and cell death are the major challenges in today's drug discovery portfolio. While cancer drugs are on the rise, with cell killing as the principal mechanism of action of drugs, cellular injury remains the major theme of scientific research. In most diseases, researchers focus on cellular damage and cell death and investigate the underlying mechanisms that may help us understand how to interfere with the process. Unfortunately, this approach is not that successful in the discovery of new drug targets, but provides us with a multitude of cellular and animal models of various diseases [28]. These models usually allow only low throughput assays to be performed but may represent a good starting point for phenotypic screens.

In many diseases, the question arises whether reduction of the damage will be possible if currently there is no therapeutic drug for the disease in clinical practice. If, under experimental conditions, protection of the injured cells is accomplished by gene silencing or by gene therapy, there will be greater chance for establishing a pharmacological intervention in the future since it indicates the existence of disease-linked genes. It may not be necessary to induce orders-of-magnitude changes or to fully suppress the expression of a disease-linked gene to attain cell survival benefit, because the cell fate in an injury may be modified by small changes in the level of interacting proteins. Also, the existence of other experimental methods (as it was the case with ischemic pre- and post-conditioning) that induce cell protection may indicate the existence of potential targets prior to the identification of a disease-linked gene. Since phenotypic screening is a target-agnostic methodology, the outcome is of primary importance and not the underlying mechanism.

The mechanism of cytoprotection may not be identical with the blockage of known cell death pathways. Apoptosis and necrosis represent the two major cell death processes and they were long regarded as examples of "programmed" and "unprogrammed" cell death. Distinguishing a clear pathway or program in the mechanism of cell death allows us to interfere with specific components of the process and to block the execution of the program. In this respect, caspase inhibitors are the prototypical inhibitors of apoptosis [29]. However, necrosis can also be blocked by poly(ADP-ribose) polymerase (PARP) inhibitors and thus its unprogrammed classification is no longer valid, even if it took us longer to fully understand the process because of its rapid execution [30–32]. Many other regulated forms of cell death (autophagy, pyroptosis, necroptosis, parthanathos and mitoptosis) have been identified and various drugs that block these cell-based processes played a key role in their discovery [33]. Since cell death may occur simultaneously via multiple pathways, our classification of the dominant cell death form may change over time in various diseases as we understand more details about an injury [34]. Understanding the key features of a disease or an injury and reproduction of these mechanistic details in a cellular model may be of higher value than close mimicking the cell death process, as the latter often represents the final steps in the damage that we have to prevent and not to interfere with. Interestingly, neither caspase inhibitors nor PARP inhibitors went through clinical trials in their originally conceived application, but paradoxically PARP inhibitors reached clinical practice in diseases, in which they had seemed to play a lesser role. Thus while PARP was discovered as the main contributor to necrotic cell death and the first PARP inhibitor started a trial in ST-Elevation Myocardial Infarction (STEMI) [35], PARP inhibitors reached the market later as cancer drugs: currently olaparib, rucaparib and niraparib are approved for ovarian cancer [36, 37]. Similarly, caspase inhibitors were initially suggested to play a role as potential drugs in a wide array of diseases including acquired immune deficiency syndrome (AIDS), ischemic diseases (myocardial infarction, stroke), neurodegenerative diseases, myelodysplatic syndrome and toxic liver injury [38], but clinical trials were only started in epilepsy, hepatitis C virus (HCV) infection and non-alcoholic steatohepatosis (NASH) and none of the caspase inhibitors have reached FDA approval [39–41].

3. Compounds libraries

The number of compounds used in a cell-based assay is often lower than what can be screened in a simple enzymatic reaction. The cell-based models are usually more complex and the assays typically require longer time to perform. Furthermore, the maintenance of a cell culture lab for high number of assays is more costly than what is needed for simple biochemical assays, thus it is worth considering whether the associated costs can be limited by testing fewer compounds. Also, the measurement results may show higher variance in cell-based assays than in biochemical assays and may require higher number of repeats that will considerably increase the expenses. Since there is limited information about the number of compounds that may protect the cells against an injury, we can start the screening with a validation set of compounds that may contain compounds that are known to reduce the cellular injury in that model and also include various other compounds to see the data variability. This can give us information about the expectable number of hits in larger sets of compounds and help us plan the screening strategy. A reference compound that protects against the injury may not be available when we study a new disease model, thus we may need to consider the use of controls in which the injury has not been induced and introduce the use of positive controls in the assay once we identified drugs that protect against the injury.

A two-step procedure may be preferred in the majority of phenotypic screens: starting with a smaller set of compounds with higher expectable hit ratio followed by a second screen of larger sets of compounds that may achieve a lower hit ratio. The number of hits is higher in sets of compounds that mostly contain biologically active compounds than in sets of drug-like molecules. It is easily understandable that drugs that interfere with biological processes definitely possess binding sites, whereas those compounds that only show resemblance to other compounds do not necessarily have any targets in a cell. However, many of the biologically active compounds may show higher level of toxicity in the cells, since their known activity may not be related to cytoprotection and it may increase the data variability.

Hit selection may also include two steps in cell-based screens: (1) identification of hits in the primary screening and (2) a secondary confirmation assay of the hit molecules. Because of the higher variability of the assays and measurement values, the active compounds may show less cytoprotection in a single measurement than their average effect, thus it is better to use cut-off values that allow us to select a broader set of initial hits. These compounds will include many false positives, which will fail to show protection in repeated tests. If we expect a hit ratio around 1 in 100 molecules in the primary screen, and run confirmatory tests in repeats (e.g. in 3–6 repeats), it gives an the assay burden of ~50% for the hit confirmation step, which is substantially less than running the primary screen in duplicates. In many cases, the number of confirmed hits will be around or below 1 in 1000 compounds tested, so the set of test compounds should include a few thousand compounds in the first primary screen to produce a meaningful set of data. Fewer compounds may not contain protective molecules at all and the lack of confirmed hits often results in discontinuation of the project.

Clinical compounds can be used for initial screening efforts and a repurposing approach can speed up the drug discovery process. The number of drugs approved for human use is around 2400 in the USA and there are no more than 4000 molecular entities approved worldwide (including the US market) [24]. There are various sets available from a few vendors that contain a selection of clinically used drugs and may also include other compounds that went through toxicology studies but failed in the clinical phases (**Table 1**). If multiple of these sets are obtained from different companies, there is usually substantial overlap in the provided drugs but the vendors mostly use independent sources for the drugs and various salts of the same compound might be included in the different sets. Another option is to use a compound library of biologically active drugs. In this case, the majority of the drugs will have an annotated target in the cells but not all compounds will possess a binding site: for example, the drug target may not be expressed in the cell type in use or an anti-infective compound may not have a mammalian homolog. In general, these libraries mostly contain a similar number of potentially cytoprotective drugs as clinical libraries but there is a huge difference between them in the subsequent steps. Those compounds that have gone through formal toxicology studies, may be directly reused for other diseases, but those compounds whose toxicity have never been investigated will require more follow-up work.

Larger chemical libraries comprising 10,000–100,000 drugs may be screened as a second step following the screen of small libraries. The number of possible drug-like molecules is not indefinite, but it is certainly large enough to forget about testing all possible compounds. Virshup et al. estimated that the set of all synthetically feasible organic molecules of 500 Da molecular weight or less contained over 10^{60} structures ("the small molecule universe") [42]. Depending on the disease and target tissue, it might be possible to exclude certain chemistries and by using chemoinformatics filtering methods, the composition of the library might be limited to a set that is easier to handle [43]. A key concept is druglikeness, prediction of

Compound library	Number of drugs	Short description	Link
NIH Clinical Collection	450	Compounds that have already been in clinical use or in clinical trials	http://www.nihclinicalcollection.com/index.php?cPath=21
LOPAC (Library of pharmacologically active compounds)/ TocriScreen collection	1280/1120	Known receptor agonists, antagonists, modulators of cellular responses and signal transduction	http://www.sigmaaldrich.com/catalog/ProductDetail.do?lang=en&N4=LO12 80 I SIGMA&N5=SEARCH_CONCAT_PNO I BRAND_KEY&F=SPEC http://www.tocris.com/dispprod.php?ItemId=5381
US Drug Collection	1140	Compounds that have reached the stage of clinical trials in the USA	http://www.msdiscovery.com/usdrugs.html
International Drug collection	240	Compounds that have reached the stage of clinical trials in other countries	http://www.msdiscovery.com/
Killer Plates	160	Compounds with known effects on cellular viability	http://www.msdiscovery.com/killer.html
New Prestwick Chemical Library	1200	Drugs that are in clinical use	http://www.prestwickchemical.com
FDA Approved Drug Library	640	Compounds selected from another library of clinically used compounds	http://www.enzolifesciences.com/BML-2841/fda-approved-drug-library/
Apexscreen Library	5000	Diverse compound library, representative set of various chemotypes for screening	http://www.timtec.com/apexscreen.html
Chembridge Diversity Library	10,000	Drug-like diverse compound library for screening library	http://www.chembridge.com/screening_libraries/diversity_libraries/#DIVERSet
Myriascreen Library	10,000	Library of drug-like diverse compounds	http://www.timtec.com/myriascreen-diversity-collection.html
Actitarg-K library	6600	Library of kinase modulators and similar structures	http://www.timtec.com/kinase-modulators-actitarg-k-library.html
Natural Product Libtrary	640	Purified natural compounds, products	http://www.timtec.com/natural-compound-library.html
AMRI Diverse sample library	10,000	Diverse selection of 'lead-like' compounds that covers Albany Molecular Research Institutes' small molecular compound collections	http://www.amriglobal.com/products_and_services/products_detail_sub.cfm?prodID=1&subServID=4&subServID2=5

Table 1. Examples of compound libraries for cell-based screening projects.

the properties of a molecule based on the physicochemical properties of approved drugs and filtering the compound library according to these parameters [44]. The absorption, distribution, metabolism and excretion (ADME) of drug-like compounds may be predicted and subsets of drugs can be chosen for a specific organ or disease based on these data [45]. Lipinski introduced his "rule of five" concept, the filtering of molecules by solubility and permeability prediction using the following parameters: the molecular weight is less than 500 daltons, CLog P is less than 5, the number of H-bond donors (the sum of OHs and NHs) is less than 5 and the number of H-bond acceptors (all nitrogen and oxygen atoms) is less than 10, that greatly reduces the number of potential drug-like molecules [46, 47]. This approach suggests that the number of drug-like molecules that we potentially use is closer to 10,000 than to a million drugs, since these compounds are sparsely distributed through "the small molecule universe" [47]. The use of a targeted library, which consists of drugs that are known to bind to certain types of targets and also contains highly similar molecules, is commonly used in chemical genomics and may prove useful in phenotypic screening, as well [43, 48].

The concentration of drugs used in cell-based screening is mostly determined by practicability and not by the effective or toxic concentrations of the individual compounds. The majority of compound libraries supplied compounds in solution at a fixed 1 or 2 mg/ml concentration in the past and nowadays, compounds are offered, mostly at 10 mM concentration in dimethyl sulfoxide (DMSO) [49]. The majority of the libraries are available in 96- or 384-well microplates, deep well plates or microtube racks. To simplify processing, dilutions of the compounds are best prepared at the same concentration for all drugs. While it would make more sense to use each clinical compound at a clinically relevant, effective concentration, equimolar concentrations are used most often to simplify and speed up the dilution steps. Compounds are usually screened at a concentration between 1 and 10 μmol/l, which might present dilution problems and may cause toxicity. Since the amount of DMSO must be limited as much as possible, dilutions of the drugs may be prepared in water-based solutions for cell-based assays and drug precipitation may occur as a result of poor water-solubility during dilution. Compound libraries are usually stored at −20°C in an upright position and compounds may settle down in the bottom of microtubes or wells during freeze-thaw cycles and some of the drugs may also precipitate. As a result, the cells may be treated with lower concentration of drugs than expected either due to incomplete mixing or dissolution of drugs. Also, compounds may lose activity during freezing and thawing, or due to an oxidative reaction with DMSO, which will also have various effects on the cells and may interfere with the assay [50]. Thus, hit compounds, if a fresh resupply is used in the confirmation studies, may show similar activity at a lower concentration than in the primary screen or even display higher activity.

Drug combinations may provide a further option to reduce the number of assays to be run [51, 52]. If you expect that the number of active compounds is low, you may consider pooling multiple compounds and testing them in combination. The number of assay runs may be reduced by an order of magnitude, if 8–12 compounds are pooled and only low number of "hits" is expected. Re-testing of the individual compounds will be necessary for each of the initial hits but since the expected hit ratio is low, it may not present excessive follow-up work. However, potential toxicity of the compounds needs to be considered: a toxic compound can mask the cytoprotective effect of an active compound if the cells are simultaneously treated with both drugs. Thus, the number or ratio of cytotoxic drugs might be the determining factor whether drug pooling is possible or not in a cellular model. On the other hand, this approach may allow us to search for potentiating compounds in a model if the test compounds are used in combination with a drug that provides limited protection [20, 53, 54].

4. Mammalian cell culture

Cell-based screening requires adaptation of cell culture techniques to higher throughput than what is typical in cellular assays and may present unexpected problems associated with the specific cell types or models [55]. The majority of these issues could have been sorted out by automation but the cost of robotic systems that handle cell cultivation remains extravagant. The first automated cell culture stations appeared in the market a decade ago, but these monstrous instruments remained outrageously expensive and very few units have been sold [56, 57]. Highly complex, cell-based models often include procedures that may not be automated and will require manual handling for specific steps. In this case, purchasing an expensive instrument that cannot fully replace the laboratory technician may increase the overall costs. Whereas training technicians specifically for higher throughput cell culture may be advantageous: provides flexibility, predictable costs and allows the introduction of newer models when needed.

Choosing the right cell type for the primary screen might be the key for discovering novel drugs or drug actions. Primary cells are often propagated for cell-based screening projects, assuming that they more closely mimic the processes of the cells in whole organisms than cell lines. However, primary cells are usually more difficult to grow and their division potential is limited to a few passages, during which they may not maintain their original characteristics. Whereas cell lines are well-characterized, immortalized cells that are easy to maintain and can be resupplied at reasonable costs, if necessary. The reagent and cell maintenance costs are lower for cell lines, as they can be cultured in classic cell culture media and typically grow faster. Human cells may be better suited for drug discovery, since the potential drug targets may not have orthologs in other species or the dissimilarity between the representative proteins may change the binding of compounds to the target [5]. On the other hand, many of the cell-based models use non-human cells either because the preferred cell-line originates from rodents or because the primary cells cannot be freshly isolated from humans. Either way, choosing the best model is more important than the use of human cells, since it is better to loose a few hits because of the differences in orthologs than to identify hits in an irrelevant model. If there are multiple options to choose from, it is worth keeping the lower cost model for the primary screening and use the other cell type as secondary model to confirm the action of hit compounds [58, 59].

Assay miniaturization is necessary to reduce the costs of cell culture and the assay-associated expenses [60]. Although, the ultimate goal is to minimize reagent costs, the power of testing treatments in larger cell populations will remain high and may be preferential depending on the model or assay type [61, 62]. Thus, 96-well cell culture plates are often used in more complex assays, while 384- and 1536-well plates can be used for simple assays when the assay readout is expected to change considerably with the treatments. In a simple cell viability assay, if the cellular injury reduces the viability by 50% and we expect that our drug treatment may provide a partial protection against the injury (e.g. 20% survival benefit) then the pipetting error and imprecision of the measurement may not allow us to downsize the assay. It should be noted that in cell culture, miniaturization involves a more complex adaptation of the cell cultivation process than proportional scaling down of the number of seeded cells and all the reagents. Differences in aeration and temperature fluctuations occur between the wells based on their respective position on a plate: typically the edges are exposed to excessive temperature changes, evaporation and better oxygenation, while the inner wells are more homogeneous in this respect but they do not have comparable gas exchange and the cells may grow slightly slower in them. As a result, the outer wells may be excluded from analysis, leaving only 60 wells on a 96-well plate or 308 wells on a 384-well plate, thus 5-times higher number of treatments might be tested on a 384-well plate.

Contamination is a major issue in cell-based screening, because of the higher throughput of assays and steps that may not be carried out in an aseptic environment [63–65]. Compound libraries are often provided in solutions that are not sterile, though the drugs are dissolved in DMSO and there is little chance for bacterial contamination. The dilution step of compounds may be associated with contamination risk, partly because the storage plates often use tube caps that require manual handling and cannot be removed by a robotic system or because the pipetting station used for the dilution step does not fit in a biosafety cabinet. Also, experimental devices that are necessary to induce cellular injury may be utilized in some models and these instruments may exceed the size limits of a laminar flow cabinet [59]. While contamination risk may be minimized by careful planning of experiments, it is often impossible to eliminate all sources of bacterial contaminants. If the cell cultivation procedure is longer because the cells require longer differentiation steps, or the assay investigates the long-term survival of cells, the risk of contamination will also increase. In general, assays terminated within 3–4 h following the injury or drug treatment, may allow that some of the steps are carried out on the benchtop and may not require to work in a biosafety cabinet, since the bacterial growth becomes exponential after a lag phase and within this time-frame the low level of contaminants impose little risk of interfering with the assay [66]. However, longer exposures or assay runs requisite that all the steps are performed in a biosafety cabinet using sterile technique. It is essential to plan regular decontamination and sterilization of the instruments to avoid generating false data because of contaminants [67].

5. Assay-related issues

The readout of the screening assay that may be a viability assay or another functional test plays an important role in the identification of hit compounds and it is a key contributor to the expenses of the project. A high sensitivity, low cost assay is the obvious choice for primary cell-based screening of compound libraries [68, 69]. High sensitivity does not mean that we need to use luminescence measurements, because it is not the detection sensitivity what is important but the sensitive detection of the changes in cellular function or viability. A simple, colorimetric lactate dehydrogenase (LDH) assay may be capable to measure minor changes in cell viability that costly methodologies cannot detect. Reagent cost makes a huge difference if the number of runs is high, thus a less expensive assay may be preferable. A custom-tailored assay with "home-made" reagents may be a better choice than a commercial assay, depending on the model, and may save on supplies.

Specificity of the assay and the instrumentation necessary to read the plates are of similar importance but reproducibility and higher sensitivity may allow more flexibility in these parameters. Since we expect that the number of cytoprotective compounds is low in most models, it is better to have fewer false negatives and more false positives among the initial hits, thus sensitivity may overcome the limitations of specificity. Endpoint assays are typically preferred, since the measurement time can severely limit the number of runs in kinetic assays. If a plate is read for 30 min in a kinetic assay, and the endpoint measurement lasts 1 min, it will take more than 2 days to read 100 plates kinetically, while the endpoint measurement can be finished within 2 h. (And no more than 6000–8000 compounds are tested on 100 plates if 96-well plates are used and the outer wells are excluded.) Thus, if an endpoint assay can replace a kinetic read with no or little loss in sensitivity, it remains the preferred choice in cell-based screening.

Viability assays are obvious choices for identification of protective compounds in a cytotoxic injury and many simple assays are available to choose from [70–72]. The most commonly used assays depend on substrates that are converted to easily detectable products by metabolic enzymes in living cells and the results are linear with the number of viable cells within a limited range [73–75]. The least expensive options are colorimetric or fluorescent tests that requisite less costly plate readers. However, assay interference is a common problem with these methods: many of the test compounds are colored or fluorescent substances and they may produce false results. The metabolic pathways or enzymes may be up or down-regulated in the studied injury model, thus careful selection of the assay is necessary [53, 71, 72]. Homogeneous assays may be preferred, since fewer steps allow less processing error, and easier automation, robotic integration of the assay.

Simultaneous use of multiple viability assays can help compensate for the weaknesses of individual tests but makes the data analysis more complex [53, 58, 71]. For example, in a cellular injury model, when the methylthiazolyldiphenyl-tetrazolium bromide (MTT) assay is the primary viability assay, LDH release may be used as a secondary measurement from the simultaneously sampled cell culture supernatant [20, 53, 71, 72]. Thus, cytoprotection (increased viability) will be detectable as an increased signal in the MTT assay and also as a reduced LDH signal (diminished cell death) in the respective supernatant sample. Whereas the simultaneous increase or decrease of both the MTT and LDH signals indicates a false positivity in one of the assays and may not be of further interest.

In cell-based assays, differences occur in the assay results depending on the respective position of individual wells, since the activity of metabolic enzymes is affected by the temperature fluctuations, inhomogeneity of gas exchange and potential pH variations. These effects may affect the results considerably in many injury models and corrections may be necessary to compensate for their impact. But even with the best compensations, the chances to find protective compounds in middle or outer wells may not be equal [53]. It is worth testing, that with the use of a positive control compound, our assay can similarly detect protection in all wells of the plate. Alternatively, we may confirm that mock-treated or vehicle treated (negative control) wells show similar results throughout the whole plate. If the measurements show larger variation, it may be necessary to run measurements in duplicates. In this case, duplicates need to be allocated to various positions and not to neighboring wells on a plate, so that the average protection will be similar for all test positions [53].

Independent repeats are expected in all cell culture experiments but running cell-based screens repeatedly several times would unnecessarily increase the expenses [76–79]. We can assume that only a handful of drugs may protect the cells and the majority of the compounds will have little effect in the injury model. It is unnecessary to confirm the lack of effect for those drugs that exert no protection. The goal of the screen is to find potentially active drugs, thus screening a compound library needs a single measurement, even if we use a cell-based assay. The primary screen will not provide necessary data to state that the initial hits exert significant protection, we need to confirm the protective effect of potential hit compounds in repeated experiments to conclude that the effect is significant [77–79].

6. Data analysis

Hit identification is the main aim of data analysis in cell-based screening and this process may not follow the rules of statistics to the letter. In high-throughput screening, Z-factor has been used as the gold standard method to analyze the assay and data set quality [80]. This methodology assumes that the identification of hit compounds requisite good separation of positive and negative controls. However, the power of this methodology was questioned later, since higher background or noise values are typically present in several assays, and poor signal-to-background or signal-to-noise separation still allow the identification of "true hits" [81, 82]. Larger variation occurs in a cell-based assay than in biochemical assays, even so cell culture experiments have been successfully used to study the effects of drug treatments. Thus, the variable damage induced in many injury models is an acceptable feature of the experimental methodology but may require more flexibility during data analysis.

The ultimate goal is to identify compounds that provide protection against an injury, which means less damage or increased viability of the cells depending on the specific model. A Z-score, the number of standard deviations from the mean vehicle treated wells undergoing the injury, may be calculated using the whole dataset and it easily shows the outliers [83]. Based on the assumptions that (1) the wells treated with various ineffective drugs will show similar response to the vehicle-treated wells and (2) there are very few active drugs, the compound-treated wells can quasi replace the negative control wells in the analysis. However, if the dataset shows larger variation, the Z-scores will be smaller values, thus meaningful cut-off values should be chosen individually for the selection of hits in each experimental model [54, 58, 59]. Apart from the more complex procedures, like Z-score calculation, there are various other options to identify cytoprotective compounds. Selection of the wells, in which diminished cell death occurred, is often easier on a single plate than in a large dataset, thus it might be useful to establish cut-off values based on the results of each plate separately. Data may be categorized immediately at plate reading and the outliers can be labeled as potential hit compounds or toxic molecules depending on the changes in viability. In this way, you can start up the hit confirmation before the completion of the primary screen, which may be preferable if the primary screen of a larger compound library requisites longer time.

Hit selection may be overly complex if dual or multiple readouts are used to identify active compounds. In the simplest case, one of the parameters is used only at a fixed cut-off value and the second parameter is ranked according to the activity to find the protective compounds. In a cell injury model, viability values may be used for preliminary classification of drugs as toxic and non-toxic compounds, and the other parameter (e.g. ROS production or an inflammatory signal) may be used to determine the protective effect of test compounds [54, 58]. Alternatively, the measurement values may be ranked separately for the individual parameters and cut-off Z-scores may be established for each of them. If a test compound performs above the cut-off values for each of the parameters, we may classify it as a hit that proceeds to the confirmation step. A further option is to streamline the decision making to the usual single parameter analysis: a new factor may be derived from the two primary measurement values, and the newly generated parameter can be ranked by the Z-scoring method.

Hit confirmation is the next step, following the identification of preliminary hits [83]. This procedure can take the usual steps of cell culture experiments. Independent repeats are needed and data analysis should be performed following the generally accepted rules of *in vitro* assays [79]. If more assays are available to test the activity of potential hits, it is worth including them at this step as secondary assays [83]. The cellular target of confirmed hits often represents new challenges, since the identification may not be a straightforward process in many of the disease models. However, the new targets are of high value for structure activity relationship (SAR) analysis and may shed new light on the mechanisms of disease development and progression.

7. Conclusion

Recent tendency in drug discovery suggests that target-based research will be complemented with target-agnostic approaches in the future. As opposed to classical target-based drug discovery approaches phenotypic assays may be necessary to identify novel compounds that show activity in orphan diseases or in common medical conditions that currently lack effective therapeutics. Cell-based models are often used to study various aspects of illnesses and many of these may be modified for powerful tools in drug discovery. The use of these models for cell-based screening may allow identification of potential drug candidates and chemical genomics approaches can promote reverse identification of novel drug targets [84].

Acknowledgements

D.G. received funding from the People Programme (Marie Curie actions) of the European Union's Seventh Framework Programme under the grant agreement number 62810.

Author details

Domokos Gerő[1,2*]

*Address all correspondence to: gerodomokos@yahoo.com

1 Institute of Pathophysiology, Semmelweis University Medical School, Budapest, Hungary

2 University of Exeter Medical School, Exeter, UK

References

[1] U. S. Food and Drug Administration. Summary of NDA Approvals & Receipts, 1938 to the present. Available from: https://www.fda.gov/aboutfda/whatwedo/history/productregulation/summaryofndaapprovalsreceipts1938tothepresent/default.htm

[2] Pennisi E. Human Genome Project. And the gene number is...? Science. 2000;**288**(5469): 1146-1147

[3] Drews J. Drug discovery: A historical perspective. Science. 2000;**287**(5460):1960-1964

[4] Ewing B, Green P. Analysis of expressed sequence tags indicates 35,000 human genes. Nature Genetics. 2000;**25**(2):232-234

[5] Santos R et al. A comprehensive map of molecular drug targets. Nature Reviews. Drug Discovery. 2017;**16**(1):19-34

[6] Chi KR. The dark side of the human genome. Nature. 2016;**538**(7624):275-277

[7] Hopkins AL, Groom CR. The druggable genome. Nature Reviews. Drug Discovery. 2002; **1**(9):727-730

[8] Swinney DC. Phenotypic vs. target-based drug discovery for first-in-class medicines. Clinical Pharmacology and Therapeutics. 2013;**93**(4):299-301

[9] Swinney DC, Anthony J. How were new medicines discovered? Nature Reviews. Drug Discovery. 2011;**10**(7):507-519

[10] Zheng W, Thorne N, McKew JC. Phenotypic screens as a renewed approach for drug discovery. Drug Discovery Today. 2013;**18**(21-22):1067-1073

[11] Eder J, Sedrani R, Wiesmann C. The discovery of first-in-class drugs: Origins and evolution. Nature Reviews. Drug Discovery. 2014;**13**(8):577-587

[12] Kotz J. Phenotypic screening, take two. Science-Business eXchange. 2012;**5**(15):1-3

[13] Strovel JS, Sittampalam NP, Coussens M, Hughes J, Inglese A, Kurtz A, Andalibi L, Patton C, Austin M, Baltezor M, Beckloff M, Weingarten M, Weir S. Early drug discovery and development guidelines: For academic researchers, collaborators, and start-up companies. In: Sittampalam GS. et al., Editors. Assay Guidance Manual. Bethesda (MD): 2004. p. 3-44

[14] Hughes JP et al. Principles of early drug discovery. British Journal of Pharmacology. 2011;**162**(6):1239-1249

[15] Writing Group, M et al. Executive summary: Heart disease and stroke statistics-2016 update: A report from the American Heart Association. Circulation. 2016;**133**(4):447-454

[16] Kinch MS et al. Target selection for FDA-approved medicines. Drug Discovery Today. 2015;**20**(7):784-789

[17] Kinch MS, Merkel J, Umlauf S. Trends in pharmaceutical targeting of clinical indications: 1930-2013. Drug Discovery Today. 2014;**19**(11):1682-1685

[18] Munos B. A forensic analysis of drug targets from 2000 through 2012. Clinical Pharmacology and Therapeutics. 2013;**94**(3):407-411

[19] Rang HP. The receptor concept: Pharmacology's big idea. British Journal of Pharmacology. 2006;**147**(Suppl 1):S9-16

[20] Gero D et al. Oxidant-induced cardiomyocyte injury: Identification of the cytoprotective effect of a dopamine 1 receptor agonist using a cell-based high-throughput assay. International Journal of Molecular Medicine. 2007;**20**(5):749-761

[21] Baldovino S et al. Rare diseases in Europe: From a wide to a local perspective. The Israel Medical Association Journal. 2016;**18**(6):359-363

[22] Montserrat Moliner A, Waligora J. The European union policy in the field of rare diseases. Public Health Genomics. 2013;**16**(6):268-277

[23] Taruscio D et al. National registries of rare diseases in Europe: An overview of the current situation and experiences. Public Health Genomics. 2015;**18**(1):20-25

[24] Huang R et al. The NCGC pharmaceutical collection: A comprehensive resource of clinically approved drugs enabling repurposing and chemical genomics. Science Translational Medicine. 2011;**3**(80):80ps16

[25] EURORDIS: European Organisation of Rare Diseases. Rare Diseases: Understanding this Public Health Priority. 2005; Available from: https://www.eurordis.org/IMG/pdf/princeps_document-EN.pdf

[26] Dharssi S et al. Review of 11 national policies for rare diseases in the context of key patient needs. Orphanet Journal of Rare Diseases. 2017;**12**(1):63

[27] Gammie T, Lu CY, Babar ZU. Access to orphan drugs: A comprehensive review of legislations, regulations and policies in 35 countries. PLoS One. 2015;**10**(10):e0140002

[28] Horvath P et al. Screening out irrelevant cell-based models of disease. Nature Reviews. Drug Discovery. 2016;**15**(11):751-769

[29] Pronk GJ et al. Requirement of an ICE-like protease for induction of apoptosis and ceramide generation by REAPER. Science. 1996;**271**(5250):808-810

[30] Gero D, Szabo C. Poly(ADP-ribose) polymerase: A new therapeutic target? Current Opinion in Anaesthesiology. 2008;**21**(2):111-121

[31] Gero D et al. Modulation of poly(ADP-ribose) polymerase-1 (PARP-1)-mediated oxidative cell injury by ring finger protein 146 (RNF146) in cardiac myocytes. Molecular Medicine. 2014;**20**:313-328

[32] Jagtap P, Szabo C. Poly(ADP-ribose) polymerase and the therapeutic effects of its inhibitors. Nature Reviews. Drug Discovery. 2005;**4**(5):421-440

[33] Duprez L et al. Major cell death pathways at a glance. Microbes and Infection. 2009;**11**(13): 1050-1062

[34] Pasparakis M, Vandenabeele P. Necroptosis and its role in inflammation. Nature. 2015; **517**(7534):311-320

[35] Morrow DA et al. A randomized, placebo-controlled trial to evaluate the tolerability, safety, pharmacokinetics, and pharmacodynamics of a potent inhibitor of poly(ADP-ribose) polymerase (INO-1001) in patients with ST-elevation myocardial infarction undergoing primary percutaneous coronary intervention: Results of the TIMI 37 trial. Journal of Thrombosis and Thrombolysis. 2009;**27**(4):359-364

[36] Davar D et al. Role of PARP inhibitors in cancer biology and therapy. Current Medicinal Chemistry. 2012;**19**(23):3907-3921

[37] Brown JS, Kaye SB, Yap TA. PARP inhibitors: The race is on. British Journal of Cancer. 2016;**114**(7):713-715

[38] Thompson CB. Apoptosis in the pathogenesis and treatment of disease. Science. 1995; **267**(5203):1456-1462

[39] O'Brien T, Linton SD. Design of Caspase Inhibitors as Potential Clinical Agents. CRC Enzyme Inhibitors Series. Boca Raton: CRC Press/Taylor & Francis Group; 2009. xii 299 p

[40] Kaur H, Kumar B, Medhi B. Antiepileptic drugs in development pipeline: A recent update. eNeurologicalSci. 2016;**4**(Supplement C):42-51

[41] Linton SD. Caspase inhibitors: A pharmaceutical industry perspective. Current Topics in Medicinal Chemistry. 2005;**5**(16):1697-1717

[42] Virshup AM et al. Stochastic voyages into uncharted chemical space produce a representative library of all possible drug-like compounds. Journal of the American Chemical Society. 2013;**135**(19):7296-7303

[43] Dandapani S et al. Selecting, acquiring, and using small molecule libraries for high-throughput screening. Current Protocols in Chemical Biology. 2012;**4**:177-191

[44] Bickerton GR et al. Quantifying the chemical beauty of drugs. Nature Chemistry. 2012; **4**(2):90-98

[45] Tao L et al. Recent progresses in the exploration of machine learning methods as in-silico ADME prediction tools. Advanced Drug Delivery Reviews. 2015;**86**:83-100

[46] Lipinski CA. Drug-like properties and the causes of poor solubility and poor permeability. Journal of Pharmacological and Toxicological Methods. 2000;**44**(1):235-249

[47] Lipinski CA et al. Experimental and computational approaches to estimate solubility and permeability in drug discovery and development settings. Advanced Drug Delivery Reviews. 2001;**46**(1-3):3-26

[48] Downey W, Liu C, Hartigan J. Compound profiling: Size impact on primary screening libraries. Drug Discovery World. 2010;(Spring)

[49] Chan JA, Hueso-Rodríguez JA. Compound library management. In: Janzen WP. editor. High Throughput Screening: Methods and Protocols. Humana Press: Totowa, NJ; 2002 pp. 117-127

[50] Jacob SW, Herschler R. Pharmacology of DMSO. Cryobiology. 1986;**23**(1):14-27

[51] Kainkaryam RM, Woolf PJ. Pooling in high-throughput drug screening. Current Opinion in Drug Discovery & Development. 2009;**12**(3):339-350

[52] Elkin LL et al. Just-in-time compound pooling increases primary screening capacity without compromising screening quality. Journal of Biomolecular Screening. 2015;**20**(5):577-587

[53] Szoleczky P et al. Identification of agents that reduce renal hypoxia-reoxygenation injury using cell-based screening: Purine nucleosides are alternative energy sources in LLC-PK1 cells during hypoxia. Archives of Biochemistry and Biophysics. 2012;**517**(1):53-70

[54] Gero D et al. Identification of pharmacological modulators of HMGB1-induced inflammatory response by cell-based screening. PLoS One. 2013;**8**(6):e65994

[55] Maddox CB, Rasmussen L, White EL. Adapting cell-based assays to the high throughput screening platform: Problems encountered and lessons learned. JALA Charlottesv Va. 2008;**13**(3):168-173

[56] Lehmann R et al. Biomek cell workstation: A variable system for automated cell cultivation. Journal of Laboratory Automation. 2016;**21**(3):439-450

[57] Ozturk SS. Equipment for large-scale mammalian cell culture. Advances in Biochemical Engineering/Biotechnology. 2014;**139**:69-92

[58] Gero D et al. Cell-based screening identifies paroxetine as an inhibitor of diabetic endothelial dysfunction. Diabetes. 2013;**62**(3):953-964

[59] Lopez-Garcia I, Gero D, Szczesny B, Szoleczky P, Olah G, Modis K, Zhang K, Gao J, Wu P, Sowers LC, DeWitt D, Prough DS, Szabo C. Development of a stretch-induced neurotrauma model for medium-throughput screening in vitro: Identification of rifampicin as a neuroprotectant. Br J Pharmacol. 2018;1**75**(2):284-300

[60] Sundberg SA. High-throughput and ultra-high-throughput screening: Solution- and cell-based approaches. Current Opinion in Biotechnology. 2000;**11**(1):47-53

[61] Maffia AM 3rd, Kariv II, Oldenburg KR. Miniaturization of a mammalian cell-based assay: Luciferase reporter gene readout in a 3 microliter 1536-well plate. Journal of Biomolecular Screening. 1999;**4**(3):137-142

[62] Mayr LM, Bojanic D. Novel trends in high-throughput screening. Current Opinion in Pharmacology. 2009;**9**(5):580-588

[63] Cote RJ. Aseptic technique for cell culture. Current Protocols in Cell Biology. 2001;Chapter 1: Unit 1. 3

[64] Stacey GN. Cell culture contamination. Methods in Molecular Biology. 2011;**731**:79-91

[65] Phelan K, May KM. Mammalian cell tissue culture techniques. Current Protocols in Pharmacology. 2016;**73**:12.1.1-12.1.23

[66] Naveen V, Hsiao CD. NrdR transcription regulation: Global proteome analysis and its role in *Escherichia coli* viability and virulence. PLoS One. 2016;**11**(6):e0157165

[67] Callaway E. Contamination hits cell work. Nature. 2014;**511**(7511):518

[68] Fernandes PB. Technological advances in high-throughput screening. Current Opinion in Chemical Biology. 1998;**2**(5):597-603

[69] Kelkar M, De A. Bioluminescence based in vivo screening technologies. Current Opinion in Pharmacology. 2012;**12**(5):592-600

[70] Chan GK et al. A simple high-content cell cycle assay reveals frequent discrepancies between cell number and ATP and MTS proliferation assays. PLOS One. 2013;**8**(5):e63583

[71] Modis K et al. Cytoprotective effects of adenosine and inosine in an in vitro model of acute tubular necrosis. British Journal of Pharmacology. 2009;**158**(6):1565-1578

[72] Modis K et al. Adenosine and inosine exert cytoprotective effects in an in vitro model of liver ischemia-reperfusion injury. International Journal of Molecular Medicine. 2013;**31**(2):437-446

[73] Prabst K et al. Basic colorimetric proliferation assays: MTT, WST, and Resazurin. Methods in Molecular Biology. 2017;**1601**:1-17

[74] Stoddart MJ. Cell viability assays: Introduction. Methods in Molecular Biology. 2011;**740**:1-6

[75] Riss TL, Moravec RA, Niles AL, Duellman S, Benink HA, Worzella TJ, Minor L. Cell viability assays. In: Sittampalam GS. et al., Editors. Assay Guidance Manual. Bethesda (MD): 2004. p. 355-385

[76] How robust are your data? Nature Cell Biology. 2009;**11**(6):667

[77] Curtis MJ, Abernethy DR. Advice on statistical analysis, and new journal guidance for experimental design and analysis. Pharmacology Research & Perspectives. 2015;**3**(1):e00095

[78] Curtis MJ et al. Experimental design and analysis and their reporting: New guidance for publication in BJP. British Journal of Pharmacology. 2015;**172**(14):3461-3471

[79] Lazic SE. Experimental Design for Laboratory Biologists : Maximising Information and Improving Reproducibility. Cambridge, United Kingdom: Cambridge University Press; 2016. xv 412 p

[80] Zhang JH, Chung TD, Oldenburg KR. A simple statistical parameter for use in evaluation and validation of high throughput screening assays. Journal of Biomolecular Screening. 1999;**4**(2):67-73

[81] Shun TY et al. Identifying actives from HTS data sets: Practical approaches for the selection of an appropriate HTS data-processing method and quality control review. Journal of Biomolecular Screening. 2011;**16**(1):1-14

[82] Sui Y, Wu Z. Alternative statistical parameter for high-throughput screening assay quality assessment. Journal of Biomolecular Screening. 2007;**12**(2):229-234

[83] Malo N et al. Statistical practice in high-throughput screening data analysis. Nature Biotechnology. 2006;**24**(2):167-175

[84] Jones LH, Bunnage ME. Applications of chemogenomic library screening in drug discovery. Nature Reviews. Drug Discovery. 2017;**16**(4):285-296

7

Application of Computer Modeling to Drug Discovery: Case Study of PRK1 Kinase Inhibitors as Potential Drugs in Prostate Cancer Treatment

Abdulkarim Najjar, Fidele Ntie-Kang and Wolfgang Sippl

Abstract

Computer modeling of natural products (NPs) and NP scaffolds is increasingly gaining importance in drug discovery, particularly in hit/lead discovery programs and at the lead optimization stage. Even though industry had lost interest in the implication of NPs in hit/lead searches, recent reports still show that computer modeling could be a useful assert for the identification of starting scaffolds from nature, which could be further exploited by synthetic modifications. In this chapter, the focus is on some useful tools for computer modeling aimed at the discovery of anticancer drugs from NP scaffolds. We also focus on some recent developments toward the identification of potential anticancer agents by the application of computer modeling. The chapter will lay emphasis on natural sources of anticancer compounds, present some useful databases and computational tools for anticancer drug discovery, and show some recent case studies of the application of computational modeling in anticancer drug discovery, as well as some success stories in virtual screening applications in anticancer drug discovery, highlighting some useful results on the application of on lead discovery (including promising NP scaffolds) against an interesting anticancer drug target, the protein kinase C-related kinase (PRK1).

Keywords: anticancer, molecular modeling, natural products, virtual screening, QSAR

1. Introduction

1.1. Cancer and natural products

Cancer is one of the most feared causes of death, as it represents several disease forms and treatments possibilities are still limited for late stages of the disease [1]. Among the known drugs for cancer treatment, camptothecin, vinblastine, vincristine, podophyllotoxin, and taxol are of natural origin [2]. Nature is known to be an immense repository of natural products (NPs), constituting the source of about half of the anticancer drugs currently in the market [3]. Inspite of the drop in interest for NPs in drug discovery projects, from an industrial point of view, recent reports still show that NPs could constitute a useful assert for the identification of starting scaffolds for further discovery [4–6]. The quest for anticancer drugs of natural origin or with NP scaffolds has resulted in the development of NP databases, the most promising one being the naturally occurring plant-based anti-cancer compound activity-target database (NPACT), with ~1500 NPs, including experimentally verified *in vitro* and *in vivo* biological activities (in the form of IC_{50}s, ED_{50}s, EC_{50}s, GI_{50}s, etc.), along with physical, elemental, and topological properties of the compounds, the tested cancer types, cell lines, protein targets, commercial suppliers, and drug-likeness classification for each compound [7].

1.2. Prostate cancer

Among the many diverse cancer forms, prostate cancer is the second leading cause of cancer deaths in men worldwide [8]. Two different types of prostate cancer were identified: androgen-dependent prostate cancer and androgen-independent prostate cancer [9]. Androgen hormones (testosterone or dihydrotestosterone) are known to activate the androgen receptors located in the cell nucleus. The main function of these receptors is to modify gene expressions, thus controlling several biological activities in the cells, including cell growth and differentiation, development, and function of male reproductive and accessory sex tissues [10, 11]. It was found that the androgen receptors signaling pathway plays an important role in the progress and development of prostate cancer. In the first stage of androgen-dependent prostate cancer, the survival and growth of the cancer cells are mainly dependent on androgen hormones [11]. The initial treatment of androgen-dependent cancer, based on androgen ablation, is called hormone therapy. This procedure aims to stop the cell growth of cancer cells, which, in most cases, respond to this therapy. The recurring prostate cancer cells from hormone therapy would further not respond to androgen ablation, thus leading to the development of androgen-independent prostate cancer, which can further progress to metastasis [11]. The molecular mechanism of tumor recurrence is not completely clear. For the second stage of prostate cancer, there is no efficient therapy available.

1.3. Protein kinase C–related kinase

Protein kinase C–related kinase (PRK1, also known as PKN1) is a serine/threonine kinase known to play a role in controlling the activity of androgen receptors in prostate cancer.

It was shown that the activation of PRK1 stimulates the activity of androgen receptors and is involved in tumorigenesis [12]. In 2008, Schüle et al. showed that PRK1 phosphorylates histone H3 upon ligand-dependent recruitment to androgen receptor target genes [12]. The phosphorylation of histone H3 at threonine 11 (H3T11) increases demethylation of Lys-9 by Jumonji C (JmjC)-domain-containing protein (JMJD2C), which promotes androgen receptor-dependent gene expression and tumor cell proliferation [13]. Additionally, PRK1 may directly phosphorylate JMJD2C, thereby stimulating its activity [14]. Meanwhile, the role of PRK1 in androgen-independent prostate cancer is unknown. PRK1 can be activated by the Rho family GTPases, thus mediating several processes related to the migration and cancer cell invasion and consequently playing a major role in the formation of metastases [15, 16]. Thus, PRK1 is considered to be a promising therapeutic target, and the discovery of novel potent and selective inhibitors could supply a meaningful tool for the treatment of prostate cancer. On the other hand, the discovery of selective and potent inhibitors would provide a tool for understanding particular biological roles of PRK1. In spite of the importance of PRK1 in the targeted therapy of cancer, only a few known inhibitors have been identified. The known PKC inhibitors (**Figures 1** and **2**) include staurosporine (PubChem CID: 44259) and its analogue (Ro-318220; PubChem CID: 5083), bisindolylmaleimide I (BIM I; PubChem CID: 2396), and lestaurtinib (PubChem CID: 126565), as well as the nonselective Akt inhibitor GSK-690693 (PubChem CID: 16725726) and Pfizer's JAK nonselective inhibitor CP-690550 (tofacitinib; PubChem CID: 9926791) [17, 18]. In a previous work, several novel PRK1 inhibitors were identified containing different scaffolds, using a homology model, with varying potencies [19]. In the present work, the focus is to search for new small molecules and natural products, which could inhibit PRK1 by using the recently published crystal structures.

1.4. Structural analysis of PRK1

PRK1 kinase belongs to the protein kinase C (PKC) superfamily and was first identified in 1994 from a human hippocampal cDNA library [20]. Three isoforms are found in mammals (called PRK1, PRK2, and PRK3). They possess different enzymatic properties and are distributed among different tissues [21]. The PRK1 structure is divided into three conserved regions:

- an N-terminal lobe (which includes a regulatory region containing three homologous stretches and is rich in charged amino acids),
- an auto-inhibitory domain called C2-like region (which is sensitive to arachidonic acids), and
- a C-terminal lobe (which contains the catalytic domains or called kinase domain).

Both lobes are connected by a hinge region. The catalytic domain is located between both terminal lobes and shows high conservation and similarity to the PKC family kinase domain [21, 22]. Moreover, PRK1 and PKC are members of AGC kinase family [23]. The characteristic feature of these kinases is a C-terminal regulatory region (C-tail). The C-tails regulate the enzymatic activity and insert conserved phenylalanine residues into the ATP-binding site [23–25].

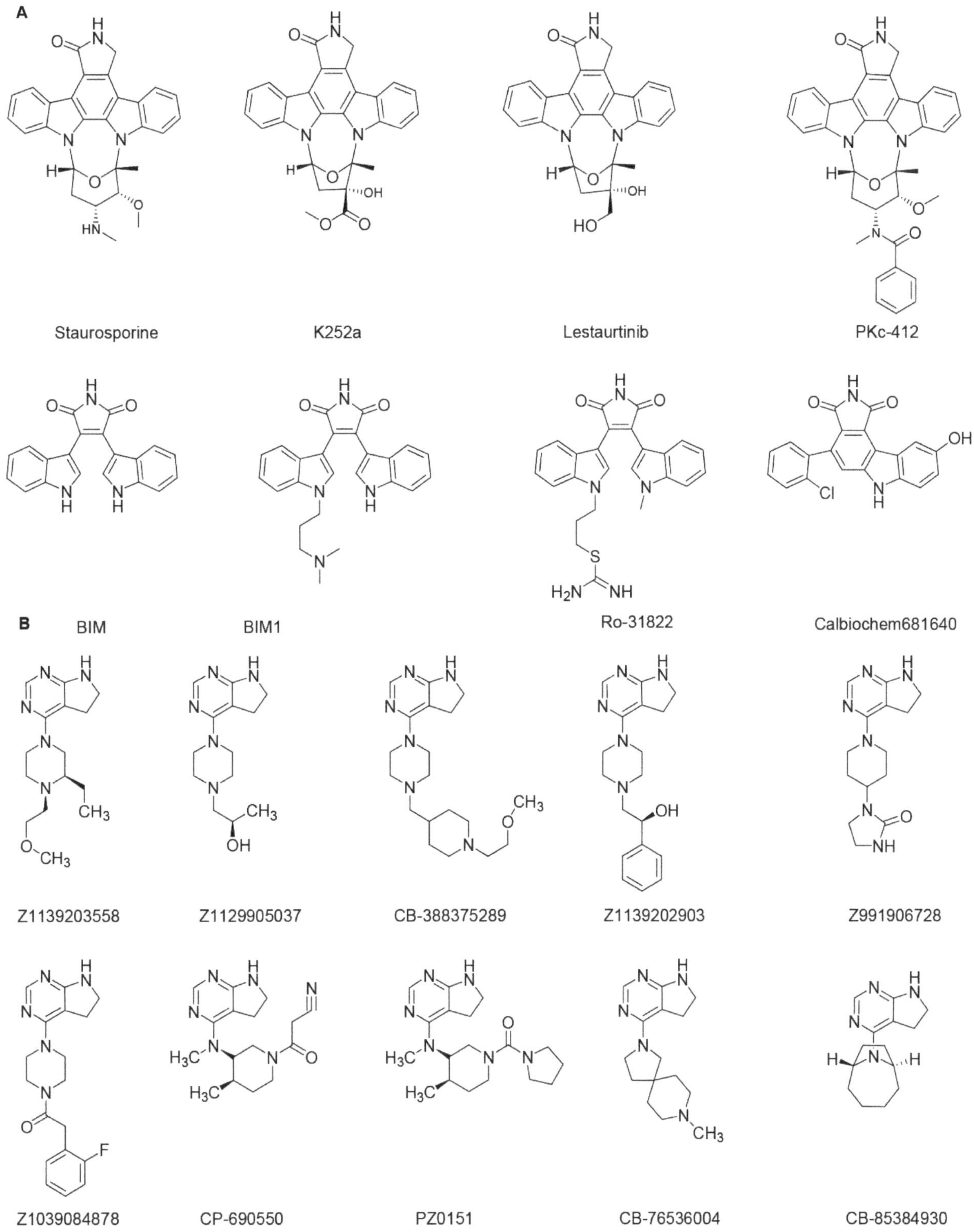

Figure 1. Chemical structures of PRK1 active compounds: (A) staurosporine and derivatives, (B) tofacitinib and other pyrrolopyrimidine derivatives [18].

1.5. Computational approaches in drug discovery

Virtual screening (VS) was first used at the end of the last century to refer to computational algorithms and techniques used to identify novel hit/lead compounds for biological target

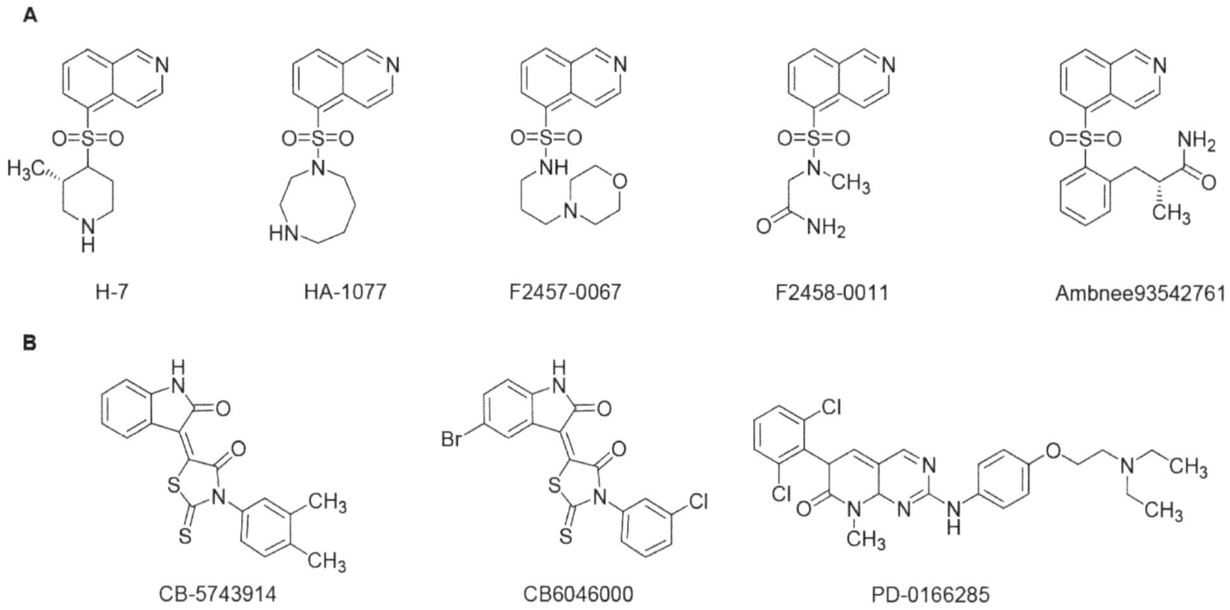

Figure 2. Chemical structures of more PRK1 active compounds. (A) Isoquinoline derivatives, (B) PD-0166285 and structurally diverse compounds identified by VS [18].

from large chemical libraries, depending on the known structure or the drug target or active ligands [26–29]. The VS approach is considered as a complementary approach to experimental or physical screening or high-throughput screening (HTS). VS has been fully integrated to most modern day drug discovery projects [30]. However, VS does not require the physical existence of the compounds to be tested. It is only based on computer models or the three-dimensional (3D) structures of the drug target, also known as structure-based VS (SBVS) or on the chemical structure of known active ligand(s), also known as ligand-based VS (LBVS) [31]. The fundamentals of the SBVS approach depend on the availability of the 3D structure of the biological target and a database of small molecules. The SBVS approach often uses molecular docking to generate the protein-ligand complexes of small molecules from a database into the target active site. The aim is to identify the compounds, which interact favorably with the target binding site [32]. Meanwhile, LBVS methods utilize chemical similarity analysis of structurally diverse or known active ligands, with the view of identifying novel small molecules, which could show similar biological activities [33–35]. However, both approaches have practical limitations. Therefore, researchers often combine SBVS and LBVS, with the aim that this might improve the efficiency of the VS results [36, 37]. Computational approaches for the prediction of biological activity also include quantitative structure-activity relationships (QSAR) analysis, which is aimed at finding a correlation between predicted and experimental biological activities of small molecules. This approach incorporates the influence of the molecular descriptors. QSAR models can be used initially to predict the activity of untested hits from a virtual screening campaign [38]. On other hand, QSAR modeling is useful tool during lead optimization, which is aimed at the improvement of the biological activities of the identified hits [39]. Recently, many crystal structures of the PRK1 drug target have been published [24]. Due to the flexibility of the biding site of the PRK1 structure, which adapts to different conformations, each protein-ligand complex was individually analyzed to reveal the important intermolecular interactions responsible for ligand binding that are useful for the identification new hits. The aim of this research project is to analyze ligand binding to PRK1 and to identify novel-specific inhibitors that could block the activity of PRK1, using structure-based VS. In a preliminary study, the applied docking methods were validated and used to investigate its ability to predict the experimental conformations of the co-crystallized ligands. Second, several QSAR models were generated in order to find the significant correlations between the computational and experimental biological activity data. The constructed QSAR models contain different scoring functions, including computed binding-free energy (BFE) values for the protein-ligand complexes, in addition to molecular descriptors of the isolated ligands. To investigate the predictive ability of the generated QSAR models, internal and external methods were performed. Moreover, an enrichment study was performed, in order to assess the ability of the scoring functions to identify known binders or actives in large databases containing actives and inactives. By focusing on kinase data sets, GSK data sets 1 and 2 were screened to search for novel lead compounds, employing virtual screening methods. A NP library including compounds isolated from African flora was also screened. This chapter begins by presenting database tools (small molecule libraries) useful in VS campaigns, with a focus on small molecule libraries and NPs with anticancer properties. This is followed by some recent success stories on VS for the identification of inhibitors and/or modulators of some anticancer drug targets. The end of the chapter shows the case study of VS for the identification of PRK1 inhibitors.

2. Databases of small molecule libraries and some recent success stories in anticancer drug discovery using computer-based methods

2.1. Small molecule databases for virtual screening

A summary of small molecule libraries utilizable in virtual screening experiments has been provided in **Table 1**. Known cancer drugs have been included in several databases, including ChEBI [43], ChEMBL [44], DrugBank [46], EpiDBase [48], NANPDB [51], NCI-DIS, NCI-DTP, and NCI-FDA [52], along with SANCDB [54], SuperDrug [55], p-ANAPL [58], PubChem [59], and ZINC15 [60]. However, those with tested and proven *in vitro* activities against known cancer cell lines and/or with known *in vivo* activities only include CancerDR [41], OAA [53], and SYFPEITHI [56], along with the NP libraries: AfroCancer [40], CancerHSP [42], CHMIS-C [43], InPACdb [49], MAPS [50], NPACT [7], and TIPdb [57].

2.2. Some recent success stories

Computational modeling has been applied to understand drug-target interactions in several validated anticancer drug targets, for the identification of novel inhibitors from small molecule databases and/or for the elucidation of modes of action. We here present some few recent cases. A typical example is the recent discovery of new inhibitors of CXC chemokine receptor 2 (CXCR2) by applying ligand-based pharmacophore models [61]. It should be mentioned that CXCR2 and its ligand, CXCL8, are known to be implicated in a number of inflammation-mediated diseases, including cancer [62–65]. In the study, Ha et al. generated a pharmacophore

Database	Description	Web accessibility	Reference
AfroCancer	A data set of natural anticancer products from African flora	http://www.african-compounds.org/about/afrocancer/	[40]
Cancer drug resistance database (CancerDR)	A database of 148 anticancer drugs and their effectiveness against around 1000 cancer cell lines	http://crdd.osdd.net/raghava/cancerdr/#thumb	[41]
CancerHSP	An anticancer herbs database of systems pharmacology	http://lsp.nwsuaf.edu.cn/CancerHSP.php/	[42]
ChEBI	A database for chemical entities of biological interest	http://www.ebi.ac.uk/chebi/	[43]
ChEMBL	An open large-scale bioactivity compound database	https://www.ebi.ac.uk/chembl/	[44]
CHMIS-C	A herbal medicines database for cancer	http://sw16.im.med.umich.edu/chmis-c/	[45]
DrugBank	A resource that combines detailed drug data with comprehensive drug target information	https://www.drugbank.ca/	[46]
DUDE datasets	Benchmarking data sets of actives and decoys for diverse targets, including proteins, GPCRs and ion channels, clustered ligands, etc. drawn from ChEMBL	http://dude.docking.org/	[47]
EpiDBase	A database for small molecule epigenetic modulators	http://www.epidbase.org/	[48]
InPACdb	Indian plant anticancer compounds database	http://www.inpacdb.org/	[49]
MAPS Database	A database of phytochemicals, including the data of >500 medicinal plants	http://www.mapsdatabase.com/	[50]
NANPDB	A natural products database for compounds of Northern African origin, with a significant number of bioactive metabolites exhibiting anticancer activity	http://www.african-compounds.org/nanpdb/	[51]
NCI Drug Information System (DIS)	A searchable database of 3D structures (mainly organic compounds) from the NCI Drug Information System (DIS)	https://cactus.nci.nih.gov/ncidb2.2/ http://dtp.nci.nih.gov/docs/3d_database/dis3d.html	[52]
NCI-DTP database	Tested compounds from the National Cancer Institute (NCI) Developmental Therapeutics Program (DTP)	https://dtp.cancer.gov/databases_tools/data_search.htm	[52]
NCI-FDA	Several sets of FDA-approved anticancer drugs to enable cancer research	https://wiki.nci.nih.gov/display/NCIDTPdata/Compound+Sets	[52]
NPACT	A database for plant-based anticancer compounds	http://crdd.osdd.net/raghava/npact/	[7]
Oral anticancer agents (OAA) from Singapore	A database of 39,772 oral anticancer agents prescribed to 8837 patients in Singapore, with 55 clinically significant drug-drug interactions for the evaluation of drug interaction facts	https://www.ncbi.nlm.nih.gov/pubmed/22795926/	[53]

Database	Description	Web accessibility	Reference
SANCDB	A database of natural products from South Africa, containing also anticancer agents from the flora and fauna of this ecologically diverse country	https://sancdb.rubi.ru.ac.za/	[54]
SuperDrug	A database of 3D-structures of active ingredients of essential marketed drugs	http://bioinf.charite.de/superdrug/	[55]
SYFPEITHI	A database of major histocompatibility complex (MHC) ligands and peptide motifs	http://www.syfpeithi.de/	[56]
TIPdb	A database of anticancer, antiplatelet, and antituberculosis phytochemicals from indigenous plants in Taiwan	http://cwtung.kmu.edu.tw/tipdb/	[57]
p-ANAPL	A collection of samples of natural products from African sources	http://www.african-compounds.org/about/p-anapl/	[58]
PubChem	A public repository for information on chemical substances and their biological activities	https://pubchem.ncbi.nlm.nih.gov/	[59]
ZINC15	A free database of over 100 million purchasable compounds for virtual screening	http://zinc15.docking.org/	[60]

Table 1. Summary of some small molecule libraries currently available for anticancer drug discovery.

model based on known CXCR2 antagonists and used it to screen a database of 5 million commercially available compounds from different vendors. The authors were able to identify small molecule hits, which were further tested by *in vitro* screening in a cell-based CXCR2-mediated β-arrestin-2 recruitment assay, followed by several other cell-based assays. *In vivo* studies were conducted by lipopolysaccharide (LPS)-induced lung inflammation in mice. It was also shown that one of the compounds inhibits CXCR2 signaling through down regulation of surface CXCR2.

Moreover, the same compound was shown to inhibit CXCL8-mediated neutrophil migration and LPS-induced lung inflammation in mice significantly. The identified compounds were shown to also inhibit CXCR2/β-arrestin-2 association, cell migration and proliferation, and acute inflammation in mouse models. Another study combined structure-based docking and pharmacophores to design novel indole and chromene analogues, which were cyclin-dependent kinase 2 (CDK2) inhibitors. The identified compounds proved to be active against MCF-7 and HeLa cell lines. The study was conducted by exploiting stereo-specific information obtained from crystal structures of CDK2, substituting the pharmacophores on their moiety and docking the target protein to calculate the binding affinities [66]. Other recent successful cases, where docking, QSAR, machine learning, and pharmacophore-based screening were combined to search for small molecules targeting cancer, are abundant in the literature [67–70].

3. Case study: structure-based virtual screening and QSAR studies on PRK1 inhibitors

3.1. Structure-based design studies (X-ray target structures and cross docking)

Four crystal structures of PRK1 are available in the protein data bank (PDB), **Table 2**. The PRK1 binding site is reported to exhibit either intrinsic or induced flexibility [17, 24]. Moreover, different bound inhibitors are known to induce different conformational changes in the binding site residues [71]. Furthermore, chemical characteristics of the co-crystallized ligands play an important role in the applicability of the X-ray structure for virtual screening. Therefore, a cross-docking procedure was carried out, as a retrospective study aimed at determining the appropriate structure for the virtual screening. The selected structure should be able to bind the nonnative ligands with low root mean square deviation (RMSD), with respect to the reference binding conformation. On the other hand, the performance of the docking power and scoring functions is varying for different targets [32]. The docking power measures the ability of docking algorithms to predict the correct conformation of the ligands [72].

The four X-ray structures of PRK1, including the apo-form, were used for a cross-docking study [24]. The co-crystallized ligands were docked toward the target binding sites, using the Glide cross-docking script, implemented in Schrödinger Suite (2014 version) with standard precision (SP) for flexible ligand docking. In order to optimize the docking solution, an option was selected to perform post-docking minimization and includes number of poses up to 5 per ligand. The structures were prepared using the default setting implemented in Protein Preparation Wizard (Schrödinger 2014). The co-crystallized water molecules were deleted. Hydrogen atoms and partial charges were assigned. Finally, the structure energy minimized applying the OPLS 2005 force field. The binding site was defined using Grid Generation of Schrödinger suite 2014 and sets the co-crystallized ligand as a center of the binding pocket. In the case of apo-structure 4OTD, the binding site was defined by applying centroid of selected residues Leu650 and Lys753 with box size 14 Å. A hydrogen bond constraint was defined at PRK1 hinge region reside Ser704. In addition, all ligands were prepared using LigPrep implemented in Schrödinger utility 2014 involving generation of ionization and tautomeric states at pH 7.4 with less than 10 low-energy ring conformations. The ligands were energy minimized using MMFFs force field.

Ligand	4OTD		4OTG		4OTH		4OTI	
	RMSD	SP	RMSD	SP	RMSD	SP	RMSD	SP
Lestaurtinib-4OTG	6.56	−4.29	0.24	−11.67	4.65	−7.82	7.56	−4.29
Ro-318220-4OTH	6.79	−7.01	2.98	−11.4	0.64	−11.76	6.47	−6.55
Tofacitinib-4OTI	3.14	−4.54	6.11	−8.09	2.7	−8.18	0.55	−8.8
Average RMSD	5.5		3.11		2.67		4.86	

Table 2. RMSD values (Å) for the top-ranked docking solutions (using Glide SP as scoring function).

The RMSD values were calculated, with respect to the respective reference ligand conformations. **Table 2** shows the RMSD values and Glide SP scores for the top-ranked poses in the corresponding structures. It was observed that none of the available structures had a binding site conformation, which allowed all the three different ligands to be docked with RMSD < 2.0 Å. Furthermore, the calculated average RMSD values for each structure were high. However, the applied docking method performed well by reproducing the binding mode of the co-crystallized inhibitor in self-docking. Moreover, the docking method correctly scored the co-crystallized inhibitors at the top of the list (**Table 2**), e.g., the X-ray structure of the ligand lestaurtinib was re-docked with an RMSD = 0.24 Å into its co-crystallized structure (PDB: 4OTG), being also ranked as the top scoring pose (Glide SP = −11.67 kcal/mol). Similar results were observed with the other inhibitors when X-ray structures were docked toward their respective co-crystallized target structures. Meanwhile, the binding pocket conformation for the apo-form of PRK1 was not found to be suitable for docking when using any of the current inhibitor structures. RMSD values were high and the docking scores were low when compared with those obtained in the rest PRK1 structures (**Table 2**). Therefore, an ensemble of PRK1 structures was proposed for the further virtual screening study.

3.2. Docking of active inhibitors

The data set DS1 includes 28 active (**Figures 1** and **2** [18]) and 300 inactive compounds. First, the active compounds were docked toward the ensemble of the three PRK1 structures using the previously described docking methods. The docking solutions were first inspected, with the aim of comparing them with the experimental conformations (the co-crystallized ligands in other kinases). The active compounds could be divided into four subsets, the first set being staurosporine derivatives (10 actives, including the co-crystallized inhibitors lestaurtinib and Ro-318220). The second subset is made of the tofacitinib or pyrrolopyrimidine family (nine actives, in addition to the inhibitor tofacitinib in PDB ID: 4OTI). The third set was made of two isoquinoline derivatives, forming a group of five actives. The last subset contains the remaining inhibitors, with diverse scaffolds. The binding mode for each compound was analyzed and compared with the experimental data. As previously seen in the cross-docking for the co-crystallized inhibitors (**Table 2**), the binding modes for lestaurtinib and Ro-318220 were correctly reproduced. The binding modes for the further staurosporine derivatives were compared with these two analogues. Since the ensemble docking procedure was applied to dock the actives, eight compounds were docked toward the 4OTG structure target site, while the others (Ro-318220 and BIM1) were docked toward the 4OTH site. It was interesting to notice that the top-ranked active poses had a quite conserved binding mode, which shares two H bonds, interacting with the hinge region of PRK1. The obtained binding modes for all staurosporine derivatives were identical to the published structure (in the PRK1 X-ray structure 4OTG). Since a part of the C-terminal regulation region (C-tail) is not resolved, resulting in a more open and accessible ATP binding pocket, most of the staurosporine derivatives could be docked into it. Furthermore, all staurosporine derivatives were docked into both PRK1 structures, which are co-crystallized with one of staurosporine derivatives (4OTG or 4OTH). For pyrrolopyrimidine and tofacitinib derivatives, the inhibitors were docked into three X-ray structures of PRK1. Tofacitinib was co-crystallized in the structure 4OTI. The RMSD value of re-docking tofacitinib was 0.55 Å. The binding modes for the other analogues were compared with the experimental data (4OTI). Additionally, several other analogues were co-crystallized with the Akt1 kinase (PDB IDs: 3MV5, 3MVJ, and 3OCB).

Each active compound forms 2 H bonds with the hinge region, besides additional H bonds with the surrounding residues in the binding pocket. There are also some isoquinoline derivatives that were co-crystallized with other kinases, e.g., cAMP-dependent kinase (PDB IDs: 1YDS and 1YDR) and Rho kinase (PDB IDs: 2GNI). This subset of actives interacts with the PRK1 hinge region by mediating 1 H bond. A former virtual screening campaign had identified several actives, including CB-6046000 and CB-5743914, which were docked using the same previously described docking method. The binding mode showed two H bonds between the dihydroindol-2-one and the backbone of the hinge region, mainly Ser704 and Glu702. Furthermore, the binding mode of PD-0166285 matched the experimental data observed for the LCK kinase (PDB ID: 3KMM).

3.3. Scoring power

The rescoring for the derived docking poses was performed by calculating BFEs and using different solvation models implemented in the AMBER12 package. IC_{50} values had been previously determined for 26 of the active compounds (**Table 3**), with only percentage inhibitions available for two others) [19]. Thus, the correlation coefficient (R^2) between the experimental pIC_{50} and the calculated enthalpy changes (ΔH) for protein-ligand binding was calculated (**Table 3** and **Figure 3**). The BFE calculation was carried out using one snapshot after two consecutive minimizations steps and applying the Generalized Born solvation model [73, 74]. First, the minimization was carried out for water and counterion molecules without the ligand-protein complex, which was restrained to their initial coordinates with a force constant of 500 kcal/mol/Å^2. In this step, there were 2000 iterations (beginning with 1000 steepest descent and followed by 1000 conjugate gradient). The second minimization step was applied for the whole system through 10,000 iterations (first 5000 steepest descent and then 5000 conjugate gradients). A significant correlation was found when using the Nguyen and Simmerling (igb = 8) version of the Generalized Born solvation model [73, 74] and applying the two minimizations steps. The cross-validated R^2 was found to be 0.60, with a root mean square error (RMSE) of 0.89. To understand the effect of the chemical modification on the main scaffold, the binding mode of the actives and the interactions in the binding pocket was analyzed. As mentioned previously, PRK1 actives can be divided into four subsets (**Table 3**). The docking score (Glide SP) and the MM/GBSA BFE values were employed to explore the differences in the inhibitory activity. However, there was a weak correlation between the pIC_{50} and Glide SP scores (R^2 of 0.43, see **Table 4**).

It was observed, from docking, that the isoquinoline derivatives are able to form an H bond between the N atom of the isoquinoline motif and the NH backbone of Ser704 located in the hinge region. The isoquinoline motif occupied the adenine binding site; meanwhile, the substituents were located in the sugar-binding site, which is surrounded by several hydrophilic residues (e.g., Asp708, Asp750). Rescoring, using MMGBSA, showed that H-7 (IC_{50} = 658 μM and ΔH = −34.51 kcal/mol) had a higher score than HA-1077 (IC_{50} = 1.95 μM and ΔH= −29.42 kcal/mol), **Table 3**. The more favorable value resulted from the additional

Compound	IC_{50} (nM)	Exp. pIC_{50}	Target structure	Glide SP	MM/GBSA**	PEOE_PC-	Pred. pIC_{50}*
Ro-318220	78.3	7.11	4OTH	−11.36	−45.97	−2.71	7.16
BIM1	579	6.24	4OTH	−9.82	−46.10	−2.29	6.58
PKC-412	14.2	7.85	4OTG	−10.98	−55.52	−3.26	8.26
Lestaurtinib	8.6	8.07	4OTG	−11.43	−46.92	−2.77	7.30
K252a	3.2	8.49	4OTG	−11.38	−51.40	−2.95	7.80
Staurosporine	0.81	9.10	4OTG	−11.83	−60.86	−2.72	8.59
Calbiochem681640	1441	5.84	4OTG	−10.61	−47.90	−1.96	6.71
BIM	154.2	6.81	4OTG	−9.16	−38.70	−1.96	5.58
K252c			4OTG	−10.53	−40.12		
Quercetin			4OTG	−8.43	−48.23		
CP-690550 **(tofacitinib)**	129	6.89	4OTI	−8.81	−38.88	−2.01	5.55
Z1139203558	55730	4.25	4OTG	−8.52	−27.91	−1.84	4.41
Z1129905037	53380	4.27	4OTI	−9.61	−35.25	−1.82	5.29
CB-38374289	42560	4.37	4OTI	−10.49	−33.36	−2.11	5.49
CB-85384930	34020	4.47	4OTH	−9.04	−35.48	−1.48	4.98
Z1139202903	31470	4.50	4OTI	−9.37	−37.77	−2.09	5.62
Z991906728	26400	4.58	4OTG	−9.18	−28.92	−2.02	4.75
CB-76536004	13090	4.88	4OTG	−9.43	−33.02	−1.45	4.83
Z1039084878	6210	5.21	4OTG	−8.76	−29.13	−2.10	4.73
PZ0151	1060	5.97	4OTI	−8.54	−43.19	−2.16	5.97
H-7	658.5	6.18	4OTH	−8.68	−34.51	−1.43	4.78
HA-1077	1945	5.71	4OTI	−8.71	−29.42	−1.39	4.31
F2457-0067	70300	4.15	4OTH	−8.49	−36.31	−1.76	5.10
F2458-0011	53730	4.27	4OTI	−8.07	−29.18	−1.70	4.34
Ambnee93542761	29330	4.53	4OTH	−9.12	−30.33	−1.68	4.66
CB-6046000	5350	5.27	4OTG	−7.39	−47.01	−1.57	5.70
CB-5743914	2940	5.53	4OTG	−9.89	−41.07	−1.72	5.81
PD-0166285	5517	5.26	4OTG	−7.48	−39.17	−2.41	5.53

Comparison of experimental pIC50 versus predicted pIC50 values calculated by QSAR_3 for the 26 training set molecules [18].

The BFE values were calculated according to the docked structure (target structure), which are supplied with the PDB ID.

Table 3. Biological activity, calculated BFE and docking scores of the active compounds.

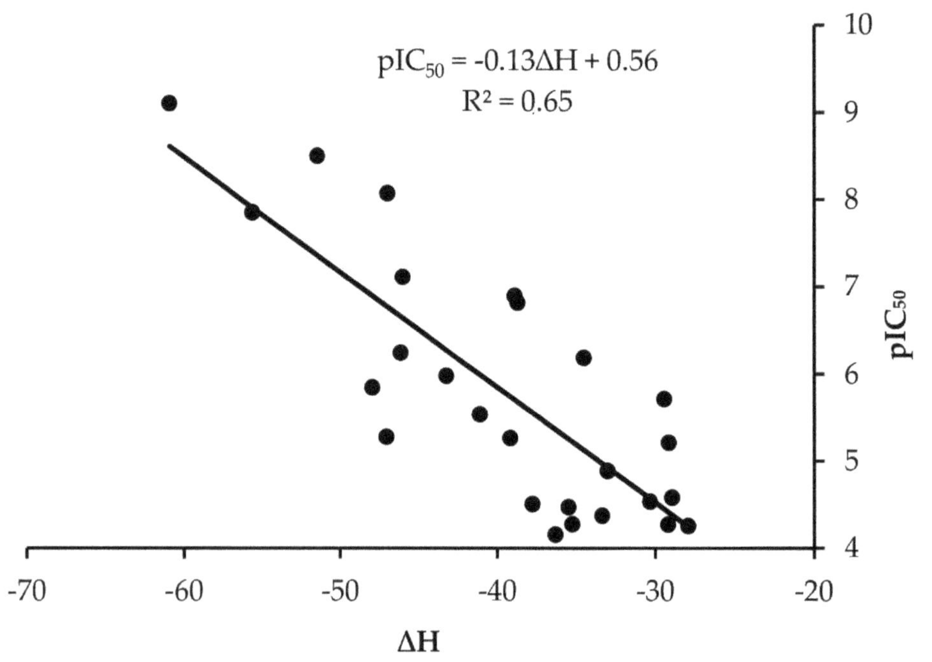

Figure 3. Correlation curve of pIC50 versus Δ*H* scores of actives using MM/GBSA.

hydrophobic interactions between the front hydrophobic pocket residues and Phe910 (from the C-tail) and the methyl substituent on the piperazine ring. Meanwhile, the van der Waals interaction became weaker in the case of HA-1077. This could be explained by the shifting of the position of the substituent, since its seven-membered ring is bulkier. Both derivatives contain a positively charged ring nitrogen, which consequently forms an additional H bond in the ATP-sugar binding pocket (**Figure 4**). Meanwhile, the interaction between Asp708 and the piperazine ring enables the methyl group to get closer to Phe910 and its surrounding residues. Moreover, the sulfonyl moiety of both compounds is located under the P-loop, where it forms hydrophilic and hydrophobic interactions.

	GLIDE		Δ*H*
	SP	**XP**	**GB8**
R^2	0.43	0.27	**0.65**
EF1%	**100**	**100**	25
EF3%	**30.3**	**33.33**	9.1
AUC*	**0.90**	**0.88**	0.66

*AUC = area under the ROC curve.

Table 4. Enrichment study results using an ensemble of PRK1 structures, where the available scoring functions in Schrödinger and BFE methods were considered. Where **SP**: Standard Precision; **XP**: Extra Precision and **ΔH**: enthalpy score; GB8: Generalized Born theory model.

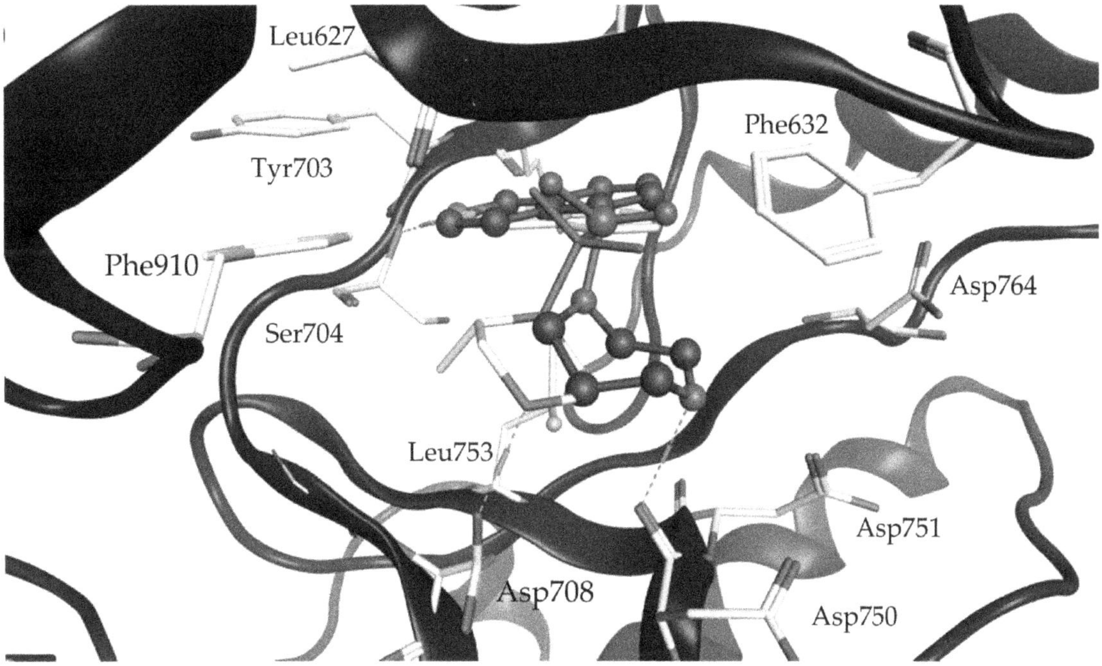

Figure 4. Comparison between the docking poses of two isoquinoline derivatives H-7 (magenta) and HA-1077 shown as green sticks (PRK1 PDB code: 4OTH). The figure was designed using MOE.

The remaining compounds share common interactions (as previously mentioned), but the biological activities of these compounds could not be predicted using the derived BFE model. However, the lower activity of compound ambnee93542761 could be explained by the loss of the interaction between of the sulfonyl moiety and weak hydrophobic interactions with Phe910. Nonetheless, it forms a hydrogen bond with the catalytic Asp764 (IC_{50} = 29.33 μM and $\Delta H = -30.32$ kcal/mol). The results of this subset show the importance of the hydrophobic interactions with the Phe910 of the C-tail and its surrounding residues. However, the BFE values and docking scores failed to predict the affinity of F2457-0067, which shows a favorable BFE value but a low IC_{50} value (**Table 3**). This could probably result from the long linker between the isoquinoline motif and the positively charged morpholine ring. The generated conformations show additional van der Waals interactions. On the other hand, the morpholine ring shows more polar properties compared to the other compounds.

The second subset of actives is made of staurosporine derivatives. Most of these compounds form two H bonds between the pyrrole ring and the hinge backbone (NH of Ser704 and CO of Glu702). The docking results for staurosporine derivatives were compared with two PRK1 crystal structures (4OTG and 4OTH). The favorable BFE values of staurosporine derivatives could be attributed to the strong hydrophobic interactions with residues from the P-loop, e.g., Val635 and Leu627, in addition to the interactions with Leu753. The only observed deviation was with parts of the docked ligand interacting with the sugar pocket, e.g., staurosporine (the most active compound) showed a BFE value of $\Delta H = -60.85$ kcal/mol and an IC_{50} = 0.0008 μM (**Table 3**). The favorable BFE value and activity of staurosporine could be estimated through the targeting of both hydrophobic pocket residues (behind the gatekeeper Met701 and near Phe910); on the other hand, several polar groups occupied the sugar polar pocket. By comparison with lestaurtinib (IC_{50} = 0.0086 μM and ΔH= −46.92 kcal/mol), the differences in the activity and BFE values could be attributed to the smaller ring/shorter linker in lestaurtinib for targeting Asp708 and Asp750 (**Figure 5**).

The third subset of PRK1 inhibitors is made of tofacitinib analogues. Ten compounds belong to this subset (**Table 3**). All derivatives interact with the hinge region by forming two H bonds through the pyrrolopyrimidine scaffold (**Figure 6**). The major substituents, which influence notably the BFE values and the biological activity of tofacitinib, are the N-methyl of the pyridine ring. Any chemical modification changing these interactions will consequently change the BFE value and the activity. A comparison of the calculated BFE values of tofacitinib with those of the other derivatives could clarify the effects of these interactions. As previously mentioned, the loss of the interactions made with the P-loop residues clearly influences the calculated BFE values and, therefore, affects the biological activities. Consequently, Z1129905037 (IC_{50} = 55.73 μM and ΔH = −27.92 kcal/mol) possesses a BFE value lower than tofacitinib (IC_{50} = 0.129 μM and ΔH = −38.88 kcal/mol) (**Table 3**). Furthermore, contrary to tofacitinib, the binding mode of Z1129905037 does not show hydrophobic interactions with the residue located at the bottom of the binding pocket. The ATP-sugar binding site is occupied by non-polar substituents in the case of Z1129905037, which is unfavorable and consequently reduces the activity. The other tofacitinib analogues, which do not contain any tertiary amine as the linker, show higher BFE values and obviously lower biological activities. One exception is PZ0151 (IC_{50} = 1.06 μM and ΔH= −43.19 kcal/mol) which displays the same binding mode with tofacitinib. The pyrrolidine

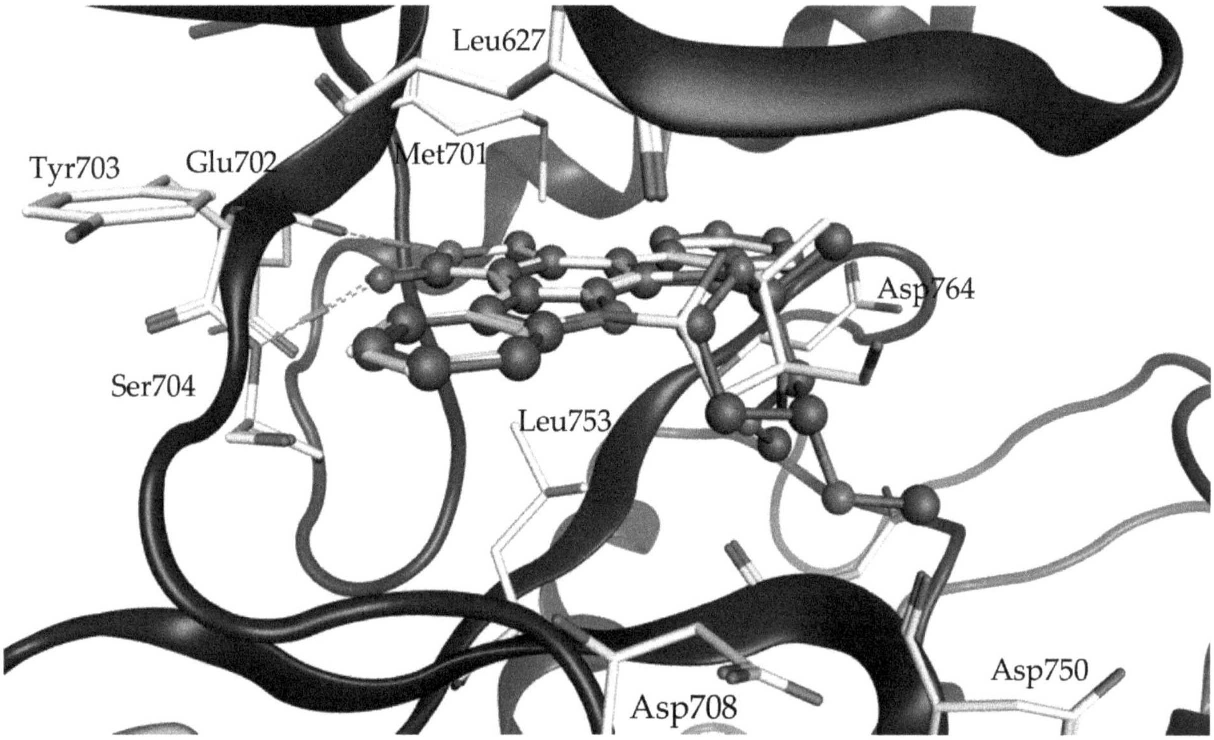

Figure 5. Comparison between the docking pose of staurosporine (seen in cyan sticks) and the binding mode of lestaurtinib (shown in white brown sticks) at PRK1 structure 4OTG. The figure was designed using MOE.

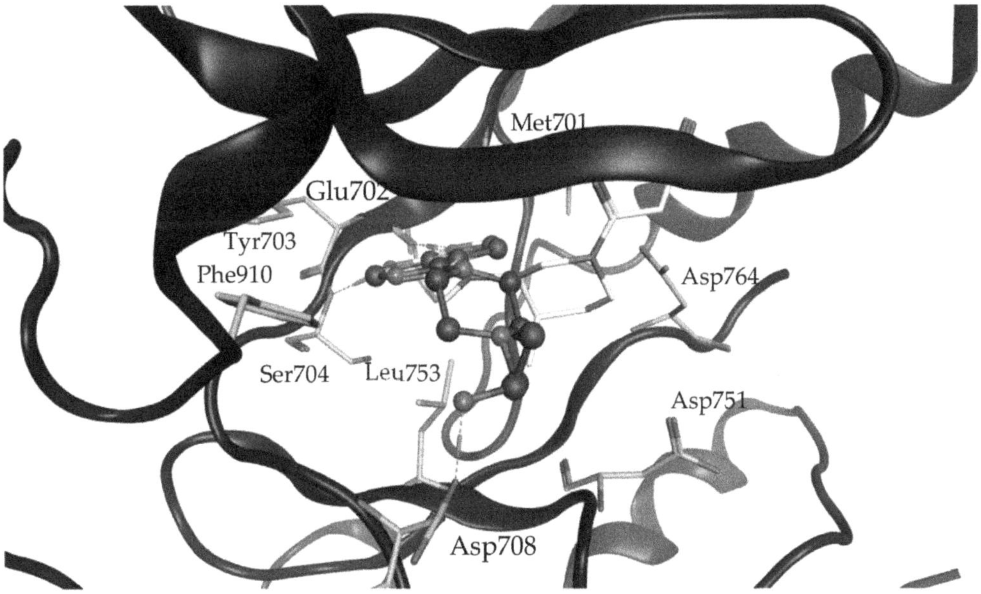

Figure 6. Comparison of the docking pose of Z1129905037 (shown as cyan sticks) and the binding mode of tofacitinib seen in magenta, at the binding site of PRK1 structure 4OTI. The figure was designed using MOE.

ring in PZ0151 takes the position of the CN group of tofacitinib but rather shows a lower activity. This could be as a result of the small size of the binding site under the P-loop residues, which is not suitable for large substituents. In general, it is difficult to explain the changes of the BFE values caused by chemical modification of all compounds under study. The observed correlation coefficient ($R^2 = 0.65$) could only be used to explain major differences in biological activities. However, it could be used as an indicator to identify the interactions, which play major roles in the determination of biological activity.

3.4. Ranking power

An enrichment study was performed in order to measure the ability to identify known binders or actives in large databases of inactives. The previously mentioned data set (named DS1), containing 28 actives and 300 inactives, was used to perform the enrichment study. The ligands were docked using the same ensemble and rescored depending on the previous findings. The results are presented in a BOX-PLOT and receiver operating characteristic (ROC) curves (**Figures 7** and **8**). **Table 4** shows enrichment study results, using an ensemble of PRK1 structures, where the available scoring functions in Schrödinger and BFE methods were considered (ΔH, Glide SP and Glide XP). As seen in **Figure 7**, Glide SP was able to discriminate between actives and inactives better than the BFE scoring (ΔH).

The median values of the pair active/inactive were −9.17/7.23 and −38.79/34.02 for Glide SP and ΔH, respectively. The area under the curve (AUC) and enrichment factors (EF) at two different percentages were calculated. **Table 4** shows the enrichment study results. It is interesting to note that at EF1%, all screened hits were actives when using both Schrödinger's scoring functions (Glide SP and XP). Interesting, it was also observed that for the EF3% (for Glide SP and XP), the rate of true positives was 100% (**Table 4**). The main factor to measure the ranking

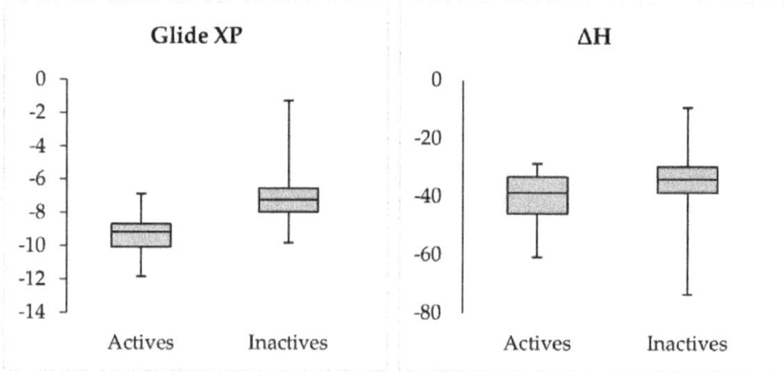

Figure 7. Box plots for the active and inactive compounds using the respective score values.

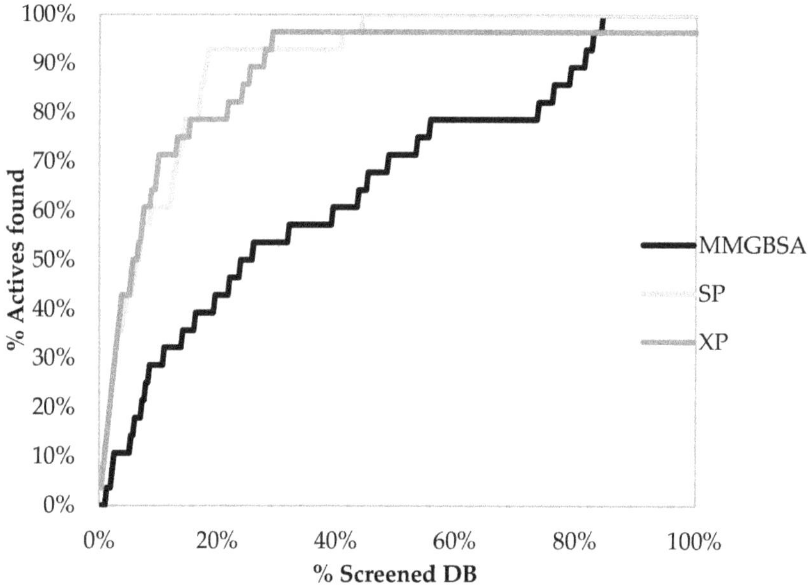

Figure 8. Enrichment plot showing comparison of the % actives found at a given percentage of the ranked database for DS1, using GLIDE SP, XP, and Δ*H* (MMGBSA).

power of the applied docking methods was the AUC value (**Table 4**). It is clear that the Glide scoring functions performed better to discriminate between the actives of inactives, having AUC = 0.90 and 0.88 for SP and XP, respectively.

3.5. QSAR model generation

Several QSAR models were generated to identify a possible correlation between experimentally obtained pIC_{50} values and calculated BFE or descriptor values (for the compounds on **Figures 1** and **2**). Calculated BFE (obtained by the MM/GBSA approach) from the previous study and 2D molecular descriptors, e.g., different descriptors referring to the partial charge and number of rotatable bonds, were considered. Since the Glide SP score showed a significant discrimination power between the active and inactive compounds, further scoring functions were also tested to optimize the QSAR models.

The best correlation coefficient in the previous study was found by applying Nguyen and Simmerling (igb = 8) Generalized Born solvation model [73, 74], after a minimization step (R^2 = 0.65, RMSE = 0.89 and cross-validated q^2 = 0.60, n = 26). In order to improve the correlation, partial charges of the ligands were calculated to compute several molecular descriptors for generating PLS models [75]. The inclusion of the PEOE_VSA-0 descriptor improved the correlation coefficient value only slightly (model QSAR_, R^2 = 0.68, RMSE = 0.8, and q^2 = 0.61, n = 26). This descriptor indicates the partial equalization of electronegativities with approximated accessible van der Waals surface area (in Å^2) of the molecule [76]. Furthermore, the inclusion of another descriptor based on ligand partial charges (PEOE_PC-) [76], which indicates to the total negative partial charge, was used instead of PEOE_VSA-0 to generate QSAR_2 (R^2 = 0.70, RMSE = 0.78 and q^2 = 0.62, n = 26; Eq. (1)). The model QSAR_3, containing three descriptors, showed a slightly better correlation coefficient (R^2 = 0.71, RMSE = 0.76 and q^2 = 0.63, n = 26; Eq. (2)). The relative importance of the individual descriptors was MM-GBSA: 1, GLIDE_SP: 0.417, and PEOE_PC-: 0.371. The other tested descriptors were not helpful and were not considered for the final models.

Further internal validation of the generated QSAR models was carried out by means of bootstrapping, in which the samples are randomly selected from the used inhibitors to form training and test sets [77, 78]. The respective models are generated, and their statistical parameters (R^2 and q^2) are calculated and compared with those of the original QSAR models (which had been generated from the whole data set). The random selection of the samples was performed within each cluster generated by hierarchical clustering, depending on the structural similarity or within activity distribution clusters of PRK1 inhibitors (low, moderate, and high active inhibitors) [77]. PRK1 inhibitors can be divided into four subsets depending on the chemical scaffolds (**Figures 1** and **2**). In the next step, hierarchical clustering using maximum common substructure (MACCS) keys and calculation of Tanimoto coefficients were carried out using the molecular operator environment (MOE) software tool (chemical computing group, Montreal, Canada, version 2014). Then, several samples within each cluster were taken, considering their activities. From 26 compounds, the sample subset contains only 20 inhibitors. The statistic parameters of the obtained QSAR models are presented in **Table 5**. The goal of the bootstrapping is to perturb the training set while not considering the statistical parameters of the test set. Since the obtained QSAR models were built from subset of the total data set, the values of R^2_{BT} and q^2_{BT} satisfy the minimum acceptable statistical parameters when

	Training set (20 inhibitors)			Test set (6 inhibitors)		
	R^2	RMSE	q^2	R^2_{BT}	$RMSE_{pred}$	q^2_{pred}
QSAR_BT_1	0.71	0.73	0.65	0.43	1.11	0.06
QSAR_BT_2	0.72	0.72	0.63	0.58	0.95	0.19
QSAR_BT_3	0.72	0.71	0.60	0.67	0.84	0.28

Table 5. Statistical parameters of obtained QSAR models in bootstrap validation.

compared with the three original QSAR models. These values also revolve around the values of the original QSAR models, generated from 26 PRK1 inhibitors (**Table 5**). It was observed that the obtained QSAR models possess acceptable statistic parameters ($q^2 > 0.5$) and were comparable with those found in the original QSAR models. However, the QSAR_BT_3 model showed poor correlation when compared with the results found in the whole data set ($q^2 =$ 0.60, **Table 5**). The remaining six inhibitors were used as the external test set to verify the ability of the obtained QSAR models (QSAR_BTs) to predict the biological activities of the test set compounds. The values of R^2_{pred} between the calculated and measured pIC_{50} are 0.43, 0.58, and 0.67 for QSAR_BT_1, QSAR_BT_2, and QSAR_BT_3, respectively (**Table 5**). These results may confirm the ability of the model QSAR_3 and its derivatives (QSAR_BT_3) to predict the biological activities of novel compounds.

Interestingly, QSAR_3 have predicted pIC_{50} values higher or close to 7 for the most potent PRK1 inhibitors (IC_{50} < 100 nM). Moreover, QSAR_3 possessed the ability to distinguish between weak, moderate, and highly potent compounds (**Table 3**). Thus, the model could be used as a filter for the prioritization of specific compounds (hits) for synthesis and testing. **Figure 9** displays the graph of the correlation between the observed and predicted pIC_{50} values using QSAR_3 model.

3.6. Validation of the generated QSAR models and GSK databases screening

It has previously been demonstrated that considering only the statistic parameters (R^2, RMSE, and q^2) to validate QSAR models is insufficient and sometimes misleading [78–82]. Therefore, it is important to validate QSAR models by testing the ability to accurately predict the biological activities of ligands not used for QSAR model generation. In the current study, two data

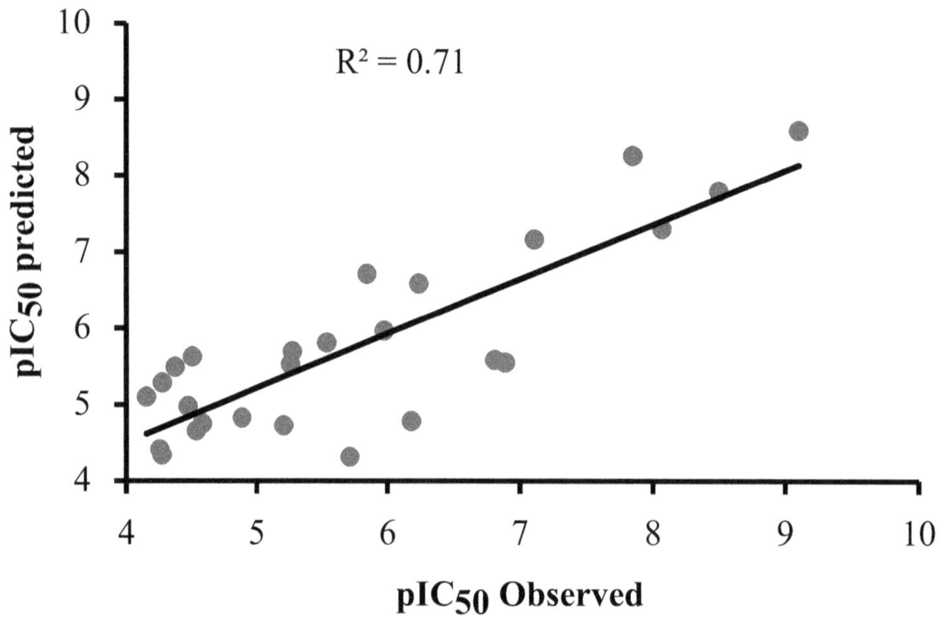

Figure 9. Correlation plot of the observed versus predicted pIC_{50} values of the training set ($n = 26$) using QSAR_3 model.

sets of compounds were available: the first set containing 26 PRK1 inhibitors with IC_{50} values was used as a training set for QSAR model generation (**Figures 1** and **2**). The second set was used as an external test set to validate the QSAR model. These compounds were identified from an *in vitro* screening (GSK PKIS1) and contain 35 compounds including 14 active compounds and 21 inactive compounds (**Figures 10** and **11**) [18]. Seven of the active compounds, for which IC_{50} values were measured (0.04–4.9 μM, **Table 6**), were taken as external test set to further evaluate the predictive power of the QSAR models.

Table 5 provides a comparison of the calculated pIC_{50} versus experimental pIC_{50} values. The calculation of pIC_{50} values was performed by using the QSAR_1, 2, and 3 models. An important statistic parameter to test the predictive power of the QSAR models is the correlation coefficient R^2_{pred} between the predicted and observed pIC_{50} values for the test set [82]. The correlation coefficients between the experimental and predicted pIC_{50} values for the seven test set compounds were quite weak ($R^2_{pred} = 0.49$, $n = 7$) when using QSAR_3 model. The predictive power of the QSAR_1 and 2 models was investigated. The correlations of both models were within a similar range ($R^2_{pred} = 0.58$ and 0.37, $n = 7$). A further analysis was performed to detect the outliers depending on Z-score values. The Z-score values were calculated using MOE, for QSAR_3. Golbraikh et al. mentioned that at least five compounds are required for a test set to validate a QSAR model [80]. After the analysis of the correlation and Z-scores, compound SB-750140 found to negatively affect the correlation coefficients. The correlation using QSAR_3 shows an improvement ($R^2_{pred} = 0.95$, RMSD = 0.17 and $q^2 = 0.89$, $n = 6$). A similar observation was made for the two other QSAR models (QSAR_1: $R^2_{pred} = 0.93$, RMSD = 0.21 and $q^2 = 0.82$, $n = 6$; QSAR_2: $R^2_{pred} = 0.98$, RMSD = 0.12 and $q^2 = 0.95$, $n = 6$). The outcomes confirm that the generated

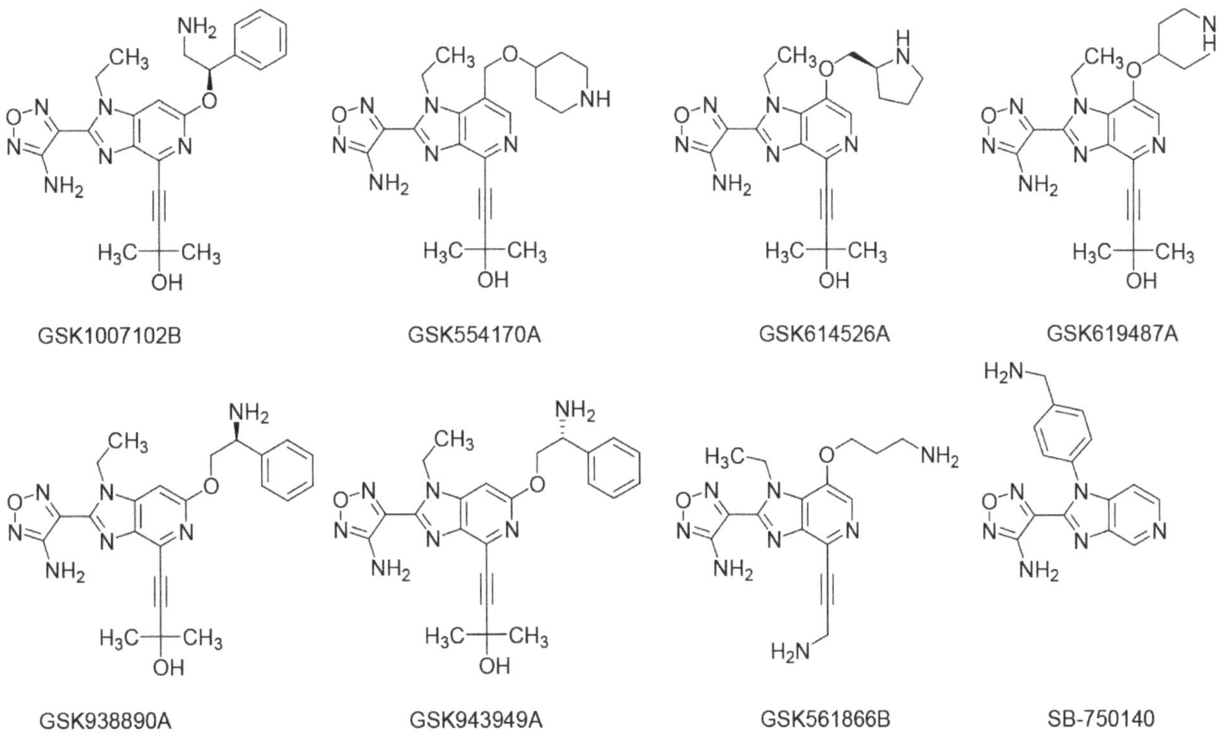

Figure 10. Chemical structures of PRK1 14 actives identified from screening the GSK PKIS1 [18].

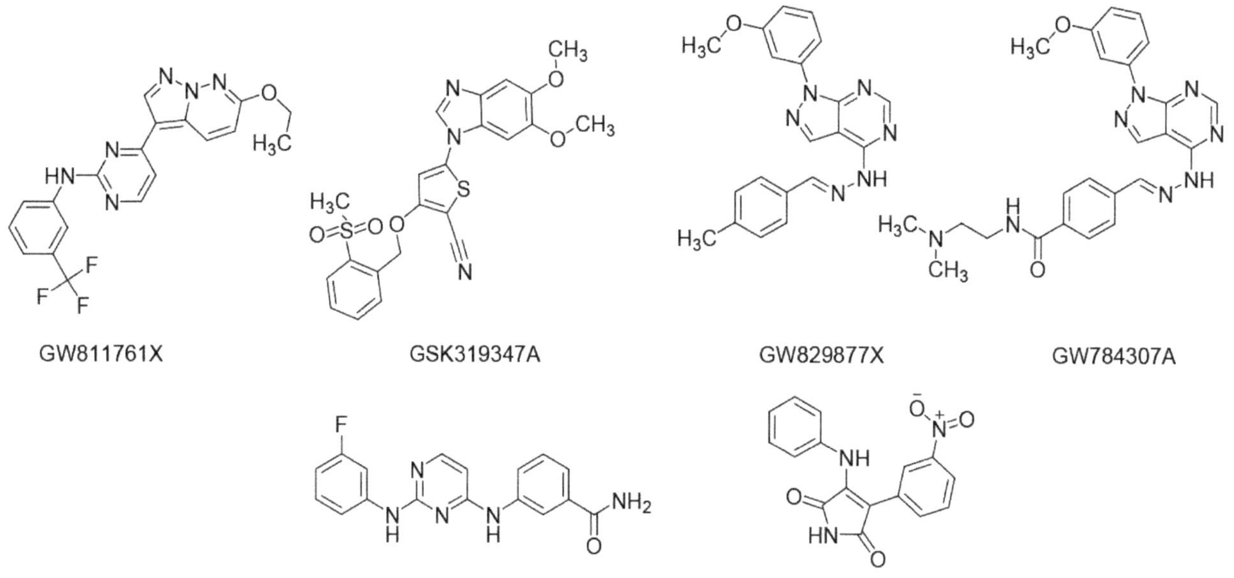

Figure 11. Chemical structures of PRK1 14 actives identified from screening the GSK PKIS1 (continued) [18].

Compound	Binding 1 μM	IC_{50} nM	pIC_{50}	Pred. pIC_{50} QSAR_3	Pred.pIC_{50} QSAR_1	Pred. pIC_{50} QSAR_2
GSK943949A	Yes	40	7.40	7.33	7.79	7.99
GSK614526A	Yes	68.1	7.17	7.09	7.68	7.69
SB-750140	Yes	120	6.92	5.70	6.06	5.88
GSK619487A	Yes	181.3	6.74	7.11	7.62	7.65
GSK554170A	Yes	710	6.15	6.34	6.76	7.02
GSK938890A	Yes	3600	5.44	5.67	5.77	6.49
SB-358518	Yes	4900	5.31	5.84	6.16	6.24
GW811761X	Yes	No IC_{50}		5.72	5.97	6.05
GW784307A	Yes	No IC_{50}		6.86	7.03	7.36
GSK1007102B	Yes	No IC_{50}		6.34	6.72	7.21
GSK561866B	Yes	No IC_{50}		5.82	6.10	6.45
GSK319347A	Weak	No IC_{50}		6.77	6.26	6.96
GW759710A	Weak	No IC_{50}		4.99	5.26	5.41
GW829877X	Weak	No IC_{50}		5.26	5.52	5.53
GSK1030059A	No			7.66	8.08	7.98
GSK625137A	No			4.16	4.43	4.47
GW290597X	No			6.52	5.67	6.53
GW513184X	No			5.27	5.25	5.55

Compound	Binding 1 μM	IC_{50} nM	pIC_{50}	Pred. pIC_{50} QSAR_3	Pred.pIC_{50} QSAR_1	Pred. pIC_{50} QSAR_2
GW643971X	No			5.27	5.19	5.60
GW794607X	No			5.44	5.66	5.71
SB-409514	No			5.13	5.56	5.48
GSK994854A	No			5.93	5.90	6.50
GW874091X	No			5.26	5.65	5.56
GW693481X	No			3.25	3.80	3.92
GSK1000163A	No			6.21	7.02	6.91
GSK1220512A	No			6.03	5.51	6.58
GSK317314A	No			5.94	6.64	6.48
GSK579289A	No			5.14	4.89	5.60
GSK949675A	No			7.20	7.99	7.89
GW580496A	No			6.18	5.37	6.77
SB-476429-A	No			4.68	4.67	4.92
SB-744941	No			4.73	5.52	5.22
GSK571989A	No			6.26	6.42	6.75
GW779439X	No			4.83	4.76	5.35
GSK978744A	No			7.76	7.75	8.10

Table 6. Comparison of the experimental pIC_{50} versus the calculated pIC_{50}, using the generated models QSAR_1, 2 and 3 [18].

QSAR models show satisfactory ability to predict the biological activities of the test set compounds. Thus, they could be accepted having an R^2_{pred} value > 0.5 [82]. Moreover, taking the last consideration of the threshold for the predicted $pIC_{50} > 7$ found in case of actives to refer to potent compounds was clearly in the test set, since the most potent inhibitors in the test set ($IC_{50} < 100$) were identified with predicted $pIC_{50} > 7$ (**Table 6**). Meanwhile, the biological activities of the moderately active compounds were predictive with calculated pIC_{50} in the range 5.5–7 (**Table 6**). Among the inactive compounds in the test set, three compounds were predicted to be highly potent compounds, but these compounds were inactive in the assay. The visualization of the false positives could not clarify the absence of activity of both compounds. However, GSK978744A and GSK1030059A, which mainly target the PLK kinase, possess the same chemical scaffold, and their binding modes were investigated and compared with the binding modes of analogues co-crystallized with other kinases (CDK2; PDB ID: 2I40, NEK2; PDB ID: 2XNN). However, it is not clear, from structural interactions, why this compound is not active. Additionally, it might possible that the exclusion of entropy changes or solvation of the binding pocket could play a role in the wrong estimation of the biological activity.

Since the QSAR_2 model shows high value of R^2_{pred} in the test set (QSAR_2: $R^2_{pred} = 0.98$, RMSD = 0.12 and $q^2 = 0.95$, $n = 6$), the discrimination performance was therefore discussed. Similar to QSAR_3, the most potent inhibitors in the test set ($IC_{50} < 100$) were identified with predicted $pIC_{50} > 7$

(**Table 6**). Furthermore, between the remaining active compounds, two of them were predicted to be high potent inhibitors $pIC_{50} > 7$ (GW784307A: predicted $pIC_{50} = 7.36$; GSK1007102B: predicted $pIC_{50} = 7.21$). However, the IC_{50} values of these two compounds have not been measured yet, but it reported to be active since it binds to PRK1 at 1 μM. Thus, the consideration of the threshold for the predicted $pIC_{50} > 7$ could also be applicable in the QSAR_2 model. The weak active compounds GSK319347A, GW759710A, and GW829877X (shown in **Table 6**) also predicted as moderate or low active compounds where predicted pIC_{50} values were less than 7. Among the inactive compounds, three compounds (the same compounds as in the case of the QSAR_3 model) were predicted to be highly potent compounds, but these compounds were inactive in the assay.

$$\begin{aligned} &\text{QSAR\_2}: pIC_{50} = 0.15509 - 0.09778 \\ &{*}\text{PEOE\_PC} - -0.09778 * \text{MM-GBSA} \\ &(R^2 = 0.70, \text{RMSE} = 0.78\ q^2 = 0.62,\ n = 26) \end{aligned} \tag{1}$$

$$\begin{aligned} &\text{QSAR\_3}: pIC_{50} = -1.37129 – 0.56938 * \text{PEOE\_PC-} \\ &–0.08688 * \text{MM-GBSA} – 0.26312 * \text{GLIDE\_SP} \\ &(R^2 = 0.71,\ \text{RMSE} = 0.76 \text{ and } q^2 = 0.63, n = 26) \end{aligned} \tag{2}$$

By comparing the three generated QSAR models (QSAR_1, 2, and 3) depending on the predicted pIC_{50} values among them to the measured ones, it was found the predicted pIC_{50} values when using QSAR_3 model were closer to the experimental values (**Table 6**), but QSAR_2 model showed the highest value of R^2_{pred} in the test set. Furthermore, in bootstrap validation, it was found that the QSAR_3 model had the ability to predict the biological activity of the test set compounds more accurately than the models QSAR_1 and 2 (**Table 6**). Thus, the QSAR_3 model could be used to predict the biological activities of the highly potent compounds, which should exhibit biological activities power in the nanomolar range and differentiate between the active compounds, according to their activity (low, moderate, and high).

3.7. Virtual screening using the p-ANAPL library

The above protocol was further used to virtually screen for possible PRK1 inhibitors from the p-ANAPL library [58]. As previously applied, ensemble docking was performed to dock the compounds to the X-ray structures of PRK1 stored in the PDB. Both data sets were prepared using Schrödinger 2014.U2, including the generation of several conformations per compound. The docking solutions were visualized using MOE to explore the conserved interactions with residues at the PRK1 hinge region. The selection of the hits was based first on the displayed binding mode, followed by their scoring, then predicting the pIC_{50} values using the generated QSAR models. Depending only on docking scores was insignificant for the selection of promising hit compounds. The docking solutions for the entire data set were visualized and several hits compounds were selected. In the next step, their predicted pIC_{50} values were calculated using QSAR_1, 2, and 3. Depending on the set threshold for the predicted pIC_{50}, several top scoring compounds could be selected as promising hits for the biological assays, e.g., those in **Figure 12**. **Figure 13** displays the binding modes of the selected hits and the interaction with residues at the binding pocket of the corresponding X-ray structure of PRK1.

One of the promising hits, DBT-6b, is Bartericin B (MW = 408.49; PubChem CID: 12136210) from *Dorstenia barteri* [83]. The binding mode of DBT-6b is shown in **Figure 13A**. The compound is predicted to interact with hinge region residue Ser704 with one H bond. The phenol ring forms an additional H bond with the backbone of Asp764 from the DFG-motif. The interaction with the front polar pocket and the ribose binding pocket is mediated by two H bonds between Asp708 and propanol substituent in DBT-6b. The calculated pIC_{50} values were 7.85, 7.64, and 7.45 using the generated QSAR models QSAR_1, 2, and 3, respectively. The second hit (P87), vitexin or apigenin-8-C glucoside (MW = 432.38; PubChem CID: 5280441), is a flavonoid glycoside from diverse sources, e.g., *Hyparrhenia hirta* [84]. The binding mode of P87 (**Figure 13B**) shows that the compound might form one H bond with the hinge region residue Ser704. Additionally, the substituents on the

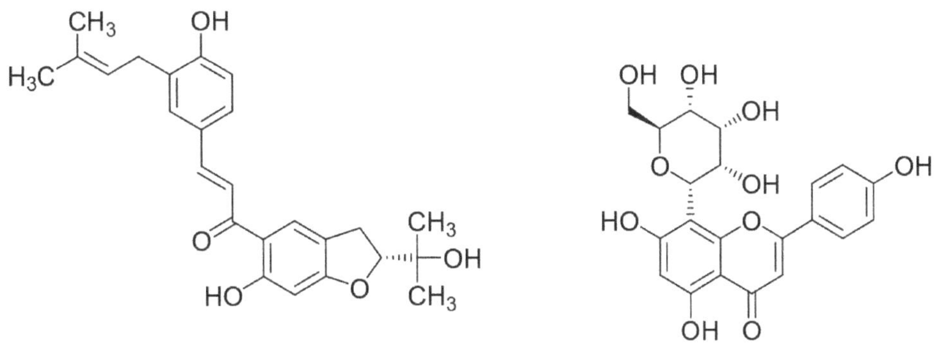

DBT-6b P87

Figure 12. Chemical structures of the selected hits.

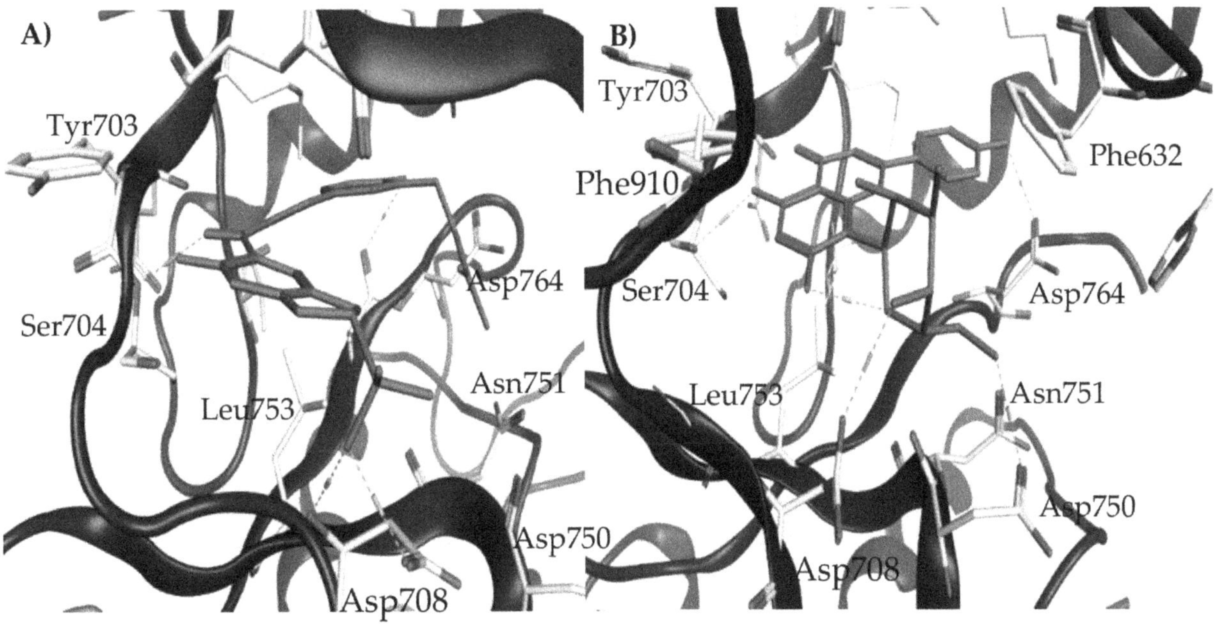

Figure 13. Docking poses of the selected hits in PRK1 binding pocket. (A) Docking poses of DBT-6b in the binding pocket of PRK1 structure 4OTG. (B) Docking pose of P87 in PRK1 structure 4OTH. The figure was designed using MOE.

oxane ring are targeting the front polar pocket and forming two H bonds with Asp708 and Asp750. The phenyl ring interacts with the back hydrophobic pocket and further forms an H bond with Asp764 in the DFG motif. P87 was predicted to be a highly potent compound, with a predicted pIC_{50} value greater than 7, using QSAR models (pred_pIC_{50}= 8.02, 8.6, and 9, respectively). Bartericin B and vitexin are the only two examples of promising compounds from natural products which could target PRK1. Among the screened databases, other hits were selected as promising compounds, which could inhibit PRK1 activity in the nanomolar range. In further investigations, the selected compounds can be submitted for biological assay to figure out their ability to bind into PRK1.

4. Conclusions

This chapter provides a brief summary of database resources for anticancer drug discovery and some recent inputs and success stories for the identification novel inhibitors of selected anticancer drug targets by the use of computer modeling. While the experimental validation of some of the natural product hits identified in the case study is ongoing, the question about the applicability domains of the derived QSAR models reported is still to be answered. Among the identified hits, 50 closely similar compounds to Bartericin B (with cut-off Tanimoto coefficient of 0.7), having reported biological activities in PubChem [59] and ChEMBL [44], with 239 biological activities and 152 published patent data. A similarity search of vitexin in PubChem gives 112 similar compounds, corresponding to 524 biological activities and 208 patents. Bartericin B is known to exhibit antimicrobial activities against *Trichomonas gallinarum*, with minimum lethal concentrations (MLCs) of 0.244 and 0.121 μg/mL after 24 H and 48 H, respectively [83], while its analogue (Bartericin A from *Dorstenia angusticornis*) is known to be very active against some bacteria and yeasts associated with human pathologies [85]. Both chalcones are known to also have potential antiprotozoal activities [86], e.g., against *Plasmodium falciparum* [87]. Vitexin, on the other hand, is known for its antioxidative and [88] spasmolytic effects [89]. The compound is known to be abundant in plants of the genus *Vitex* (Verbenaceae), which is known to exert insect antifeeding activities, among others [90]. These compounds could now be tested in biological assays for potential PRK1 inhibition.

Acknowledgements

A.N. is currently a doctoral candidate financed by the German Academic Exchange Services (DAAD), Germany. F.N.K. acknowledges a Georg Forster fellowship from the Alexander von Humboldt Foundation, Germany.

Competing interests

The authors declare that they have no competing interests.

List of abbreviations

AfroCancer	African Anticancer Natural Products Database
BFE	Binding free energy
EC_{50}	Half maximal effective concentration, i.e., the concentration of a drug, antibody or toxicant which induces a response halfway between the baseline and maximum after a specified exposure time
ED_{50}	The median effective dose, a dose that produces the desired effect in 50% of a population
GI_{50}	The growth inhibition of 50%, drug concentration resulting in a 50% reduction in the net protein increase
IC_{50}	The drug concentration causing 50% inhibition of the desired activity
NANPDB	Northern African Natural Products Database
NP	Natural product
NPACT	Naturally Occurring Plant-based Anti-cancer Compound Activity-Target Database
p-ANAPL	Pan-African natural products library
PDB	Protein databank
PLS	Partial least squares
PRK1	protein kinase C–related kinase
QSAR	Quantitative structure-activity relationship
RMSD	Root mean square deviation
RMSE	Root mean square error
SM	Secondary metabolite
VS	Virtual screening

Author details

Abdulkarim Najjar[1], Fidele Ntie-Kang[1,2]* and Wolfgang Sippl[1]

*Address all correspondence to: ntiekfidele@gmail.com

1 Department of Pharmaceutical Chemistry, Martin-Luther University of Halle-Wittenberg, Halle (Saale), Germany

2 Department of Chemistry, University of Buea, Buea, Cameroon and Department of Pharmaceutical Chemistry, Martin-Luther University of Halle-Wittenberg, Halle, Germany

References

[1] Hanahan D. Rethinking the war on cancer. Lancet. 2014;**383**:558-563. DOI: 10.1016/S0140-6736(13)62226-6

[2] Cragg GM, Grothaus PG, Newman DJ. Impact of natural products on developing new anti-cancer agents. Chemical Reviews. 2009;**109**:3012-3043. DOI: 10.1021/cr900019j

[3] Newman DJ, Cragg GM. Natural products as sources of new drugs from 1981 to 2014. Journal of Natural Products. 2016;**79**:629-661. DOI: 10.1021/acs.jnatprod.5b01055

[4] Harvey AL, Edrada-Ebel R, Quinn RJ. The re-emergence of natural products for drug discovery in the genomics era. Natural Reviews Drug Discovery. 2015;**14**:111-129. DOI: 10.1038/nrd4510

[5] Ntie-Kang F, Lifongo LL, Judson PN, Sippl W, Efange SMN. How "drug-like" are naturally occurring anti-cancer compounds?. Journal of Molecular Modeling. 2014;**20**:2069. DOI: 10.1007/s00894-014-2069-z

[6] Rodrigues T, Reker D, Schneider P, Schneider G. Counting on natural products for drug design. Natural Chemistry. 2016;**8**:531-541. DOI: 10.1038/nchem.2479

[7] Mangal M, Sagar P, Singh H, Raghava GP, Agarwal SM. NPACT: Naturally occurring plant-based anti-cancer compound-activity-target database. Nucleic Acids Research. 2013;**41**:D1124-D1129. DOI: 10.1093/nar/gks1047

[8] American Cancer Society, 2013. Cancer Facts & Figures. 2013. https://www.cancer.org/content/dam/cancer-org/research/cancer-facts-and-statistics/annual-cancer-facts-and-figures/2013/cancer-facts-and-figures-2013.pdf (Accessed 27-01-2017)

[9] Jilg CA, Ketscher A, Metzger E, Hummel B, Willmann D, et al. PRK1/PKN1 controls migration and metastasis of androgen-independent prostate cancer cells. Oncotarget. 2014;**5**:12646-12664. DOI: 10.18632/oncotarget.2653

[10] Heinlein CA, Chang C. Androgen receptor in prostate cancer. Endocrine Reviews. 2004;**25**:276-308. DOI: 10.1210/er.2002-0032

[11] Lonergan PE, Tindall DJ. Androgen receptor signaling in prostate cancer development and progression. Journal of Carcinogensis. 2011;**10**:20. DOI: 10.4103/1477-3163.83937

[12] Metzger E, Yin N, Wissmann M, Kunowska N, Fischer K, et al. Phosphorylation of histone H3 at threonine 11 establishes a novel chromatin mark for transcriptional regulation. Nature Cell Biology. 2008;**10**:53-60. DOI: 10.1038/ncb1668

[13] Wissmann M, Yin N, Müller JM, Greschik H, Fodor BD, et al. Cooperative demethylation by JMJD2C and LSD1 promotes androgen receptor-dependent gene expression. Nature Cell Biology. 2007;**9**:347-353. DOI: 10.1038/ncb1546

[14] Di Croce L, Shiekhattar R. Thrilling transcription through threonine phosphorylation. Natural Cell Biology. 2008;**10**:5-6. DOI: 10.1038/ncb0108-5

[15] Lachmann S, Jevons A, De Rycker M, Casamassima A, Radtke S, et al. Regulatory domain selectivity in the cell-type specific PKN-dependence of cell migration. PLoS One. 2011;**6**:e21732. DOI: 10.1371/journal.pone.0021732

[16] Turner EC, Kavanagh DJ, Mulvaney EP, McLean C, Wikström K, et al. Identification of an interaction between the TPα and TPβ isoforms of the human thromboxane A2 receptor with protein kinase C-related kinase (PRK) 1: implications for prostate cancer. Journal of Biological Chemistry. 2011;**286**:15440-15457. DOI: 10.1074/jbc.M110.181180

[17] Köhler J, Erlenkamp G, Eberlin A, Rumpf T, Slynko I, et al. Lestaurtinib inhibits histone phosphorylation and androgen-dependent gene expression in prostate cancer cells. PLoS One. 2012;**7**:e34973. DOI: 10.1371/journal.pone.0034973

[18] Slynko I, Schmidtkunz K, Rumpf T, Klaeger S, Heinzlmeir S, et al. Identification of highly potent protein kinase C-related kinase 1 inhibitors by virtual screening, binding free energy rescoring, and *in vitro* testing. ChemMedChem. 2016;**11**:2084-2094. DOI: 10.1002/cmdc.201600284

[19] Slynko I, Scharfe M, Rumpf T, Eib J, Metzger E, et al. Virtual screening of PRK1 inhibitors: Ensemble docking, rescoring using binding free energy calculation and QSAR model development. Journal of Chemical Information and Modeling. 2014;**54**:138-150. DOI: 10.1021/ci400628q

[20] Mukai H, Ono Y. A novel protein kinase with leucine zipper-like sequences: Its catalytic domain is highly homologous to that of protein kinase C. Biochemical and Biophysical Research Communications. 1994;**199**:897-904. DOI: 10.1006/bbrc.1994.1313

[21] Mukai H. The structure and function of PKN, a protein kinase having a catalytic domain homologous to that of PKC. Journal of Biochemistry. 2003;**133**:17-27. PMID: 12761194

[22] Lim WG, Tan BJ, Zhu Y, Zhou S, Armstrong JS, et al. The very C-terminus of PRK1/PKN is essential for its activation by RhoA and downstream signaling. Cell Signal. 2006 Sep;**18**(9):1473-1481. DOI: 10.1016/j.cellsig.2005.11.009

[23] Kannan N, Haste N, Taylor SS, Neuwald AF. The hallmark of AGC kinase functional divergence is its C-terminal tail, a *cis*-acting regulatory module. Proceedings of National Academy Science USA. 2007;**104**:1272-1277. DOI: 10.1073/pnas.0610251104

[24] Chamberlain P, Delker S, Pagarigan B, Mahmoudi A, Jackson P, et al. Crystal structures of PRK1 in complex with the clinical compounds lestaurtinib and tofacitinib reveal ligand induced conformational changes. PLoS One. 2014;**9**:e103638. DOI: 10.1371/journal.pone.0103638

[25] Metzger E, Müller JM, Ferrari S, Buettner R, Schüle R. A novel inducible transactivation domain in the androgen receptor: implications for PRK in prostate cancer. EMBO Journal. 2003;**22**:270-280. DOI: 10.1093/emboj/cdg023

[26] Rester U. From virtuality to reality - Virtual screening in lead discovery and lead optimization: a medicinal chemistry perspective. Current Opinion in Drug Discovery and Developments. 2008;**11**:559-568. PMID: 18600572

[27] Rollinger JM, Stuppner H, Langer T. Virtual screening for the discovery of bioactive natural products. Progress in Drug Research. 2008;**65**:211,213-249. PMID: 18084917

[28] Lavecchia A, Di Giovanni C. Virtual screening strategies in drug discovery: A critical review. Current Medicinal Chemistry. 2013;**20**:2839-2860. DOI: 10.2174/09298673113209990001

[29] Heikamp K, Bajorath J. The future of virtual compound screening. Chemical Biology and Drug Design. 2013;**81**:33-40. DOI: 10.1111/cbdd.12054

[30] Schneider G. Virtual screening: An endless staircase?. Natural Reviws Drug Discovery. 2010;**9**:273-276. DOI: 10.1038/nrd3139

[31] McInnes C. Virtual screening strategies in drug discovery. Current Opinion in Chemical Biology. 2007;**11**:494-502. DOI: 10.1016/j.cbpa.2007.08.033

[32] Cheng T, Li Q, Zhou Z, Wang Y, Bryant SH. Structure-based virtual screening for drug discovery: A problem-centric review. AAPS Journal. 2012;**14**:133-141. DOI: 10.1208/s12248-012-9322-0

[33] Sun H. Pharmacophore-based virtual screening. Current Medicinal Chemistry. 2008;**15**: 1018-1024. DOI: 10.2174/092986708784049630

[34] Ripphausen P, Nisius B, Bajorath J. State-of-the-art in ligand-based virtual screening. Drug Discovery Today. 2011;**16**:372-376. DOI: 10.1016/j.drudis.2011.02.011

[35] Anighoro A, Bajorath J. Three-dimensional similarity in molecular docking: prioritizing ligand poses on the basis of experimental binding modes. Journal of Chemical Information and Modeling. 2016;**56**:580-587. DOI: 10.1021/acs.jcim.5b00745

[36] Ballester PJ, Westwood I, Laurieri N, Sim E, Richards WG. Prospective virtual screening with ultrafast shape recognition: The identification of novel inhibitors of arylamine N-acetyltransferases. Journal of Royal Society Interface. 2010;**7**:335-342. DOI: 10.1098/rsif.2009.0170

[37] Li GB, Yang LL, Yuan Y, Zou J, Cao Y, et al. Virtual screening in small molecule discovery for epigenetic targets. Methods. 2015;**71**:158-166. DOI: 10.1016/j.ymeth.2014.11.010

[38] Verma J, Khedkar VM, Coutinho EC. 3D-QSAR in drug design - A review. Current Topics in Medicinal Chemistry. 2010;**10**:95-115. DOI: 10.2174/156802610790232260

[39] Winkler DA. The role of quantitative structure - activity relationships (QSAR) in biomolecular discovery. Briefings in Bioinformatics. 2002;**3**:73-86. PMID: 12002226

[40] Ntie-Kang F, Nwodo JN, Ibezim A, Simoben CV, Karaman B, et al. Molecular modeling of potential anticancer agents from African medicinal plants. Journal of Chemical Information and Modeling. 2014;**54**:2433-2450. DOI: 10.1021/ci5003697

[41] Kumar R, Chaudhary K, Gupta S, Singh H, Kumar S, et al. CancerDR: Cancer drug resistance database. Scientific Reports. 2013;**3**:1445. DOI: 10.1038/srep01445

[42] Tao W, Li B, Gao S, Bai Y, Shar PA, et al. CancerHSP: Anticancer herbs database of systems pharmacology. Scientific Reports. 2015;**5**:11481. DOI: 10.1038/srep11481

[43] Hastings J, Owen G, Dekker A, Ennis M, Kale N, et al. ChEBI in 2016: Improved services and an expanding collection of metabolites. Nucleic Acids Research. 2016;**44**:D1214-D1219. DOI: 10.1093/nar/gkv1031

[44] Gaulton A, Hersey A, Nowotka M, Bento AP, Chambers J, et al. The ChEMBL database in 2017. Nucleic Acids Research. 2017;**45**:D945-D954. DOI: 10.1093/nar/gkw1074

[45] Fang X, Shao L, Zhang H, Wang S. CHMIS-C: A comprehensive herbal medicine information system for cancer. Journal of Medicinal Chemistry. 2005;**48**:1481-1488. DOI: 10.1021/jm049838d

[46] Wishart DS, Knox C, Guo AC, Shrivastava S, Hassanali M, Stothard P, Chang Z, Woolsey J. DrugBank: A comprehensive resource for *in silico* drug discovery and exploration. Nucleic Acids Research. 2006;**34**:D668-D672. DOI: 10.1093/nar/gkj067

[47] Mysinger MM, Carchia M, Irwin JJ, Shoichet BK. Directory of useful decoys, enhanced (DUD-E): Better ligands and decoys for better benchmarking. Journal Medicinal Chemistry. 2012;**55**:6582-6594. DOI: 10.1021/jm300687e

[48] Loharch S, Bhutani I, Jain K, Gupta P, Sahoo DK, Parkesh R. EpiDBase: A manually curated database for small molecule modulators of epigenetic landscape. Database (Oxford). 2015;**2015**.pii: bav013. DOI: 10.1093/database/bav013

[49] Vetrivel U, Subramanian N, Pilla K. InPACdb - Indian plant anticancer compounds database. Bioinformation. 2009;**4**:71-74. PMID: 20198172

[50] Ashfaq UA, Mumtaz A, Qamar TU, Fatima T. MAPS database: Medicinal plant activities. Phytochemical and structural database. Bioinformation. 2013;**9**:993-995. DOI: 10.6026/97320630009993

[51] Ntie-Kang F, Telukunta KK, Döring K, Simoben CV, Moumbock, et al. The Northern African Natural Products Database (NANPDB); 2017. www.african-compounds.org/nanpdb/

[52] Milne GW, Nicklaus MC, Driscoll JS, Wang S, Zaharevitz D. National cancer institute drug information system 3D database. Journal of Chemical Information and Computer Science. 1994;**34**:1219-1224. DOI: 10.1021/ci00021a032

[53] Ko Y, Tan SL, Chan A, Wong YP, Yong WP, et al. Prevalence of the coprescription of clinically important interacting drug combinations involving oral anticancer agents in Singapore: A retrospective database study. Clinical Therapy. 2012;**34**:1696-1704. DOI: 10.1016/j.clinthera.2012.06.025

[54] Hatherley R, Brown DK, Musyoka TM, Penkler DL, Faya N, et al. SANCDB: A South African natural compound database. Journal of Cheminformatics. 2015;**7**:29. DOI: 10.1186/s13321-015-0080-8

[55] Goede A, Dunkel M, Mester N, Frommel C, Preissner R. SuperDrug: A conformational drug database. Bioinformatics. 2005;**21**:1751-1753. DOI: 10.1093/bioinformatics/bti295

[56] Rammensee H, Bachmann J, Emmerich NP, Bachor OA, Stevanović S. SYFPEITHI: Database for MHC ligands and peptide motifs. Immunogenetics. 1999;**50**:213-219. DOI: 10.1007/s002510050595

[57] Lin YC, Wang CC, Chen IS, Jheng JL, Li JH, et al. TIPdb: A database of anticancer, antiplatelet, and antituberculosis phytochemicals from indigenous plants in Taiwan. Scientific World Journal. 2013;**2013**:736386. DOI: 10.1155/2013/736386

[58] Ntie-Kang F, Amoa Onguéné P, Fotso GW, Andrae-Marobela K, Bezabih M, et al. Virtualizing the p-ANAPL library: A step towards drug discovery from African medicinal plants. PLoS One. 2014;**9**:e90655. DOI: 10.1371/journal.pone.0090655

[59] Kim S, Thiessen PA, Bolton EE, Chen J, Fu G, et al. PubChem substance and compound databases. Nucleic Acids Research. 2016;**44**:D1202-D1213. DOI: 10.1093/nar/gkv951

[60] Sterling T, Irwin JJ. ZINC 15 - ligand discovery for everyone. Journal of Chemical Information and Modeling. 2015;**55**(11):2324-2327. DOI: 10.1021/acs.jcim.5b00559

[61] Ha H, Debnath B, Odde S, Bensman T, Ho H, et al. Discovery of novel CXCR2 inhibitors using ligand-based pharmacophore models. Journal of Chemical Information and Modeling. 2015;**55**:1720-1738. DOI: 10.1021/acs.jcim.5b00181

[62] Zhu YM, Webster SJ, Flower D, Woll PJ. Interleukin-8/CXCL8 is a growth factor for human lung cancer cells. British Journal of Cancer. 2004;**91**:1970-1976. DOI: 10.1038/sj.bjc.6602227

[63] Rubie C, Kollmar O, Frick VO, Wagner M, Brittner B, et al. Differential CXC receptor expression in colorectal carcinomas. Scandinavian Journal of Immunology. 2008;**68**:635-644. DOI: 10.1111/j.1365-3083.2008.02163.x

[64] Murphy C, McGurk M, Pettigrew J, Santinelli A, Mazzucchelli R, et al. Nonapical and cytoplasmic expression of interleukin-8, CXCR1, and CXCR2 correlates with cell proliferation and microvessel density in prostate cancer. Clinical Cancer Research. 2005 ;**11**:4117-4127. DOI: 10.1158/1078-0432.CCR-04-1518

[65] Yang G, Rosen DG, Liu G, Yang F, Guo X, et al. CXCR2 promotes ovarian cancer growth through dysregulated cell cycle, diminished apoptosis, and enhanced angiogenesis. Clinical Cancer Research. 2010;**16**:3875-3886. DOI: 10.1158/1078-0432.CCR-10-0483

[66] Kumar AV, Mohan K, Riyaz S. Structure guided inhibitor designing of CDK2 and discovery of potential leads against cancer. Journal of Molecular Modeling. 2013;**19**:3581-3589. DOI: 10.1007/s00894-013-1887-8

[67] Al-Sha'er MA, Khanfar MA, Taha MO. Discovery of novel urokinase plasminogen activator (uPA) inhibitors using ligand-based modeling and virtual screening followed by *in vitro* analysis. Journal of Molecular Modeling. 2014;**20**:2080. DOI: 10.1007/s00894-014-2080-4

[68] Ren JX, Li LL, Zheng RL, Xie HZ, Cao ZX, et al. Discovery of novel Pim-1 kinase inhibitors by a hierarchical multistage virtual screening approach based on SVM model, pharmacophore, and molecular docking. Journal of Chemical Information and Modeling. 2011;**51**:1364-1375. DOI: 10.1021/ci100464b

[69] Li L, Khanna M, Jo I, Wang F, Ashpole NM, et al. Target-specific support vector machine scoring in structure-based virtual screening: Computational validation, in vitro testing in kinases, and effects on lung cancer cell proliferation. Journal of Chemical Information and Modeling. 2011;**51**:755-759. DOI: 10.1021/ci100490w

[70] Khanfar MA, Taha MO. Elaborate ligand-based modeling coupled with multiple linear regression and k nearest neighbor QSAR analyses unveiled new nanomolar mTOR

inhibitors. Journal of Chemical Information and Modeling. 2013;**53**:2587-2612. DOI: 10.1021/ci4003798

[71] B-Rao C, Subramanian J, Sharma SD. Managing protein flexibility in docking and its applications. Drug Discovery Today. 2009;**14**:394-400. DOI: 10.1016/j.drudis.2009.01.003

[72] Bjerrum EJ. Machine learning optimization of cross docking accuracy. Computational Biology and Chemistry. 2016;**62**:133-144. DOI: 10.1016/j.compbiolchem.2016.04.005

[73] Tan C, Yang L, Luo R. How well does Poisson-Boltzmann implicit solvent agree with explicit solvent? A quantitative analysis. Journal of Physical Chemistry B. 2006;**110**:18680-18687. DOI: 10.1021/jp063479b.

[74] Wang J, Tan C, Chanco E, Luo R. Quantitative analysis of Poisson-Boltzmann implicit solvent in molecular dynamics. Physical Chemistry Chemical Physics. 2010;**12**:1194-1202. DOI: 10.1039/b917775b

[75] Mateos-Aparicio G. Partial least squares (PLS) methods: Origins, evolution, and application to social sciences. Communications in Statistics - Theory and Methods. 2011;**40**:2305-2317. DOI: 10.1080/03610921003778225

[76] Gasteiger J, Marsili M. Iterative partial equalization of orbital electronegativity-A rapid access to atomic charges. Tetrahedron. 1980;**36**:3219-3228. DOI: 10.1016/0040-4020(80)80168-2

[77] Kiralj R, Ferreira MMC. 2009. Basic validation procedures for regression models in QSAR and QSPR studies: Theory and application. Journal of Brazilian Chemical Society. 2009;**20**:770-787. DOI: 10.1590/S0103-50532009000400021

[78] Veerasamy R, Rajak H, Jain A, Sivadasan S, Varghese CP, et al. Validation of QSAR models - Strategies and importance. International Journal of Drug Design Discovery. 2011;**2**:511-519

[79] Golbraikh A, Tropsha A. Predictive QSAR modeling based on diversity sampling of experimental datasets for the training and test set selection. Molecular Diversity. 2002;**5**:231-243. PMID: 12549674

[80] Golbraikh A, Tropsha A. Beware of q^2! Journal of Molecular Graphics and Modeling. 2002;**20**: 269-276. DOI: 10.1016/S1093-3263(01)00123-1

[81] Nahum OE, Yosipof A, Senderowitz H. A multi-objective genetic algorithm for outlier removal. Journal of Chemical Information Modeling. 2015;**55**:2507-2518. DOI: 10.1021/acs.jcim.5b00515

[82] Pratim Roy P, Paul S, Mitra I, Roy K. On two novel parameters for validation of predictive QSAR models. Molecules. 2009;**14**:1660-1701. DOI: 10.3390/molecules14051660

[83] Omisore NOA, Adewunmi CO, Iwalewa EO, Ngadjui BT, Adenowo TK, et al. Antitrichomonal and antioxidant activities of *Dorstenia barteri* and *Dorstenia convexa*. Brazilian Journal of Medical and Biological Research. 2005;**38**:1087-1094. DOI: 10.1590/S0100-879X2005000700012

[84] Bouaziz M, Simmonds MS, Grayer RJ, Kite GC, Damak M. Flavonoids from *Hyparrhenia hirta* Stapf (Poaceae) growing in Tunisia. Biochemical Systematics and Ecology. 2001;**29**:849-851. DOI: 10.1016/S0305-1978(01)00028-X

[85] Kuete V, Konga Simo I, Ngameni B, Bigoga DJ, Watchueng J, et al. Antimicrobial activity of the methanolic extract, fractions and four flavonoids from the twigs of *Dorstenia angusticornis* Engl. (Moraceae). Journal of Ethnopharmacology. 2007;**112**:271-277. DOI:10.1016/j.jep.2007.12.017

[86] Fotie J. The antiprotozoan potential of flavonoids. Pharmacognosy Reviews. 2008;**2**:6-19

[87] Ngameni B, Watchueng J, Boyom FF, Keumedjio F, Ngadjui BT, et al. Antimalarial prenylated chalcones from the twigs of *Dorstenia barteri* var. *subtriangularis*. Arkivoc. 2007;**13**:116-123

[88] Kim JH, Lee BC, Kim JH, Sim GS, Lee DH, et al. The isolation and antioxidative effects of vitexin from *Acer palmatum*. Archives of Pharmacal Research. 2005 ;28:195. DOI:10.1007/BF02977715

[89] Ragone MI, Sella M, Conforti P, Volonté MG, Consolini AE. The spasmolytic effect of *Aloysia citriodora*, Palau (South American cedrón) is partially due to its vitexin but not isovitexin on rat duodenums. Journal of Ethnopharmacology. 2007;**113**:258-266. DOI: 10.1016/j.jep.2007.06.003

[90] Hernández MM, Heraso C, Villarreal ML, Vargas-Arispuro I, Aranda E. Biological activities of crude plant extracts from *Vitex trifolia* L. (Verbenaceae). Journal of Ethnopharmacology. 1999;**67**:37-44. DOI: 10.1016/S0378-8741(99)00041-0

8

Medicinal Plants of West Godavari

Sudhakar Pola and Venkata Narasimha Kadali

Abstract

Medicinal plants are one of the nature's greatest gifts to the mankind. Each plant will have an exquisite deal of character, which can act as an antidote to various of diseases. Traditional medicine has become a vital alternative source of medicine all over the world today with some approximation of about 80% of the primary health care system in some developing countries. Medicinal plants are known to comprise of hundreds of active constituents that may be potentially useful for the development of therapeutic agents. The development of therapeutic agents involves the isolation and identification of bioactive compounds from plant materials which is crucial for drug discovery. Researchers from all around the globe have focused on drug discovery from the natures' wonder medicinal plants, forming an important group of complementary and alternative medicine (CAM) therapy. West Godavari is a part of Andhra Pradesh, India, which hosts several plants that have high therapeutic significance. Each of the plants has a unique feature which can be employed for healing of various lethal diseases. The present examination intends to review the therapeutic plant assets of West Godavari area Andhra Pradesh. This evaluation also offers the critical elements which include medicinal properties of various medicinal plants found in West Godavari district of Andhra Pradesh, India.

Keywords: drug discovery, traditional medicine, West Godavari district, nature, antidote

1. Introduction

The great thing that nature has given us is the medicinal plants. Each plant will have a great deal of character, which can act as an antidote against different types of diseases.

Traditional medicine has become a vital alternative source of medicine all over the world today with some approximation of about 80% of the primary health care system in some developing countries (e.g., Nigeria, Ghana, China, and India [1, 2]).

India has a recognized traditional system of medicine, that is, Ayurveda, Siddha, Unani, Homeopathy, Yoga, and Naturopathy which placed India in a unique position in the world [3].

As the growth of knowledge has increased, the number of new plant-derived drugs grow at an accelerated pace. India has an enormous wealth of medicinal plants, and often it has been referred to as the Medicinal Garden of the world [4].

Medicinal plants are known to comprise hundreds of active constituents that may be potentially useful for the development of therapeutic agents. The development of therapeutic agents involves Identification and segregation of bioactive compounds from plant materials that are crucial for drug discovery [5].

Researchers from all around the globe have focused on drug discovery from the nature's wonder medicinal plants, an important group of complementary and alternative medicine (CAM) therapy [5].

The man has acclimated himself with plants and utilized them in an assortment of courses all through the ages. Primitive man looking for nourishment and to adapt efficiently to human sufferings started to recognize those plants appropriate for restorative reason from others with complete pharmacological activity. This connection between plants and man has developed, and many plants came to be utilized as medicines. The development of information to cure infections proceeded at a quick pace and various new plant-derived drugs expanded in this manner.

Herbs employed in ancient medicines represent a tiny, low portion of present plants solely. With the advances in informative innovation and science, many bioactive concoction substances are distinguished in plants or foodstuffs through phytochemical and pharmacological studies.

The clinical utilization of plants portrayed in Indian Vedas for curing distinctive maladies. In the present setting, the conventional arrangement of pharmaceutical is broadly acknowledged and drilled by individuals around the world.

The natural solution is drilled around the world. For a considerable length of time, individuals have swung to natural solutions for basic cure illnesses, for example, colds, sensitivity, annoy stomachs, and toothaches, and the pattern is continually expanding. In this way, there has been a move in general pattern from manufactured to homegrown solutions.

The advancement of plant-derived drugs began when improvement of science. The homegrown drug is compelling, minor symptom, and moderate than the medications purchased from an allopathic pharmaceutical. Homegrown medications incorporate herbs, homegrown materials, natural arrangements, and homegrown items that contain diverse parts of plants or other plant materials as dynamic fixings.

As the worldwide utilization of homegrown therapeutic items keeps on developing and numerous, the newest items are brought into the market, general medical problems and concerns encompassing their well-being are likewise progressively perceived. Although some homegrown herbs have promising potential and are utilized, a considerable lot of them stay untested and their utilization likewise not observed.

It has turned out to be fundamental, subsequently, to outfit the overall population incorporating human services experts with adequate data to encourage better comprehension of the dangers related to the utilization of these items and to guarantee that all solutions are protected and of reasonable quality. Discussion in this review is restricted to lethality-related issues, and significant well-being concerns are emerging from the utilization of homegrown drugs and additional factors advancing them. Some essential difficulties related to the successful checking of security of these homegrown cures are additionally featured to refocusing appropriate administrative offices on the requirement for viability and guaranteeing sufficient assurance of general well-being and advancing well-being.

The worldwide acknowledgment and utilization of natural medicines and related items keep on assuming exponential increment. Issues identifying with unfavorable responses as of late are additionally ending up more distinctive, expanding in common and no longer accessible to refute as a result of prior misguided judgment with regards to or classifying homegrown restorative items as "protected" because they are getting from "characteristic" source. In this manner, regulatory approaches on homegrown pharmaceuticals should be institutionalized and reinforced on a worldwide scale. Pertinent administrative experts in various nations of the world should be proactive and keep on putting proper set up measures to secure the general well-being by guaranteeing that every single natural prescription endorsed available to be purchased sheltered and of reasonable quality. Suppliers of pharmaceuticals, for example, doctors, attendants, and drug specialists, regularly have little preparing in and comprehension of how homegrown solutions influence the well-being of their patients. Satisfactory preparation is present extremely basic since most patients are regularly on different sorts of the solution or non-professionally prescribed drugs. Additionally, it is vital that all suppliers of natural solutions are adequately enabled to assume a part in observing well-being of homegrown prescriptions. This, be that as it may, ought to be in a joint effort with the traditional healers. For this to be successful, it is basic to make a climate of trust to encourage satisfactory sharing of information about the utilization and well-being of homegrown solutions. Truth be told to suppliers of homegrown solutions, and patients/shoppers are imperative for the version of possibly genuine dangers from misuse of natural medications. The supplier must demonstrate adequate responsibility toward understanding the utilization of homegrown drugs.

West Godavari is a part of Andhra Pradesh, India, which hosts several plants that have high medicinal importance. Each of the plants has a unique feature which can heal lethal diseases. Some researchers have drawn some plants into attention from lots of surveys. It also hosts traditional healers who can efficiently cure some of the deadly diseases.

The traditional plant healing has brought a significant breakthrough in curing diseases very efficiently. The nutraceutical companies have isolated plant compounds based on the knowledge provided by the traditional healers. An adequate amount of knowledge is still to be known from the traditional healers. There is a substantial increase in the use of Ayurvedic medicines and medicines derived from plant sources. The reason being its efficacy and lack of side effects, and there is an economic point of view as well. Based on the information given by the traditional healing system, several modern scientific studies are being conducted on the various medicinal plants.

Some of the medicinal plants have been perished because of urbanization. The ancient knowledge about medicinal plants had not been documented, and many of the valuable plants are at the edge of extinction. The government and NGO should take necessary conservatory steps to avoid extinction of valuable medicinal plants.

Several bioactive compounds isolated from medicinal plants are in excess demand in nutraceutical companies.

The present study aims to review the medicinal plant resources of West Godavari district, Andhra Pradesh. This review also deals with the critical aspects such as medicinal properties of various medicinal plants present in West Godavari district of Andhra Pradesh, India. This article deals with the medicinal properties of plants which are implicated in various diseases such as jaundice, cardiac diseases, asthma, cancer, skin diseases, diarrhea, conjunctivitis, ulcers, diabetes, leprosy, syphilis, and neural diseases.

This article also deals with the scientific studies conducted by the researchers on numerous medicinal plants present in West Godavari.

2. Medicinal plants of West Godavari

2.1. *Annona reticulata* L.

Annona genus (Annonaceae) has about 119 species [6]. *Annona reticulata* belongs to the plant family Annonaceae and is a semi-evergreen and small deciduous tree [7]. *Annona* species are having a place in custard apple family and is cultivated everywhere in India for its fruit. All components of genus *Annona* are employed in natural medication within the tropics. It is thought to be a smart supply of natural antioxidants for various diseases.

It is being cultivated in Peru and Brazil and is grown mostly in the Bahamas and occasionally in southern Florida, Bermuda, the east coast of Malaysia, and throughout Southeast Asia and the Philippines [8, 9].

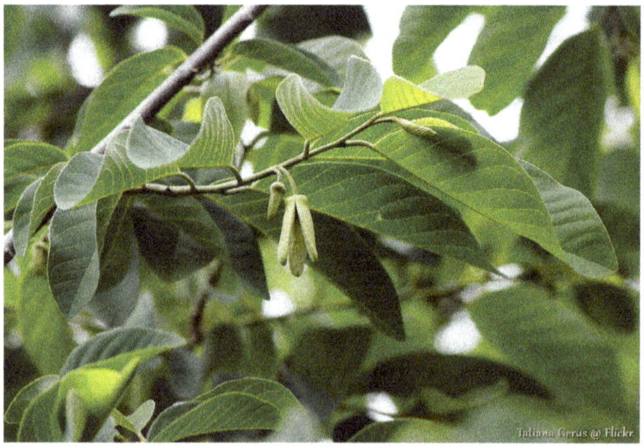

2.1.1. Scientific evidences

This plant is known to possess antioxidant activity [7], anticancer activity [10–13], anti-helminthic activity [14], anti-inflammatory activity [6], analgesic, and CNS depressant activity [15].

2.2. *Abutilon indicum*

Abutilon indicum (Linn.) belong to family Malvaceae and it is scattered throughout Andhra Pradesh, India, and it is being used for treating various diseases like diabetes, leprosy, ulcer, and jaundice [16].

In Siddha System of Medicine, it has been using as a remedy for jaundice, piles, ulcers, and leprosy [17].

2.2.1. Scientific studies on Abutilon indicum

This plant is proved to have diuretic activity [18], antimycotic activity [19], anti-arthritic activity [20], anti-inflammatory and anti-asthmatic activity [21], hypoglycemic activity [22], anticonvulsant activity [23], wound healing activity [24], antidiarrhoeal activity [25], antimalarial [26], and hepatoprotective activity [27].

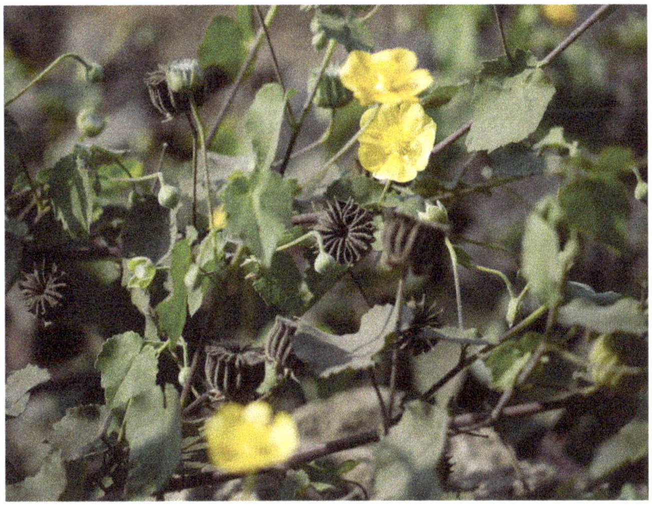

2.3. *Abrus precatorius*

Abrus precatorius belongs to family Fabaceae. *Abras precatorius* is a plant originating from Southeast Asia. The name *Abrus*, means beautiful or graceful, is used to describe the appearance of the seed [28]. The seeds of *Abrus precatorius* have a history in a variety of roles because they have uniform size and weight. They were once called as Rati, and utilized as weights for measuring gold and silver [28].

2.3.1. Scientific studies on Abrus precatorius

This plant is demonstrated to have antibacterial activity [29], diuretic activity [30], nephroprotective activity [31], neuroprotective activity [32], bronchodilator activity [33], effect on neuromuscular antioxidant activity [34], anticonvulsant activity [35], antispasmodic activity [36].

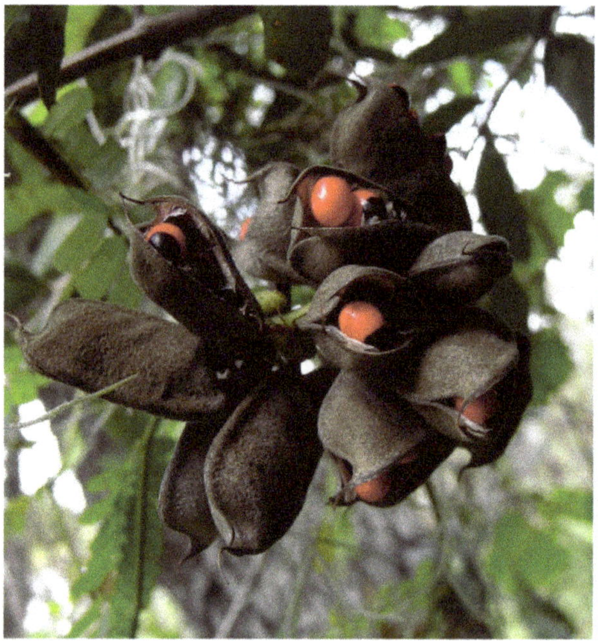

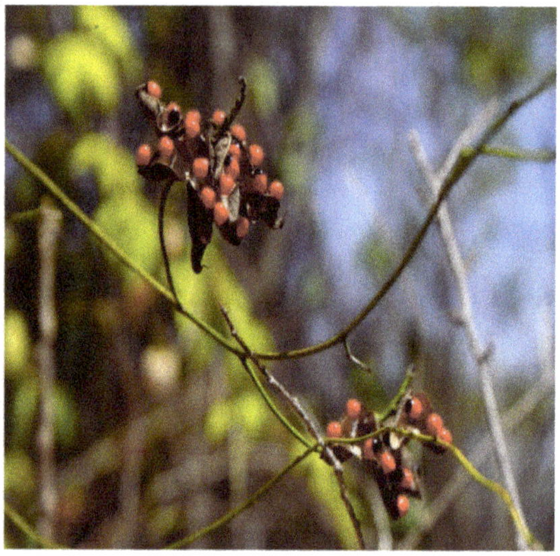

2.4. *Acacia Arabica*

Acacia is the most remarkable variety of family: Leguminosae, as a matter of first importance, portrayed by Linnaeus in 1773. It is assessed that there are approximately 1380 types of Acacia around the world, and two-thirds of them local in Australia and rest of spread around tropical and subtropical districts of the world [37–39].

2.4.1. *Scientific studies on Acacia Arabica*

This plant is proved to have antidiabetic activity [40], antimutagenic activity [41], antimicrobial activity [42], antifungal activity [43], antidiarrhoeal activity [44], antiviral activity [45], nematicidal activity [46], antioxidant activity [47], and abortifacient activity [48].

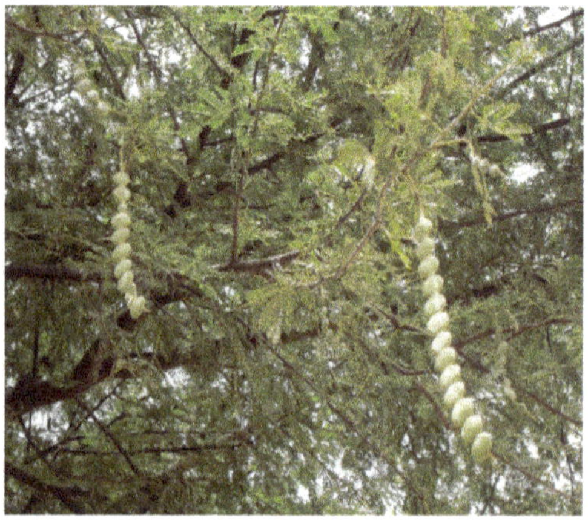

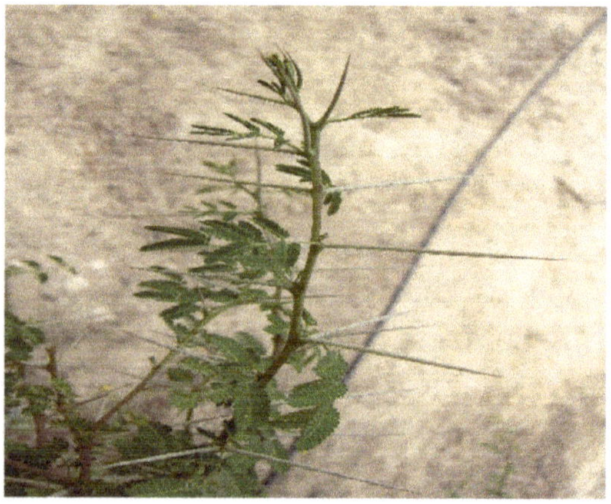

2.5. *Bambusa arundinacea*

Bambusa arundinacea, belong to Gramineae family, is a highly reputed Ayurvedic tree commonly known as the Bamboo [49]. Bamboos contrast from alternate individuals from the grass family because of the nearness of branches at every node. A bamboo culm comprises of an internode (which is empty for most bamboo) and a node, which is robust and gives basic structural integrity to the plant. The buds on the node later develop into side branches [50].

2.5.1. *Scientific evidences*

This plant is demonstrated to have antifertility activity [51], anti-bacterial activity [52], anti-inflammatory [53], and anti-ulcer activity [54].

2.6. *Boerhavia diffusa* L.

Boerhaavia diffusa L. (Nyctaginaceae), generally known as "Punarnava" in the Indian arrangement of medicine, is a perennial creeping herb found all through the wastelands of India [55]. The roots are reputed to be diuretic and laxative and are given for the treatment of anasarca, ascites, and jaundice [56].

2.6.1. *Scientific evidences*

This plant is verified to have antidiabetic activity [57], antibacterial activity [58], hepatoprotective activity [56], analgesic/anti-inflammatory activity [59], antitumor activity [60], anticonvulsant activity [61], antiproliferative and antiestrogenic activity [62], cytological activity [63], bronchial asthma [64], and anti-fibrinolytic activity [65].

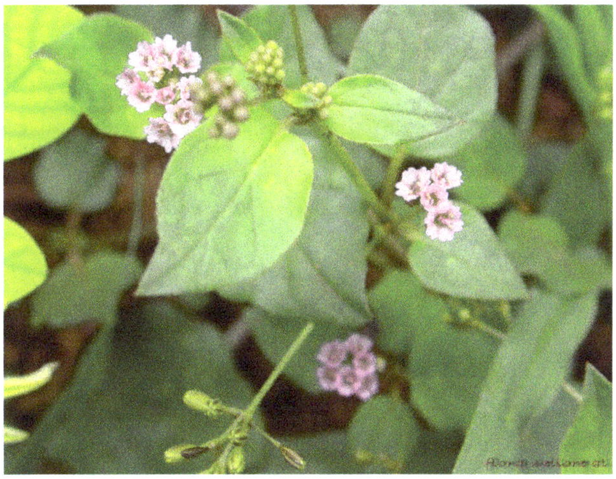

2.7. *Calotropis procera*

Calotropis procera belong to family Asclepiadaceae is a tropical plant growing wild in warm climate up to an altitude of about 1050 m. It is a native plant of North Africa, and it is well distributed throughout India, particularly it is abundantly found in Rajasthan. It also found in Pakistan, Africa, Mexico, Australia, Egypt, Central and South America, and Caribbean islands [66, 67].

2.7.1. *Scientific evidences*

This plant is verified to have hepatoprotective activity [68], antioxidant activity [69], antipyretic activity [70], anthelmintic activity [71], anti-inflammatory activity [72], antidiarrhoeal activity [73], spasmolytic activity [74], antidiabetic activity [75], antiulcer activity [76], and wound healing activity [77].

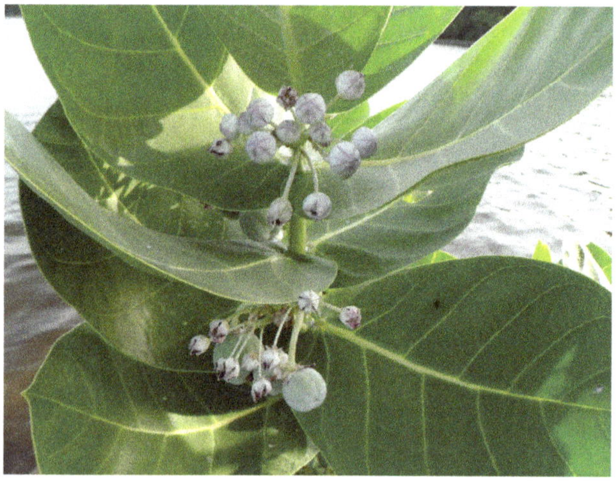

2.8. *Momordica charantia*

Momordica charantia is a climber that have its place in family Cucurbitaceae, is commonly known as bitter gourd or bitter melon. This plant typically grows in tropical areas of Asia, Amazon, East Africa, and the Caribbean and it is being cultivated throughout the world for its use as a vegetable as well as medicine [78].

2.8.1. Scientific evidences

This plant is demonstrated to have antioxidant activity [79], antidiabetic activity [80], anticancer and antitumoral activity [81], antiviral activity [82], antifertility activity [83], and antineoplastic activity [78].

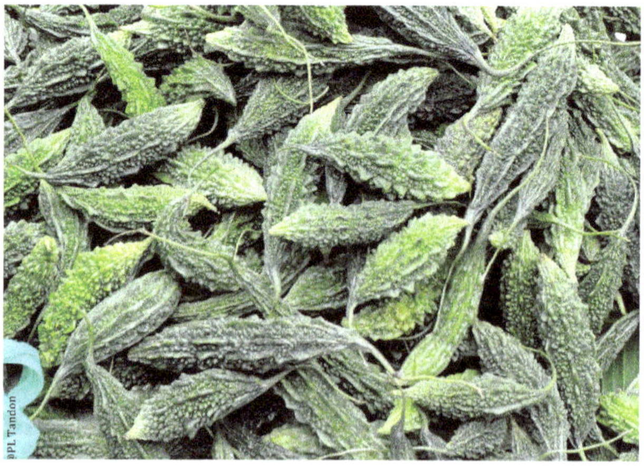

2.9. *Punica granatum*

Punica granutam is widely known as pomegranate. It belongs to Punicaceae family, which is a large deciduous shrub or small tree native to Asia. *Punica granutam* have been used in folk medicine for centuries in the Middle East, India, and China, and it has been used to treat disorders ranging from inflammation and rheumatism to the pain of a simple sore throat. The most famous usage worldwide has been as a vermifugal or taenicidal agent [84–87].

2.9.1. Scientific evidences

This plant is verified to have healing activity [88], anti-inflammatory activity [89], antidiabetic activity [90], and anticancer activity [91].

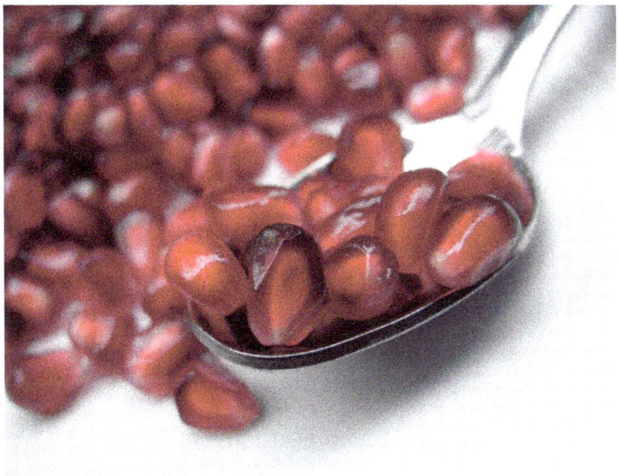

2.10. *Pongamia pinnata*

It is a medicinal plant native to the Western Ghats and is chiefly found in tidal forests of India. *Pongamia pinnata* also was known as *Derris indica*, is a monotypic genus and grows profusely along the coasts and riverbanks in Myanmar and it has multi-purpose benefits and as a potential source of biodiesel [92, 93].

2.10.1. Scientific evidences

This plant is proved to have antihyperglycemic and antilipidperoxidative effects [94], antihyperammonemic effect [95], anti-inflammatory activity [96], antiviral activity [97], antifilarial potential [98], ulceroprotective activity [99], nootropic activity [100], and antinociceptive activity [101].

2.11. *Piper longum*

Piper longum Linn. has been named under the family Piperaceae is a flowering plant in the *Piper* family. *Piper longum* commonly known as long Indian pepper, it is widely being used as a spice and flavoring agent in various foods and herbal formulations. It is widely cultivated in India, Nepal, Indonesia, Malaysia, Sri Lanka, Timor, and the Philippines. In India, it is extensively grown in the central Himalayas to Assam, Khasi and Mikir hills, lower hills of West Bengal and evergreen forests of the Western Ghats from Konkan to Kerala and also from Car Nicobar Islands because of its therapeutic potential [102–105].

2.11.1. Scientific evidences

This plant is shown to have anti-apoptosis and antioxidant [106], analgesic activity [107], immunomodulatory activity [108], anticancer and antitumor activity [109], antidiabetic activity [110], antifertility activity [111], anti-snake venom activity [112], melanin-inhibiting activity [113], and antiulcer activity [114].

2.12. *Ricinus communis*

Ricinus communis, belong to a family Euphorbiaceae and it is most commonly known as castor oil plant. *Ricinus communis* as a tropical plant, known as castor bean, distributed widely across the world, and it is a local of India and developed all through the nation in greenery enclosures and fields and furthermore develops wild in squandering places [115, 116].

2.12.1. Scientific evidences

This plant is shown to have antimicrobial and antifungal [117], antioxidant activity [118], anti-implantation activity [119], anti-inflammatory and free radical scavenging activity [120], central analgesic activity [121], anti-tumor activity [122], larvicidal and adult emergence inhibition activity [123], antiulcer activity [124], molluscicidal, insecticidal and larvicidal activity [125], antidiabetic activity [126], cytotoxic activity [127], and antihistaminic activity [128].

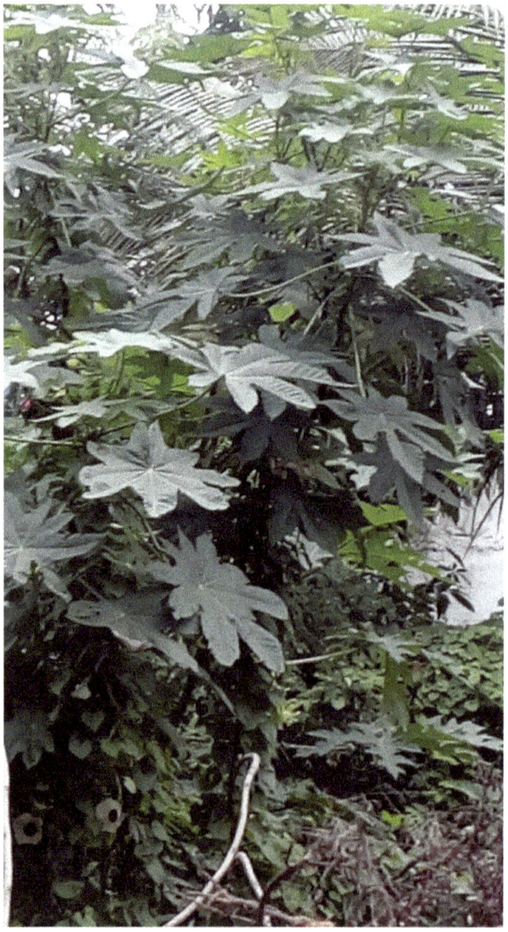

2.13. *Syzygium cumini* (L.)

Syzygium cumini Linn. is a huge evergreen tropical tree belongs to the family Myrtaceae, and this plant is also mentioned in literature as Jamun, synonym as black plum or jambolana, since ancient age this plant is very well-known for their pharmacological properties [129, 130].

2.13.1. Scientific evidences

This plant is revealed to have antiallergic activity [131], gastroprotective activity [132], antioxidant activity [133], CNS activity [134], anti-inflammatory activity [135], antihyperlipidemic activity [136], antidiarrhoeal activity [137], antipyretic activity [138], antispasmodic activity [139], and antiviral activity [140].

2.14. *Sida cordifolia*

Sida cordifolia L. belongs to family Malvaceae and commonly called as Country Mallow and Bala (Sanskrit). This herb is extensively spread throughout the tropical and subtropical regions of India [141].

In Ayurvedic practices, *Sida cordifolia* has three basic applications: Mashabaladi Kvatha, where the plant seeds are blended with different fixings to soothe relieve muscular pain; Balataila, a procedure for the treatment of sensory system grievances and stomach issues and as a heart tonic; and the squashed leaves of the plant as an astringent for the treatment and dressing of wounds or skin wounds [142].

2.14.1. Scientific evidences

This plant is shown for its antioxidant activity [143], anti-inflammatory activity [144], anti-ulcer activity [145], antidiabetic activity [146], nephroprotective activity [147], cytotoxicity [148], anti-hypercholestrolemic activity [149], hepatoprotectivity [150], cardiovascular activity [151], and anticancer activity [152].

2.15. *Sapindus mukorossi*

Sapindus mukorossi belongs to family Sapindaceae and has some common names such as soapnut, soapberry, washnut, reetha, aritha, dodan, and doadni. It is an attractive medium-sized deciduous tree found in diverse geographical provinces like Gangetic Plains, Western Ghats, and Deccan Plateau in India [153].

2.15.1. Scientific evidences

This plant is proved to have an anti-mosquito activity or larvicidal activity [154], cytotoxic activity [155], tyrosinase inhibition and free radical scavenging [156], antigonorrhoeal activity [157], antifungal activity [158], and molluscicidal activity [159].

2.16. *Tribulus terrestris* L.

Tribulus terrestris L. is a well-known plant that belongs to genus Tribulus. The genus *Tribulus*, having a place with family Zygophyllaceae, involves around 20 species on the world. Among them, *T. terrestris* is a well-practiced medicinal herb by Ayurvedic practitioners as well as by modern herbalists [160].

2.16.1. Scientific evidences

This plant is demonstrated to have diuretic activity [161], aphrodisiac activity [162], anti-urolithic activity [163], immunomodulatory activity [164], antidiabetic activity [165], hypo-lipidemic [166], central nervous system (CNS) activity [167], anticancer activity [168], and larvicidal activity [169].

2.17. *Terminalia chebula*

Terminalia chebula is a moderate plant which is being utilized as a part of conventional solutions. It has a place in the Combretaceae family. It is typically called as Black Myrobalan, Ink tree (or) Chebulic myrobalan and furthermore known as "Ruler of the drug." It is widely utilized as a part of Unani, Ayurveda, and homeopathic prescription. *Terminalia chebula* is a well-known conventional plant utilised in the pharmaceutical industry in India as well as in different countries of Asia and Africa [170]. It stimulates the liver and ensures it is promote by removing the excretory waste items from the digestion tracts. It is shown in protracted loose bowels with hematochezia and prolapse of rectum. It is a decent nervine, utilized as a part of anxious shortcoming, apprehensive crabbiness.

2.17.1. Scientific evidences

This plant is demonstrated to have antibacterial activity [171], antiamoebic and immunomodulatory activities [172], antianaphylactic and adaptogenic activities [173], antiviral activity [174], antimutagenic and anticarcinogenic activities [175], anti-arthritic activity [176], antidiabetic and retinoprotective activities [177], and hepatoprotective activity [178].

2.18. *Tephrosia purpurea*

Tephrosia purpurea or Sharpunkha has its place in the family Leguminosae (subfamily-Papilionaceae). The genus *Tephrosia* encompasses between 300 and 400 species of annual and perennial woody herb, scattered in the tropical and subtropical local of the world. This plant has excessive economic cost due to the presence of phytochemicals like flavonoids, sugars, gums tannins and phenols, alkaloids and glue, settled oils and fats, and saponins and lipids [179, 180]. As per Ayurveda writing, this plant has additionally given the name of "Sarwa Wranvishapaka" which implies that it has the property of mending a wide range of wounds. It is an imperative part of a few arrangements, for example, Tephroli and Yakrifitused for the liver issue. In the Ayurvedic arrangement of different pharmaceutical parts of this plant, they are utilized as a solution for impotency, asthma, diarrhea, gonorrhea, ailment, ulcer, and urinary issue.

2.18.1. *Scientific evidences*

This plant is verified to have anticarcinogenic and anti-lipid peroxidative [181], anti-inflammatory and analgesic [182], in vitro antioxidant [183], anticancer activity [184], and in vitro anthelmintic activity [185].

2.19. *Tectona grandis*

T. grandis Linn. belongs to family Verbenaceae is one of the most well-known timbers in the world and is famous for its dimensional stability, extreme durability, and hardness which also resists decay even when unprotected by paints and preservatives. This plant is commonly called as teak. It is one of the most famous heartwood of the world. Timber value of teak has been well-known for decades [186, 187].

2.19.1. *Scientific evidences*

This plant is verified to have hair growth activity [188], cytotoxic activity [189], anti-hemolytic anemia activity [190], hypoglycemic activity [191], anti-inflammatory activity [192], diuretic activity [193], and gastroprotective activity [194].

2.20. *Tamarindus indica* L.

Tamarindus indica or tamarind regarded as a tropical fruit tree native to the African savannahs and it is found in numerous tropical nations. It is arranged as a monospecific class in the group of Leguminosae. The sweet and harsh taste of its natural product mash is utilized to add flavor to neighborhood cooking styles. Other than culinary, tamarind is likewise utilized as a part of the conventional drug as purgative, diuretic, antibacterial operators and also in the treatment of fever and malarial contaminations [195, 196].

2.20.1. *Scientific evidences*

This plant is verified to have antipyretic activity [197], laxative activity [195], anticancer activity [198], antiemetic activity [199], antimicrobial [200], hepatoprotective [201], and analgesic activity [202].

2.21. *Withania somnifera*

Withania somnifera (WS) belongs to the Solanaceae family, commonly known as Ashwagandha. Traditionally this plant was named for its potential to calm the mind, the capacity to improve learning ability, memory power, and to improve poor eyesight. It is also named for anti-inflammatory potential in the treatment of joint diseases and an appropriate remedy for asthma and bronchitis [203]. Ashwagandha is one among the vast assorted variety of the restorative plant, which is exploited well for its phytopharmacological impact. The restorative properties of *Withania somnifera* are accessible both in the composed and non-composed arrangement as conventional information since time immemorial. In the conventional framework, the plant has been utilized as a calming, antitumor, antistress, cell reinforcement, immunomodulatory, and adaptogenic medicate. It likewise applies a positive effect on the endocrine, cardiopulmonary, and focal sensory systems with next to zero-related poisonous quality. It has the ability to battle growths by lessening tumor size and ended up being a decent regular wellspring of a sturdy and moderately safe radiosensitizer/chemo-remedial specialist.

2.21.1. Scientific evidences

This plant is proved to have anti-inflammatory activity [204], antioxidant property [205], anticancer properties [206], immunomodulatory potential [207], neuroprotective effects [208], cardioprotective and hypocholesteremic [209], and antimalarial potential [210].

Author details

Sudhakar Pola* and Venkata Narasimha Kadali

*Address all correspondence to: sudhakarpola@gmail.com

Department of Biotechnology, Andhra University, Visakhapatnam, India

References

[1] World Health Organization Guidelines on Safety Monitoring of Herbal Medicines in Pharmacovigilance Systems. Geneva, Switzerland: World Health Organization; 2004

[2] Ekor M. The growing use of herbal medicines: Issues relating to adverse reactions and challenges in monitoring safety. Frontiers in Pharmacology. 2014;**4**;article 177. DOI: 10.3389/fphar.2013.00177

[3] Kumar N, Wani ZA, Dhyani S. Ethnobotanical study of the plants used by the local people of Gulmarg and its allied areas, Jammu & Kashmir, India. International Journal of Current Research in Bioscience and Plant Biology. 2015;**2**(9):16-23

[4] Shakya AK. Medicinal plants: Future source of new drugs. International Journal of Herbal Medicine. 2016;**4**(4):59-64

[5] Pan S-Y, Zhou S-F, Gao S-H, Yu Z-L, Zhang S-F, Tang M-K, Sun J-N, Ma D-L, Han Y-F, Fong W-F, Ko K-M. New perspectives on how to discover drugs from herbal medicines: CAM's outstanding contribution to modern therapeutics. Evidence-Based Complementary and Alternative Medicine. 2013;**2013**, Article ID 627375, 25 pages. DOI: 10.1155/2013/627375

[6] Thang TD, Kuo PC, Huang GJ, Hung NH, Huang BS, Yang ML. Chemical constituents from the leaves of *Annona reticulata* and their inhibitory effects on NO production. Molecules. 2013;**18**:4477-4486

[7] Baskar R, Rajeswari V, Kumar TS. In vitro antioxidant studies in leaves of *Annona species*. Indian Journal of Experimental Biology. 2007;**45**(5):480-485

[8] Available from: http://www.hort.purdue.edu/newcrop/nexus/Annona_reticulata_nex.html

[9] Chavan SS, Shamkuwar PB, Damale MG, Pawar DP. A comprehensive review on *Annona reticulata*. International Journal of Pharmaceutical Sciences and Research. 2014;**5**(1):45-50. DOI: 10.13040/IJPSR.0975-8232.5(1).45-50

[10] Chang FR, Wu YC, Duh CY, Wang SK. Studies on the acetogenins of Formosan annonaceous plants. II. Cytotoxic acetogenins from *Annona reticulata*. Journal of Natural Products. 1993;**56**(10):1688-1694

[11] Available from: http://www.hort.purdue.edu/newcrop/morton/wild_custard_apple_ars.html

[12] Yuan SS, Chang HL, Chen HW, Yeh YT, Kao YH, Lin KH, Wu YC, Su JH. Annonacin, a mono-tetrahydrofuran acetogenin, arrests cancer cells at the G1 phase and causes cytotoxicity in a Bax- and caspase-3-related pathway. Life Sciences. 2003;**72**(25):2853-2861

[13] Yuan SS, Chang HL, Chen HW, Kuo FC, Liaw CC, Su JH, Wu YC. Selective cytotoxicity of squamocin on T24 bladder cancer cells at the S-phase via a Bax-, Bad-, and caspase-3-related pathways. Life Sciences. 2006;**78**(8):869-874

[14] Kaleem M, Asif M, Ahmad QU, Bano B. Antidiabetic and antioxidant activity of *Annona squamosa* extract in streptozotocin induced diabetic rats. Singapore Medical Journal. 2006;**47**:670-675

[15] Bhalke RD, Chavan MJ. Analgesic and CNS depressant activities of extracts of *Annona reticulata* Linn. Bark. Phytopharmacology. 2011;**1**(5):160-165

[16] Chopra RN, Nayer SL, Chopra IC. Glossary of Indian Medicinal Plant. New Delhi, India: National Institute of Science and Communication. C.S.I.R Publications; 1956

[17] Yoganarasimhan SN. Medicinal Plants of India. Vol. II. Bangalore: Cyber Media; 2000. p. 10

[18] Gunasekaran B, Selvarajan S, Balakrishnan D, Muralidharan P. Journal of Herbal Medicine and Toxicology. 2010;**4**(1):49-52

[19] Vairavasundaram RP, Kalaiselvi S. Drug Invention Today. 2009;**1**(2):137-139

[20] Vallabh D, Jadhav Varsha M, Kadam VJ. Journal of Pharmacy Research. 2009;**2**(4):644-645

[21] Paranjape Archana N, Mehta Anita A. Global journal of Pharmacology. 2008;**2**(2):23-30

[22] Adisakwattana S, Pudhom K, Yibchokanun S. African Journal of Biotechnology. 2009; **8**(10):2011-2015

[23] Golwala Dharmesh K, Patel Laxman D, Vaidya Santosh K, Bothara Sunil B, Munesh M, Piyush P. International Journal of Pharmacy and Pharmaceutical Sciences. 2010;**2**(1):66-71

[24] Roshan S, Ali S, Khan A, Tazneem B, Purohit MG. Pharmacognosy Magazine. 2008;**4**(15): 85-88

[25] Chandrashekhar VM, Nagappa AN, Channes TS, Habbu PV, Rao KP. Journal of Natural Remedies. 2000;**4**(1):12-16

[26] Rahuman AA, Gopalakrishnan G, Venkatesan P, Kannappan G. Parasitology Research. 2008;**102**:981-988

[27] Dash GK, Samanta A, Kanungo SK, Shau SK, Suresh P, Ganpathy S. Indian Journal of Natural Products. 2000;**16**(2):25-27

[28] Meena Prabha P, Chendraya Perumal P, Praveen Kumar M, Soundarrajan S, Srinivasan M, Sampathkumar R. Pharmacological activities of *Abrus precatorius* (L.) seeds. International Journal of Medical Research and Pharmaceutical Sciences. 2015;**3**(2):195-200

[29] Wingard LB, Larner J, Schwartz A. Human Pharmacology, Molecular to Clinical. Mosby Year Book; 1991. pp. 767-774

[30] Ligha AE, Bnr J, Numere NF. Protective effect of *Abrus precatorius* seed extract following alcohol induced renal damage. European Journal of Scientific Research. 2009;**25**(3): 428-436

[31] Sohn SH, Lee H, Nam JY, Kim SH, Jung HJ, Kim Y, Shin M, Hong M, Bae H. Screening of herbal medicines for the recovery of Cisplatin induced nephrotoxicity. Environmental Toxicology and Pharmacology. 2009;**28**:206-212

[32] Wambebe C, Amosun S. Some neuromuscular effects of the crude extracts of the leaves of *Abrus Precatorius*. Journal of Ethnopharmacology. 1984;**11**:49-58

[33] Mensah AY, Bonsu AS, Fleischer TC. Investigation of the bronchodilator activity of *Abrus Precatorius*. International Journal of Pharmaceutical Sciences Review and Research. 2011;**6**(2):09-13

[34] Limmatvapirat C, Sirisopanaporn S, Kittakoop P. Antitubercular and antiplasmodial constituents of *A. Precatorius*. Planta Medica. 2004;**70**:276-278

[35] Adesina SK. Studies on some plants used as anticonvulsants in Amerindian and African traditional medicine. Fitoterapia. 1982;**53**:147-162

[36] OFC N, Botting JH. Uterotonic activity of extracts of the seeds of *Abrus precatorius*. Planta Medica. 1983;**47**(4):230-233

[37] Saurabh R, Nagori BP, Singh GK, Dubey BK, Desai P, Alok S, Jain S. A review on Acacia Arabica—An Indian medicinal plant. IJPSR. 2012;**3**(7):1995-2005

[38] Maslin BR, Miller JT, Seigle DS. Overview of the generic status of *Acacia* (Leguminosae: Mimosoideae). Australian Systematic Botany. 2003;**16**(1):1-18

[39] Orchard AE, Maslin BR. Proposal to conserve the name *Acacia* (Leguminosae: Mimosoideae) with a conserved type. Taxon. 2003;**52**(2):362-363

[40] Singh KN, Chandra V, Barthwal KC. Hypoglycaemic activity of *Acacia arabica, Acacia benthamii* and *Acacia modesta* leguminous seed diet in normal albino rats. Indian Journal of Physiology and Pharmacology. 1975;**19**:167-168

[41] Jain AK, Shimoi K, Nakamura Y, Tomita I, Kada T. Preliminary study on the desmutagenic and antimutagenic effect of some natural products. Current Science. 1987;**56**:1266-1269

[42] Chhabra S, Thakral J, Kamboj P, Paliwal Y. Comparative evaluation of antimicrobial potential of different extracts of *Cuscuta reflexa* growing on *Acacia Arabica* and *Zizyphus jujube*. Pharmacognosy Journal. 2010;**2**(9):293-296

[43] Sundrial RC. Fungitoxic properties of flower extract of some wild plants of Grahwal Himalaya. Advances in Plant Sciences. 1991;**4**:230-234

[44] Agunua A, Yusuf S, Andrewa GO, Zezi AU, Abdurahmana EM. Evaluation of five medicinal plants used in diarrhoea treatment in Nigeria. Journal of Ethnopharmacology. 2005;**101**:27-30

[45] Singh R, Singh R. Screening of some plant extract for antiviral properties. Technology (Sindri). 1972;**9**:415-416

[46] Sharma W, Trivedi PC. Nemeticial and Nematostatic response of aqueous extract of certain plants of semi-arid niche. Current Nematology. 1995;**6**:43-53

[47] Singh R, Singh B, Singh S, Kumar N, Kumar S, Arora S. Umbelliferone—An antioxidant isolated from *Acacia Nilotica* (L.) Willd. Ex. Del. Food Chemistry. 2010;**120**:825-830

[48] Nath D, Sethi N, Singh RK, Jain AK. Commonly used Indian abortifacient plants with special reference to their teratologic effects in rats. Journal of Ethnopharmacology. 1992;**36**:147-154

[49] Thamizharasan S, Umamaheswari S, Hari R, Ulagaratchagan V. Quantitative phytochemical analysis of *Bambusa arundinacea* seeds. International Journal of Pharmacognosy and Phytochemical Research. 2015;**7**(5):980-983

[50] Rathod Jaimik D, Pathak Nimish L, Patel Ritesh G, Jivani NP, Bhatt Nayna M. Phytopharmacological properties of *Bambusa arundinacea* as a potential medicinal tree: An overview. Journal of Applied Pharmaceutical Science. 2011;**01**(10):27-31

[51] Vanithakumari G, Manonayagi S, Padma S, Malini T. Antifertility effect of *Bambusa arundinacea* shoot extracts in male rats. Journal of Ethnopharmacology. 1989;**25**(2):173

[52] Zhang J, Gong J, Ding Y, Lu B, Wu X, Zhang Y. Antibacterial activity of water-phase extracts from bamboo shavings against food spoilage microorganisms. African Journal of Biotechnology. 2010;**9**(45):7710-7717

[53] Muniappan M, Sundararaj T. Antiinflammatory and antiulcer activities of *Bambusa arundinacea*. Journal of Ethnopharmacology. 2003;**88**:161-167

[54] Honga E-J, Junga E-M, Leea G-S, Kima JY, Naa K-J, Parkb M-J, Kangb H-Y, Seonga K-CCYH, Choic I-G, Jeunga E-B. Protective effects of the pyrolyzates derived from bamboo

against neuronal damage and hematoaggregation. Journal of Ethanopharmacology. 2010; **128**(3):594-599

[55] Mahesh AR, Kumar H, Ranganath MK, Devkar RA. Detail study on *Boerhaavia Diffusa* plant for its medicinal importance—A review research journal of pharmaceutical sciences res. Journal of Pharmaceutical Sciences. 2012;**1**(1):28-36

[56] Rawat AKS, Mehrotra S, Tripathi SC, Shome U. Hepatoprotective activity of *Boerhaavia diffusa* L. roots a popular Indian ethnomedicine. Journal of Ethnopharmacology. 1997; **56**:61-66

[57] Bhatia V, Kinja K, Bishnoi H. Antidiabetic activity of the alcoholic extract of the arial part of *Boerhaavia diffusa* in rats. In and Gnaneshwari D editors. Recent Research in Science and Technology. 2001;**3**(7):04-07

[58] Sharma M, Vohra S, Arnason JT, Hudson JB. Echinacea extracts contain significant and selective activities against human pathogenic bacteria. Pharmaceutical Biology. 2008;**46**:111-116

[59] Hiruma Lima CA, Gracioso JS, Bighetti EJB. Germonse'n Robineou L. and Souza Brito a.R.M., the juice of fresh leaves of *Boerhaavia diffusa* L. (Nyctaginaceae) markedly reduces pain in mice. Journal of Ethnopharmacology. 2000;**71**(1-2):267-274

[60] Bharali R, Azad MRH, Tabassum J. Chemopreventive action of *Boerhaavia diffusa* on DMBA-induced skin carcinogenesis in mice. Indian Journal of Physiology and Pharmacology. 2003;**47**(4):459-464

[61] Kaur M, Goel RK. Anti-convulsant activity of *Boerhaavia diffusa*: Plausible role of calcium channel antagonism. Evidence-Based Complementary and Alternative Medicine. 2011;**4**:1-7

[62] Sreeja S, Sreeja S. An in vitro study on antiproliferative and antiestrogenic effects of *Boerhaavia diffusa* L. extracts. Journal of Ethnopharmacology. 1923;**126**:221-225

[63] Nwakanma NMC, Okoli BE. Cytological effects of the root extracts of *Boerhaavia diffusa* on root tips of Crinum jagus. EurAsian Journal of BioSciences. 2010;**4**:105-111

[64] Sasikala M, Vijay SK, Gauthaman K. Relevance of the use of alternative medicine for bronchial asthma: A review. Journal of Young Pharmacists. 2009;**1**(2):184-189

[65] Barthwal M, Srivastava K. Histologic studies on endometrium of menstruating monkeys wearing IUDs: Comparative evaluation of drugs. Advances in Contraception. 1990;**6**:113-124

[66] Chaudhary P, Ahamad S, Khan NA. A review on medicinal utility of *Calotropis Procera*. WJPMR. 2017;**3**(1):335-342

[67] Pusapati MR, Eswara Rao G, Krishnapriya M, Nagalakshmi V, Silpa P, Anjali M. An overview of phytochemical and pharmacological activities of *Calotropis procera*. FS Journal of Pharmacy Research. 2012;**1**(2):17-25

[68] Setty SR, Quereshi AA, Viswanath Swamy AHM, Patil T, Prakash T, Prabhu K, Gouda Veeran A. Hepatoprotective activity of *Calotropis procera* flowers against paracetamol induced hepatic injury in rats. Fitoterapia. 2007;**78**(7):451-454

[69] Ahmad N, Anwar F, Hameed S, Boyce MC. Antioxidant and antimicrobial attributes of different solvent extracts from leaves and flowers of *Calotropis procera*. Journal of Medicinal Plants Research. 2011;**5**(19):4879-4887

[70] Dewan S, Kumar S, Kumar VL. Preliminary studies on the analgesic activity of latex of *Calotropris procera*. Journal of Ethnopharmacology. 2000;**32**:252-253

[71] Larhsini M, Bousaid M, Lazrek HB, Jana M. Evaluation of antifungal and molluscicidal properties of extracts of *Calotropis procera*. Fitotrapia. 1997;**68**:371-373

[72] Majumder PK, Kumar VL. Anti-inflammatory activity of fractions of latex of *Calotropis procera* in carrageenan induced rat paw oedema. Phytotherapy Research. 1997;**11**(2):166-167

[73] Kumar S, Dewan S, Sangraula H, Kumar VL. Antidiarrhoeal activity of the latex of *Calotropis procera*. Journal of Ethnopharmacology. 2001;**76**(1):115-118

[74] Kumar VL, Shivkar YM. In vivo and in vitro effect of latex of *Calotropis procera* on gastrointestinal smooth muscles. Journal of Ethnopharmacology. 2004;**93**(2-3):377-379

[75] Roy S, Sehgal R, Padhy BM, Kumar VL. Antioxidant and protective effect of latex of *Calotropis procera* against alloxan induced diabetes in rats. Journal of Ethnopharmacology. 2005;**102**(3):470-473

[76] Basu A, Sen T, Pal S, Mascolo N, Capasso F, Nag AK. Studies on the antiulcer activity of the chloroform fraction of *Calotropis procera* root extract. Phytotherapy Research. 1996;**11**(2):163-165

[77] Rasik AM, Raghubir R, Gupta A, Shukla A, Dubey MP, Srivastava S, Jain HK, Kulshrestha DK. Healing potential of *Calotropis procera* on dermal wounds in guinea pigs. Journal of Ethnopharmacology. 1999;**68**(3):261-266

[78] Grover JK, Yadav SP. Pharmacological actions and potential uses of *Momordica charantia*: A review. Journal of Ethnopharmacology. 2004;**93**(1):123-132

[79] Sathishsekar D, Subramanian S. Antioxidant properties of *Momordica Charantia* (bitter gourd) seeds on Streptozotocin induced diabetic rats. Asian Pacific the Journal of Clinical Nutrition. 2005;**14**(2):153-158

[80] Virdia J, Sivakamia S, Shahanib S, Sutharc AC, Banavalikar MM, Biyanic MK. Antihyperglycemic effects of three extracts from *Momordica charantia*. Journal of Ethnopharmacology. 2003;**88**(1):107-111

[81] Cunnick JE, Sakamoto K, Chapes SK, Fortner GW, Takemoio DJ. Induction of tumor cytotoxic immune cells using a protein from the bitter melon (*Momordica charantia*). Cellular Immunology. 1990;**126**(2):278

[82] Bourinbaiar AS, Lee-Huang S. The activity of plant derived antiretroviral proteins MAP30 and GAP31 against *Herpes simplex* virus in vitro. Biochemical and Biophysical Research Communications. 1996;**219**(3):923-929

[83] Stepka W, Wilson KE, Madge GE. Antifertility investigation on *Momordica*. Lloydia. 1974;**37**(4):645c

[84] Das AK, Mandal SC, Banerjee SK, Sinha S, Das J, Saha BP, Pal M. Studies on antidiarrheal activity of *Punica granatum* seed extract in rats. Journal of Ethnopharmacology. 1999;**68**:205-208

[85] Jafri MA, Aslam M, Javed K, Singh S. Effect of *Punica granatum* Linn. (flowers) on blood glucose level in normal and alloxan induced diabetic rats. Journal of Ethnopharmacology. 2000;**70**:309-314

[86] Zhicen L. Colour Atlas of Chinese Traditional Drugs. Vol. 1. Beijing, People's Republic of China: Science Press; 1987. pp. 75-76

[87] Kapoor LD. CRC Handbook of Ayurvedic Medicinal Plants. Boca Raton, Florida: CRC Press; 1990

[88] Murthy KN, Reddy VK, Veigas JM, Murthy UD. Study on wound healing activity of *Punica granatum* peel. Journal of Medicinal Food. 2004;**7**:256-259

[89] Nugteren DH, Christ-Hazelhof E. Naturally occurring conjugated octadecatrienoic acids are strong inhibitors of prostaglandin biosynthesis. Prostaglandins. 1987;**33**:403-417

[90] Esmaillzadeh A, Tahbaz F, Gaieni I, Alavi-Majd H, Azadbakht L. Cholesterol-lowering effect of concentrated pomegranate juice consumption in type II diabetic patients with hyperlipidemia. International Journal Vitamin Nutritional Resources. 2006;**76**(3):147-151

[91] Lansky EP, Newman RA. *Punica granatum* (pomegranate) and its potential for prevention and treatment of inflammation and cancer. Journal of Ethnopharmacology. 2007;**109**(2):177-206

[92] Krishnamurthi A. The Wealth of India. Vol. VIII. New Delhi, India: Publication and Information Directorate CSIR; 1969

[93] Naik M, Meher LC, Naik SN, Dasa LM. Production of biodiesel from high free fatty acid Karanja (*Pongamia pinnata*) oil. Biomass and Bioenergy. 2008;**32**:354-357

[94] Punitha R, Manohar S. Antihyperglycemic and anti-lipid peroxidative effects of *Pongamia pinnata* (Linn.) Pierre flowers in alloxan induced diabetic rats. Journal of Ethnopharmacology. 2006;**105**:39-46

[95] Essa MM, Subramanian P, Sudhakar G, Manivasagam T, Dakshayani KB. Protective influence of *Pongamia pinnata* (Karanja) on blood ammonia and urea levels in ammonium chloride induced hyperammonemia. Journal of Applied Biomedicine. 2005;**3**:133-138

[96] Singh RK, Joshi VK, Goel RK. Pharmacological actions of *Pongamia pinnata* seeds—A preliminary study. Indian Journal of Experimental Biology. 1996;**34**:1204-1207

[97] Rameshthangam P, Ramasamy P. Antiviral activity of bis (2-methylheptyl) phthalate isolated from *Pongamia pinnata* leaves against white spot syndrome virus of Penaeus monodon Fabricius. Virus Research. 2007;**126**(1-2):38-44

[98] Uddin Q, Parveen N, Khan NU, Singhal KC. Antifilarial potential of the fruits and leaves extracts of *Pongamia pinnata* on cattle filarial parasite. Phytotherapy Research. 2003;**17**(9):104-110

[99] Akhtar AH, Ahmad KD, Gilani SN, Nazir A. Antiulcer effects of aqueous extracts of Nigella sativa and *Pongamia pinnata* in rats. Fitoterapia. 1996;**67**(3):195-199

[100] Singh RK, Pandey BL. Anti-inflammatory potential of *Pongamia pinnata* root extracts in experimentally induced inflammation in rats. Journal Basic Applied Biomed. 1996; **4**:21-24

[101] Srinivasan K, Muruganandan S, Lal J, Chandra S, Tandan SK, Raviprakash V, Kumar D. Antinociceptive and antipyretic activities of *Pongamia pinnata* leaves. Phytotherapy Research. 2003;**17**:259-264

[102] Dorman HJ, Deans SG. Antimicrobial agents from plants: Antibacterial activity of plant volatile oils. Journal of Applied Microbiology. 2000;**88**:308-316

[103] El Hamss R, Idaomar M, Alonso-Moraga A, Muñoz Serrano A. Antimutagenic properties of bell and black pepper. Food and Chemical Toxicology. 2003;**41**:41-47

[104] Satyavati G, Gupta AK, Neeraj T. Medicinal Plants of India. Vol. 2. New Delhi: Indian Council of Medical Research; 1987

[105] Dhanalakshmi D, Umamaheswari S, Balaji D, Santhanalakshmi R, Kavimani S. Phytochemistry and pharmacology of *Piper longum*—A systematic review. World Journal of Pharmacy and Pharmaceutical Sciences. 2017;**6**(1):381-398. DOI: 10.20959/Wjpps20171-8362

[106] Natarajan KS, Narasimhan M, Shanmugasundaram KR, Shanmugasundaram ER. Antioxidant activity of a salt/ spice/herbal mixture against free radical induction. Journal of Ethnopharmacology. 2006;**105**:76-83

[107] Vedhanayaki G, Shastri GV, Kuruvilla A. Analgesic activity of *Piper longum* Linn. root. Indian Journal of Experimental Biology. 2003;**41**:649-651

[108] Yende SR, Sannapuri VD, Vyawahare NS, et al. Antirheumatoid activity of aqueous extract of *Piper longum* on freunds adjuvant-induced arthritis in rats. IJPSR. 2010;**1**(9): 129-133

[109] Bezerra DP, Castro FO, Alves APNN, et al. In vivo growth-inhibition of Sarcoma180 by piplartine and piperine, two alkaloid amides from piper. Brazilian Journal of Medical and Biological Research. 2006;**39**:801-807

[110] Nabi SA, Kasetti RB, Sirasanagandla S, et al. Antidiabetic and antihyperlipidemic activity of *Piper longum* root aqueous extract in STZ induced diabetic rats. BMC Complementary and Alternative Medicine. 2013;**13**:37

[111] Lakshmi V, Kumar R, Agarwal SK, et al. Anti-fertility activity of *Piper longum* Linn. in female rats. Natural Product Research. 2006;**20**(3):235-239

[112] Shenoy PA, Nipate SS, Sonpetkar JM, et al. Anti-snake venom activities of ethanolic extract of fruits of *Piper longum* L. (Piperaceae) against *Russell's viper* venom: Characterization of piperine as active principle. Journal of Ethnopharmacology. 2013;**147**(2): 373-382

[113] Kim KS, Kim JA, Eom SY, Lee SH, Min KR, Kim Y. Inhibitory effect of piperlonguminine on melanin production in melanoma B16 cell line by downregulation of tyrosinase expression. Pigment Cell Research. 2006;**19**:90-98

[114] Bajad S, Bedi KL, Singla AK, Johri RK. Piperine inhibits gastric emptying and gastrointestinal transit in rats and mice. Planta Medica. 2001;**67**(2):176-179

[115] de Assis Junior EM, dos Santos Fernandes IM, Santos CS, de Mesquita LX, Pereira RA, Maracaja PB, Soto-Blanco B. Toxicity of castor bean (*Ricinus communis*) pollen to honeybees. Agriculture, Ecosystems and Environment. 2011;**141**:221-223

[116] Rana M, Dhamija H, Prashar B, Sharma S. *Ricinus communis* L.—A review. International Journal PharmTech, Research. 2012;**4**(4):1706-1711

[117] Panghal M et al. In vitro antimicrobial activity of ten medicinalplants against clinical isolates of oral cancercases. Annals of Clinical Microbiology and Antimicrobials. 2011;**10**:21

[118] Singh PP et al. Activity guided isolation of antioxidants from the leaves of *Ricinus communis* L. Food Chemistry. 2009;**114**(3):1069-1072

[119] Okwuasaba FK et al. Anticonceptive and estrogenic effects of a seedextract of *Ricinus communisvar.* minor. Journal of Ethnopharmacology. 1991;**34**:141-145

[120] Ilavarasan R et al. Anti-inflammatory and free radical scavengingactivity of *Ricinus communis* root extract. Journal of Ethnopharmacology. 2006;**103**:478-480

[121] Ferraz AC et al. Pharmacological evaluation of ricinine, a central nervous system stimulant isolated from *Ricinus communis*. Pharmacology Biochemistry and Behavior. 1999;**63**(3):367-375

[122] Lin JY et al. Studies on the antitumour lectins isolated from the seeds of *Ricinus communis* (castor bean). Toxicon. 1986;**24**(8):757-765

[123] Mandal S. Exploration of larvicidal and adult emergence inhibition activities of *Ricinus communis* seed extract against three potential mosquito vectors in Kolkata, India. Asian Pacific Journal of Tropical Medicine. 2010;**3**(8):605-609

[124] Rachhadiya RM, Prasad KM, Shete Rajkumar V. Evaluation of antiulcer activity of castor oil in rats. International Journal of Research in Ayurveda & Pharmacy. 2011;**2**(4):1349-1353

[125] Elimam AM, Elmalik KH, Ali FS. Larvicidal, adult emergence inhibition and oviposition deterrent effects of foliage extract from *Ricinus communis* L. against anopheles arabiensis and Culex Quinquefasciatus in Sudan. Tropical Biomedicine. 2009;**26**(2):130-139

[126] Islam T et al. Assessment of antibacterial potential of leaves of *Ricinus communis* against pathogenic and dermatophytic bacteria. International Journal of PharmaResearch and Development. 2010;**1**(12):1-7

[127] Shokeen P et al. Antidiabetic activity of 50% ethanolic extract of *Ricinus communis* and its purified fractions. Food and Chemical Toxicology. 2008, 2008;**46**:3458-3466

[128] Valderramas AC et al. Antiinflammatory activity of *Ricinus communis* derived polymer. Brazilian Journal of Oral Sciences. 2008;**7**(27):1666-1672

[129] Wealth of Indian. A Dictionary of Indian Raw materials and Industrial Products. National Institute of Science Communication, Council of Scientific and Industrial Research, New Delhi. Raw Material. 2002;**10**:100-107

[130] Sah AK, Verma VK. *Syzygium cumini* : An overview. Journal of Chemical and Pharmaceutical Research. 2011;**3**(3):108-113

[131] Brito FA, Lima LA, Ramos MF, Nakamura MJ, Cavalher Machados SC, Henrigues MG, Sampaino AL. Pharmacological study of anti-allergic activity of *Syzygium cumini* (L) Skeels. Brazillian Journal of Medical and Biological Research. 2007;**40**:105-115

[132] Chaturvedi A, Kumar MM, Bhawani G, Chaturvedi H. Effect of ethanolic extract of *Eugenia jambolana* seeds on gastric ulceration and secretion in rats. Indian Journal of Physiology and Pharmacology. 2007;**51**(2):131-140

[133] Dasgupta N. In vivo study of antioxidant activity of *S. cumini* fruit. Food Chemistry. 2005;**90**(4):727-733

[134] Kumar A, Padmanabhan N, Krishnan MRV. Central nervous system activity of *Syzygium cumini* seed. Pakistan Journal of Nutrition. 2007;**6**(6):698-700

[135] Muruganandan S, Srinivasan K, Chandra S, Tandan SK, Lal J, Raviprakash V. Anti-inflammatory activity of *Syzygium cumini* bark. Fitoterapia. 2001;**72**(4):369-375

[136] Kasiappan R, Subbaih R, Subramanian S. Antihyperlipidemic effect of *Eugenia jambolana* seed kernel on streptozotocin induced diabetes rats. Food and Chemistry Toxicology. 2005;**43**(9):1433-1439

[137] Namba TM, Tsunezuka NK, Dissanayake UP, Hattori M. Studies on dental caries prevention by traditional medicines part VII, screening of ayurvedic medicines for anti-plaque action. Shoyakugaku Zasshi. 1985;**39**(2):146

[138] Chaudhari AKN, Pal S, Gomes A, Bhattacharya S. Anti-inflammatory and related actions of *Syzygium cumini* seed extract. Phytotherapy Research. 1990;**4**(1):5-10

[139] Dhawan BN, Patnaik GK, Rastogi RP, Singh KK, Tandon JS. Screening of Indian plants for biological activity. Indian Journal of Experimental Biology. 1977;**15**:208-219

[140] Rana NS, Joshi MN. Investigation on the antiviral activity of ethanolic extracts of *Syzygium* species. Fitoterpia. 1992;**63**(3):542-544

[141] Srinithya B, Muthuraman MS. An overview on the biological perspectives of *Sida Cordifolia* Linn. International Journal of Pharmacy and Pharmaceutical Sciences. 2014;**6**(11):15-17

[142] Pawar RS, Kumar S, Toppo FA, Lakshmi PK, Suryavanshi P. *Sida cordifolia* Linn. Accelerates wound healing process in type 2 diabetic rats. Journal of Acute Medicine. 2016;**6**:82-89. DOI: 10.1016/j.jacme.2016.08.004

[143] Sutradhar RK, Rahman AKMM, Ahmad MU, Bachar SC. Bioactive flavones of *Sida cordifolia*. Phytochemistry Letters. 2011;**1**:179-182

[144] Franzotti EM, CVF S, Rodrigues HMSL, RHV M, Andrade MR, Antoniolli AR. Anti-inflammatory, analgesic activity and acute toxicity of *Sida cordifolia* L. (Malva-branca). Journal of Ethnopharmacology. 2000;**72**:273-278

[145] Akilandeswari S, Valarmathi R, Indulatha VN, Senthamarai R. Screening of gastric anti-ulcer activity of *Sida cordifolia*. International journal of pharmaceutical and chemical sciences. 2013;**2**(3):1288-1292

[146] Kanth VR, Diwan PV. Analgesic, anti-inflammatory and hypoglycaemic activities of *Sida cordifolia* L. Phytotherapy Research. 1999;**13**(1):75-77

[147] Lovkesh B, Vivek B, Manav G. Nephroprotective effect of fresh leaves extracts of *sida cordifolia* linn in gentamicin induced nephrotoxicity in rats. International Journal of Research in Pharmaceutical Sciences. 2012;**2**(2):151-158

[148] Joseph B, Ajisha AU, Kumari S, Sujatha S. Effect of bioactive compounds and its pharmaceutical activities of *Sida cordifolia* (Linn.). International Journal of Biological and Medical Research. 2011;**2**(4):1038-1042

[149] Kaur G, Kamboj P, Kalia AN. Antidiabetic and anti-hypercholesterolemic effects of aerial parts of *Sida cordifolia* L. on Streptozotocin induced diabetic rats. Indian Journal of Natural Products and Resources. 2011;**2**(4):428-434

[150] Rao KS, Mishra SH. Isolation and assessment of hepatoprotective activity of fumaric acid obtained for the first time from *Sida cordifolia* Linn. Indian Drugs. 1997;**34**(12):702-706

[151] Medeiros IA, Santos MRV, Nascimento NMS, Duarte JC. Cardiovascular effects of *Sida cordifolia* leaves extract in rats. Fitoterapia. 2006;**77**:19-27

[152] Mallikarjuna G, Jaya Sankar Reddy V, Prabhakaran V. Evaluation of anticancer activity of *Sida cordifolia* l. against aflatoxin b1 induced hepatocellular carcinoma. International Journal of Pharmaceutical Sciences Review and Research. 2013;**23**(2):126-132

[153] Sonawane SM, Sonawane H. A review of recent and current research studies on the biological and pharmalogical activities of *Sapindus Mukorossi*. International Journal of Interdisciplinary Research and Innovations. 2015;**3**(4):85-95

[154] Arora B, Bhadauria P, Tripathi D, Sharma A. *Sapindus Emarginatus*: Phytochemistry & various biological activities. Indo Global Journal oh Pharmaceutical Sciences. 2012;**2**(3):250-257

[155] Sharma A, Sati SC, Sati OP, Kothiyal SK. Chemical Constituents and Bioactivities of Genus Sapindus. IJRAP. 2011;**2**(2):403-409

[156] Upadhay A, Singh DK. "Pharmacological Effects of *Sapindus mukorossi*" DDU Gorakhpur University, Gorakhpur, U.P. India. Revista do Instituto de Medicina Tropical de São Paulo. 2012;**54**(5):273-280

[157] Bhargava D, Shivapuri JN, Kar S, Pandit BR, Sidhiqie A, Upadhyay A, Thakur S, Mondal KC. Evaluation of antigonorrhoeal activity of saponins extract of *Sapindus Mukorossi* Gaertn. Research Journal of Pharmaceutical, Biological and Chemical Sciences. 2012; **7**(2):459-470

[158] Moghimipouri E, Handali S. Saponin: Properties, Methods of evaluation and Applications. Annual Research & Review in Biology, Science Domain International; 2015;**5**(3):207-220

[159] Huang HC, Liao SC, Chang FR, Kuo YH, Wu YC. Molluscicidal saponins from *Sapindus mukorossi*, inhibitory agents of golden apple snails *Pomacea canaliculata*. Journal of Agricultural and Food Chemistry. 2003;**51**:4916-4919

[160] Gupta SK, Zafar R, Pathak D. Review of phytochemical and pharmacological aspects of steroidal saponins from *Tribulus terrestris*. Indian Drugs. 1997;**4**(8):422-426

[161] Chhatre S, Nesari T, Somani G, Kenjale R, Sathaye S. Comparative evaluation of diuretic activity of different extracts of *Tribulus terrestris* fruits in experimental animals. International Journal of Research in Phytochemistry and Pharmacology. 2012;**3**:129-133

[162] Singh S, Nair V, Gupta YK. Evaluation of the aphrodisiac activity of *Tribulus terrestris* Linn. in sexually sluggish male albino rats. Journal of Pharmacology and Pharmacotherapeutics. 2012;**3**:43 7

[163] Sangeeta D, Sidhu H, Thind SK, Nath R. Effect of *Tribulus terrestris* on oxalate metabolism in rats. Journal of Ethnopharmacology.1994;**44**:61-6

[164] Tilwari A, Shukla NP, Devi U. Effect of five medicinal plants used in Indian system of medicines on immune function in Wistar rats. African Journal of Biotechnology. 2011;**10**:16637-45

[165] Amin A, Lotfy M, Shafiullah M, Adeghate E. The protective effect of *Tribulus terrestris* in diabetes. Annals of the New York Academy of Sciences. 2006;**1084**:391-401

[166] Tuncer MA, Yaymaci B, Sati L, Cayli S, Acar G, Altug T, Demir R. Influence of *Tribulus terrestris* extract on lipid profile and endothelial structure in developing atherosclerotic lesions in the aorta of rabbits on a high cholesterol diet. Acta Histochemica. 2009;**111**: 488 500

[167] Deole YS, Chavan SS, Ashok BK, Ravishankar B, Thakar AB, Chandola HM. Evaluation of antidepressant and anxiolytic activity of Rasayana Ghana tablet (a compound Ayurvedic formulation) in albino mice. Ayu. 2011;**32**:375 9

[168] Kumar M, Panwar M, Samarth R, Kumar A. Evaluation of radiomodulatory influence of *Tribulus terrestris* root extract against gamma radiation: Hematological, biochemical and cytogenetic alterations in swiss albino mice. Pharmacology Online. 2009;**1**: 1214-28

[169] El Sheikh TM, Bosly HA, Shalaby NM. Insecticidal and repellent activities of methanolic extract of *Tribulus terrestris* L. (Zygophyllaceae) against the malarial vector Anopheles arabiensis (Diptera: Culicidae). Egyptian Academic Journal of Biological Sciences. 2012;**5**:13-22

[170] Dinesh MD, Soorya TM, Vismaya MR, Janardhanan D, Athira TP, Nidhin KB, Ajeesh PP. Terminalia chebula A traditional herbal drug—A short review. International Journal of Pharmaceutical Science Invention. 2047;**6**(2):39-40

[171] Kannan P, Ramadevi SR, Hopper W. Antibacterial activity of *Terminalia chebula* fruit extract. African Journal of Microbiology Research. 2009;**3**(4):180-184

[172] Sohni YR, Bhatt RM. Activity of a crude extract formulation in experimental hepatic amoebiasis and in immunomodulation studies. Journal of Ethnopharmacology. 1996; **54**(2-3):119-124

[173] Shin TY, Jeong HJ, Kim DK, Kim SH, Lee JK, Kim DK, Chae BS, Kim JH, Kang HW, Lee CM, Lee KC, Park ST, Lee EJ, Lim JP, Kim HM, Leen YM. Inhibitory action of water soluble fraction of *Terminalia chebula* on systemic and local anaphylaxis. Journal of Ethnopharmacology. 2001;**74**:133-140

[174] Lin LT, Chen TY, Chung CY, Noyce RS, Grindley TB, McCormick C, Lin TC, Wang GH, Lin CC, Richardson CD. Hydrolyzable tannins (chebulagic acid and punicalagin) target viral glycoprotein-glycosaminoglycan interactions to inhibit herpes simplex virus 1 entry and cell-to-cell spread. Journal of Virology. 2011;**85**(9):4386-4398

[175] Ponnusankar S, Pandit S, Babu R, Bandyopadhyay A, Mukherjee PK. Cytochrome P450 inhibitory potential of Triphala-A Rasayana from Ayurveda. Journal of Ethnopharmacology. 2011;**133**(1):120-125

[176] Nair V, Singh S, Gupta YK. Anti-arthritic and disease modifying activity of *Terminalia chebula* Retz. in experimental models. The Journal of Pharmacy and Pharmacology. 2010;**62**(12):1801-1806

[177] Murali YK, Anand P, Tandon V, Singh R, Chandra R, Murthy PS. Long-term effects of *Terminalia chebula* Retz. on hyperglycemia and associated hyperlipidemia, tissue glycogen content and in vitro release of insulin in streptozotocin induced diabetic rats. Experimental and Clinical Endocrinology & Diabetes. 2007;**115**(10):641-646

[178] Tasduq SA, Singh K, Satti NK, Gupta DK, Suri KA. *Terminalia chebula* (fruit) prevents liver toxicity caused by sub-chronic administration of rifampicin, isoniazid and pyrazinamide in combination. Human & Experimental Toxicology. 2006;**25**:111-118

[179] Akanksha B, Avijit M, Chakraborthy GS, Seema G. Phytopharmacological uses of *Tephrosia Purpurea*—A review. Pharmacophore. 2014;**5**(4):658-665

[180] Kumari S, Srivastava M, Abbasi P. Response of *Tephrosia purpurea* to salinity stress in relation to germination, carotenoid content and proline content. An International Quarterly Journal of Biology & Life Sciences. 2014;**2**:276-281

[181] Kavitha K, Manoharan S. Anticarcinogenic and antilipidperoxidative effects of *Tephrosia purpurea* (Linn.) Pers. (tpet) on 7, 12-dimethylbenz (a) anthracene (DMBA)-induced hamster buccal pouch carcinoma. Indian Journal of Pharmacology. 2006;**38**(3):185-189

[182] Gopalakrishnan S, Vadivel E, Dhanalakshmi K. Antiinflammatory and analgesic activities of *Tephrosia purpurea* Linn. aerial and root extracts. Journal of Pharmacy Research. 2010;**3**(5):1103-1106

[183] Shah R, Kathad H, Sheth R, Sheth N. In vitro antioxidant activity of roots of *Tephrosia purpurea* Linn. International Journal of Pharmacy and Pharmaceutical Sciences. 2010;**2**(3):30-33

[184] Gulecha V, Sivakuma T. Anticancer activity of *Tephrosia purpurea* and Ficus religiosa using MCF 7 cell lines. Asian Pacific Journal of Tropical Medicine. 2011;**4**(7):526-529

[185] Manjula RR, Spandana U, Joshi AT, Sudheer M. In vitro anthelmintic activity of aqueous and methanolic leaf extract of *Tephrosia purpurea* linn. International Journal of Research in Pharmacy and Chemistry. 2013;**3**(1):12-14

[186] Keiding H, Wellendorf H, Lauridsen EB. Evaluation of an International Series of Teak Rovenance Trials. Humlebaek, Denmark: Danida Forest Seed Center; 1986

[187] Kjaer ED, Lauridsen EB, Wellendorf H. Second Evaluation of an International Series of Teak Provenance Trials. Humlebaek, Denmark: Danida Forest Seed Centre; 1995

[188] Jaybhaye D, Varma S, Gagne N, Bonde V, Gite A, Bhosle D. Effect of *Tectona grandis* Linn. seeds on hair growth activity of albino mice. International Journal of Ayurveda Research. 2010;**1**(3):163-166

[189] Rafullah MK, Suleiman MM. 5-Hydroxylapachol: A cytotoxic agent from *Tectona grandis*. Phytochemistry. 1999;**50**:439-442

[190] Aboudoulatif D, Messanvi G, Ahoefa V, Kwashie EG, Kodjo A, Amegnona A, et al. Effect of *Tectona grandis* on phenylhydrazine-induced anaemia in rats. Fitoterapia. 2008;**79**:332-336

[191] Varma SB, Jaybhaye DL. Antihyperglycemic activity of *Tectona grandis* Linn. bark extract on alloxan induced diabetes in rats. Natural Product Research. 2010;**24**(11):1059-1068

[192] Ramachandran S, Rajinikanth B, Rajasekaran A, Manisenthil Kumar KT. Evaluation of anti-inflammatory and analgesic potential of methanol extract of *Tectona grandis* flowers. Asian Pacific Journal of Tropical Biomedicine. 2011;**1**(2):S155-S158

[193] Kore KJ, Jadhav PJ, Shete RV, Shetty SC. Diuretic activity of *Tectona grandis* leaves aqueous extract in wistar rats. International Journal of Pharmaceutical Research and Development. 2011;**3**(7):141-146

[194] Neetu S, Nivedita S, Pratibha S, Rolee S, Rajendran SM, Rakesh M, et al. Verbascoside isolated from *Tectona grandis* mediates gastric protection in rats via inhibiting proton pump activity. Fitoterapia. 2010;**81**:755-761

[195] Havinga RM, Hartl A, Putscher J, Prehsler S, Buchmann C, Vogl CR. *Tamarindus indica* L. (Fabaceae): Patterns of use in traditional African medicine. Journal of Ethnopharmacology. 2010;**127**(3):573-588

[196] Bhadoriya SS, Ganeshpurkar A, Narwaria J, Rai G, Jain AP. *Tamarindus indica*: Extent of explored potential. Pharmacognosy Reviews. 2011;**5**(9):73-81

[197] Izquierdo T, Gracia-Tamayo F, Soto C, Castrillon LEA. *Tamarindus indica* Linn pulp polysaccharide inhibits fever in-vivo and IL-1β release by murine peritoneal exudates cell. Pharmaceutical Biology. 2007;**45**:22-30

[198] AL-fatimi M, Wurster M, Schroder G, Lindeiquist U. Antioxidant antimicrobial and cytotoxic activities of selected medicinal plant from Yemen. Journal of Ethnopharmacology. 2007;**111**:657-666

[199] Khan RA, Siddiqui SA, Azhar I, Ahmed SP. Preliminary screening of methanol and butanol extract of *Tamarindus indica* for anti-emetic activity. Journal of Basic and Applied Sciences. 2005;**1**:51-54

[200] Nwodo UU, Obiiyeke GE, Chigor VN, Okoh A. Assessment of *Tamarindus indica* extracts for antibacterial activity. International Journal of Molecular Sciences. 2011;**12**:6385-6396

[201] Mahesh KM, Rao KM, Rajeswari G, Ravindra Reddy KR, Jyothi B. Hepatoprotective activity of ethanolic flower extract of *Tamarindus indica* in Wistar rats hepatotoxicity induced by isoniazide and rifampicin. IJAPR. 2010;**1**(1):17-20

[202] Khalid S, Shaik Mossadeq WM, Isaraf DA, Hashim P, Rajeb S, Shaberi AM, Mohamada AS, Zakaria ZA, Sulaiman MR. *In Vivo* analgesic effect of aqueous extract of *Tamarindus indica* Linn. fruits. International Journal of the Kuwait University, Health Science Centre. 2010;**19**(4):255-259

[203] John J. Therapeutic potential of *Withania somnifera*: A report on phyto-pharmacological properties. International Journal of Pharmaceutical Sciences and Research. 2014;**5**(6):2131-2148. DOI: 10.13040/IJPSR.0975-8232.5(6).2131-48

[204] Rasool M, Varalakshmi P. Immunomodulatory role of *Withania somnifera* root powder on experimental induced inflammation: An in vivo and in vitro study. Vascular Pharmacology. 2006;**44**(6):406-410

[205] Bhattacharya A, Ghosal S, Bhattacharya SK. Anti oxidant effect of *Withania somnifera* glycowithanolides in chronic footshock stress-induced perturbations of oxidative free radical scavenging enzymes and lipid peroxidation in rat frontal cortex and striatum. Journal of Ethnopharmacology. 2001;**74**(1):1-6

[206] Muralikrishnan G, Dinda AK, Shakeel F. Immunomodulatory effects of *Withania somnifera* on azoxymethane induced experimental colon cancer in mice. Immunological Investigations. 2010;**39**(7):688-698

[207] Ziauddin M, Phansalkar N, Patki P, et al. Studies on the immunomodulatory effects of Ashwagandha. Journal of Ethnopharmacology. 1996;**50**(2):69-76

[208] Jain S, Shukla SD, Sharma K, et al. Neuroprotective effects of *Withania somnifera* Dunn. in hippocampal subregions of female albino rat. Phytotherapy Research. 2001;**15**(6): 544-548

[209] Mohanty I, Arya DS, Dinda A, et al. Mechanisms of cardioprotective effect of *Withania somnifera* in experimentally induced myocardial infarction. Basic & Clinical Pharmacology & Toxicology. 2004;**94**(4):184-190

[210] Muregi FW, Ishih A, Miyase T, et al. Antimalarial activity of methanolic extracts from plants used in Kenyan ethnomedicine and their interactions with chloroquine (CQ) against a CQ- tolerant rodent parasite, in mice. Journal of Ethnopharmacology. 2007;**111**(1):190-195

9

On the Organization of a Drug Discovery Platform

Jean A. Boutin, Olivier Nosjean and Gilles Ferry

Abstract

Some of the most exciting parts of work in the pharmaceutical industry are the steps leading up to drug discovery. This process can be oversimplified by describing it as a screening campaign involving the systematic testing of many compounds in a test relevant to a given pathology. This naïve description takes place without taking into consideration the numerous key steps that led up to the screening or the steps that might follow. The present chapter describes this whole process as it was conducted in our company during our early drug discovery activities. First, the purpose of the procedures is described and rationalized. Next follows a series of mostly published examples from our own work illustrating the various steps of the process from cloning to biophysics, including expression systems and membrane-bound protein purifications. We believe that what is described here presents an example of how pharmaceutical industry research can organize its platform(s) when the goal is to find and qualify a new preclinical drug candidate using cutting-edge technologies and a lot of hard work.

Keywords: drug discovery, validation, cloning & expression, biophysics, structural biology, organization

1. Introduction

Drug discovery involves a suite of processes as part of a program aimed at finding drug therapies for diseases. These programs encompass many different scientific steps from validation of the target (or attempts to do so) and characterization of the hits until the selection of candidates for medicinal chemistry programs. We felt that an accurate description of those steps has not previously been available and that such a description could be interesting.

In PubMed®, several thousand publications exist with the term 'drug discovery' in their titles. Most frequently, these reports share with readers how important the authors' particular area of expertise is in this domain, covering almost everything from crystallography to screening and high-content screening, origin of the screened molecules, compound libraries, sample conservation, biochemical approaches, microarrays, proteomics, and aptamers. These publications are a useful source of inspiration for each new program. Clearly, the first step in drug discovery is inspired by the state of the art, and the literature will help drive research towards the 'bench-to-bed' goal of finding a new molecule that will eradicate some disease that affects our society.

We feel, however, that the complete picture of such processes is not very often characterized. Thus, here we exemplify how we built our drug discovery (DD) platform on basic science with the goal of following, in a unique location (a set of specialized laboratories), the logical successive steps of drug discovery from ideas to first hits. An oversimplified picture of the logical progression from start to end of these processes can be seen in **Figure 1**.

This configuration did not preclude failures but probably helped forward our successes. In the pharmaceutical industry, the attrition rate is around 9 of 10 projects, meaning that only 1 project in 10 will have a slight chance of ending up in clinical development, and a further 2–3 out of 5 of these will have a chance to reach patients. Therefore, in preclinical research, scientists will try to deliver on time and with maximal rigor the tools necessary for the pathological problem to be at least partially solved. In 9 cases out of 10, the efforts will be vain, as the programs will be terminated, either for lack of results or for a change in strategy. The reasons for attrition are many, and a key to decreasing number is certainly a better characterization of molecules entering the medicinal chemistry program that will drive candidates from hit to

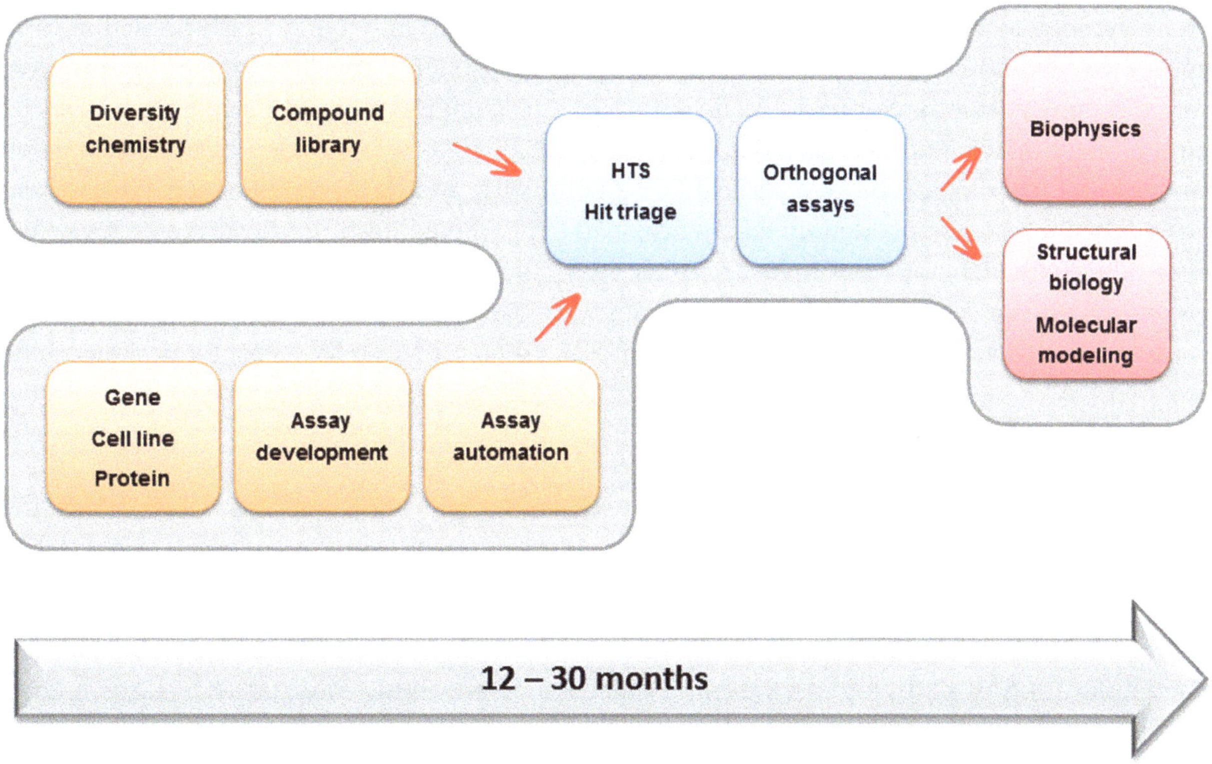

Figure 1. Schematic representation of a drug discovery process. Note that the exploratory/validation of the target process is not part of the schedule. Rather, these two steps might take several years to complete upstream.

lead. Among the characterizations that are essential is the specificity of the molecule within its class of targets (e.g., one given kinase among the 800 in the kinome) or its specificity towards the rest of the genome-encoded proteins. Another key is a better understanding of the molecule-target relationship at the atom level.

In addition to these scientific aspects, daily nonscientific aspects of business also require attention. Examples include practical questions, such as 'Can we hire new specialists to explore and assess a new field for a particular problem?'; economic questions, such as 'Can we spend the money necessary to acquire a particular technology'; and time-related questions, such as 'Can we spend the 12 to 20 months to deliver the results after the necessary assessment for a new technology/technique?'

Below, we offer our view through our experiences with all of these aspects, reflecting the work of a laboratory ultimately consisting of about 70 people, with some impressive achievements.

2. Basic sciences, organization?

Our group has a "simple" core job: the discovery of drug candidates. Programs are based on two types of knowledge: the pharmacological background linked to the various areas of therapeutics (e.g. cancer, cardiology, or neurosciences) and the techniques needed to explore the molecular side of the program (e.g. molecular biology, cellular biology, biochemistry, structural biology), in other words 'basic sciences for discovery'. That basis was a mixture of molecular and cellular pharmacology techniques that allowed starting from a protein target and finishing with a compound (or several) that interfered with this target in a reasonably specific manner. To this were added chemistry (for the compound collection) and molecular modeling (for dynamics and structural biology data interpretation). One of the major challenges was the identification of a given target in the pathological process, its role in the pathology, and its manipulation. These necessities meant that we also needed upstream access to experimental techniques such as siRNA, KO mice, alternative laboratory animals (such as yeast, flies, and zebrafish [1], and *Caenorhabditis elegans* [2]) often at a time when these techniques were barely validated. It also meant that we frequently had to make the choice of collaboration rather than pursuing these techniques internally.

2.1. Exploring pathology

"Exploring" means several things in this context, from exploring the disease to exploring the tools and the literature to validate a target. The literature is rather scarce in this context, but one resource is the essay by Scudamore, who tries to make us understand how difficult and diverse this area could be [3].

The exploration of pathology is the main objective of academia, but industry faces a challenging problem. Should it run brand-new programs using its internal research capacities or should it collaborate with academia to help them run such program? Considering that part of the work in industry is to choose relevant targets accessible to chemistry (even if chemistry has broadened its borders for the last decades) and that are truly and undoubtedly linked to a pathological situation, it cannot start several million-euro projects without a validation that convinces everyone that the end discovery will help the patient.

Thus, industry must equilibrate its efforts among internal, confidential, and secured experiments that would identify and elucidate the role of a target in a pathological process while scouting externally in academia and biotech for new ideas, concepts, targets, and even sometimes candidates. In these last cases, however, internal reproduction of key data should not be underestimated in terms of time, money, and results (see Section 2.2).

We were involved intensively in several such programs. For example, N-myristoyltransferase is a protein-modifying enzyme with a key role in addressing substrate to the membrane [4], including oncogenes or viral proteins [5, 6]. Our discovery that one isoform was associated with rough endoplasmic reticulum led us to believe that this particular isoform potentially had a role in pro-virion maturation [7]. On another front, we discovered/characterized a new activity for the enzyme autotaxin, a lysophospholipase D, the activity of which explained why that protein was previously believed to be a migration factor [8, 9]. This enzyme could be deeply involved in fat accumulation processes [10] and in metastasis [11]. We pursued this program up to the discovery and characterization of a hit compound that failed for stability reasons [12]. Another example is N-arylalkylamine acetyltransferase (AANAT), an enzyme involved in the synthesis of melatonin, of which we characterized the properties of the human isoform [13], while its importance in regulating melatonin synthesis had been demonstrated [14]. Our approach to the uncoupling proteins was similar to this. We thought that UCP3 might be a good target for diabesity, if we could find an activator of this enzyme. The challenging idea was that by accelerating proton exchange, one could reasonably enhance the heat dispersed by muscles. We thus started to study this particular enzyme in various contexts [15, 16], up to an *in vivo* model for which elegant techniques were developed [17, 18].

Opportunities are numerous for scientists in the core of a network. As noted, the challenge is always to be original enough but not too much involved in fundamental research because the time frame is simply not suitable to the business of industry, at least for the most part.

2.2. Validating targets (as actor in a pathology)

The validation of the implied involvement of a given molecular target in a pathological process requires many different approaches and technical applications. A special issue of *Current Topics in Medicinal Chemistry* was published in 2017 on this subject (see the editorial by Henderson and Gibert in [19]). Furthermore, Kaelin published an interesting paper [20] on the pitfalls in preclinical cancer target validation. Indeed, one of the main aspects of the Kaelin essay is that many experiments reported even in major journals are hard to reproduce independently, if at all, and thus validation is a difficult task. Obviously, this has been an endless debate in the scientific community, and commenting on it further here will not add to the discussion. The *primum movens* is not the same between academia and industry. Basically, it is fair to say that the protocols are not regularly described in enough detail to be easily reproducible in a different laboratory context.

Without a strong, scientific knowledge about the pathology, cures will not be found except by chance. Thus, being able to present our program in a way that is reproducible is important.

One has to be able to ensure (or be reasonably sure) that the observations made are linked to the 'pathological' situation and not to experiment-generated artifacts. Of course, achieving this goal requires a mixture of pure luck, hard work, prepared minds, curiosity, and willingness to move forward.

Most of the time, however, only a portion of these experiments is feasible, either for timescale reasons or for cost. Therefore, the choice is often made to go to primary approaches such as knockout cells or knockout animals. We reported such an approach with cells [21], knocking out the product of a gene by measuring the catalytic activity of the corresponding enzyme, spontaneously expressed in a cell line, HT22, after siRNA and shRNA treatments. It took a double transfection with a shRNA encoding a siRNA specific of QR2 to knock down only 80% of the catalytic activity of the enzyme. This result suggests that knocking out a spontaneously expressed protein in a cell line—especially in a cancer cell line, which is often pluri-nuclear—is difficult, if not impossible beyond knocking it down somehow. It is interesting to compare this type of data, including those we obtained in similar conditions but that remained unpublished, with claims that cocktails of siRNA transfected directly into (cancer) cells would kill the activity of an enzyme within hours (if not minutes). A recent review on the subject [22] emphasized the fact that RNAi studies have been used and abused, suggesting that the key role of those RNAs should be kept to a tightly verified level to gain from this outstanding technology and fix once and for all the problem of *in cellulo* identification and engagement of a target in a given pathology. Technologies involving nucleases and CRISPR have changed the technological landscape of cellular biology because these techniques lead to complete knockout and are almost universal—until exceptions to their effectiveness or accuracy start to emerge.

Cellular validations are often not complete enough to give strong support to a pathophysiological hypothesis. It is thus necessary to move to another approach: the genetic deletion of the target in mice, or, more recently, in rats. The bias of this approach, besides its cost and often the length of the process, is linked to the potential capacity of animals to compensate for the absence of a particular gene (or the absence of a particular catalytic activity). This compensation might happen often, but proofs of such situations are rare. The two main difficulties we have encountered were either the lethality of the KO in mouse embryos [23] or the complete absence of an obvious phenotype due to the loss of this particular gene [24, 25], a surprisingly frequent feature. The former example offers a rare case. When we mutated a single amino acid in the catalytic site of lysophospholipase D, which renders the enzyme completely catalytically inactive, the mouse embryos died in the very early stages of their development [23]. This outcome was unexpected but proved at least that the enzyme activity was a key player in mouse embryogenesis [26, 27]. Knockout animals can also be fantastic tools to prove that the compound engages the target. For instance, our antagonist of the melanin-concentrating hormone (MCH) receptor, S38151, has no activity in MCHR1 KO animals, while it reduces feeding wild-type ones, demonstrating that the compound exerts its expected activity only through its binding to the receptor [28]. Other examples have been generated in our DD platform, such as with the deletion of trace amine 1 receptors, revealing the involvement of those receptors in the actions of the drug Ecstasy (MDMA) [29]. Unexpected properties of the modified animals are sometimes found long after the knockout has been performed, resulting in the resuscitation of the program. For example, the knockout of Ucp2, an uncoupling protein expressed in almost all mouse tissues, confers an unexpected resistance to *Toxoplasma gondii* infection [30]. Finally, particularly difficult is the choice of the mouse strain usable for the KO line. Indeed, some examples of animals totally deprived of circulating melatonin led to slightly different observations about the impact of the knockout when compared to a strain presenting a "normal" level of circadian melatonin [31]; thus, not only are some strains partially blind but consequently their daily rhythm is profoundly affected.

Again, recent progress in cellular surgery, thanks to CRISPR techniques [32], might make the development of KO animals faster and even commonplace in the near future, but today the process remains a lengthy one.

Alternatively, in addition to these genetic manipulations *in vivo* or *in cellulo*, the pharmacological approach remains a possibility. Strategically, though, it is rare for a pharmacological set of tools for a "new" target to exist beforehand, and these molecules need to be specific and/or powerful enough to help validate the system. An upstream decision must be made about whether the high-throughput screening (HTS) approach that will probably deliver compounds can be used very early in the discovery process to bring tools rather than drug candidates to validate the target around which the program was/will be built. This theoretical situation can provide the community with very early tools to validate their activities (see reviews by [33, 34]).

Of interest, another approach has become possible in recent years, thanks to our collaborative work with the Shanghai Institute of Materia Medica (SIMM): a validation with molecules of poor specificity but engaging the target. Indeed, as soon as the first compounds are issued from this screening process, even if they are far from perfect, attempting high doses of such molecules on an animal model relevant to the pathology brings interesting and important information about the validation of the pathological hypothesis. Only a couple of examples have been published following these attempts, one with thioredoxin-interacting protein (i.e., TixNip) modulators [35] and the other with a gpr119 antagonist [36].

2.3. Cloning/expressing/purifying the targets

Obviously, targets come from independent experimental observations that have suggested their role in a given pathology in a given system through the measure of activity such as a catalytic activity or a potential binding site. Ultimately, purification should be performed and should lead to the unequivocal characterization of the protein the program targets. A recent trend is to consider that this given protein is a brick in the pathway(s) leading to the pathology. In this framework, the protein should retain its cellular context to allow for consideration of the potential role of its partners and cellular neighborhood. This situation is no doubt optimal. Nevertheless, finding compounds that will hit the target should begin with a simplification of the system. Without this simplification, one should consider the multiple interferences from the cell milieu (see also the HCS discussion below, Section 2.6.3).

This is an old debate between the pros and cons of protein purification. The pros consider that the candidate molecules should be aiming directly at the protein and that structural biology will deliver key information on the target-molecule relationship providing that the system is as simple as possible. The cons remind us that inside the cytosol, an enzyme interacts or is in proximity to many other proteins, some of which can involve interference. Rather than being an assortment of simple linear pathways, the cytosol in reality is more like a bag of marbles—proteins—rolling around and bumping into each other.

As far as enzymes are concerned, is it acceptable to work on a partially purified extract or should we aim for the pure version? For screening purposes (the *nec plus ultra* of the work of such a DD platform), the need for membranes overexpressing a receptor is key to the success of the next processes, so are there alternatives?

Cloning remains a source of novelty. Obviously, using already published sequences for new targets involves a bias because these targets are already known in the literature, so that the results with them are less novel that would be desirable for the drug market. Thus, cloning efforts of new, not already described targets, are at best a challenge. Our first attempts were to control the expression of receptors or enzymes, together with an associated protein (whether naturally associated or needed for building an assay for this target). Particularly interesting was trying to find ways by which the expression of two proteins—or two peptides—could be stoichiometric. For such a goal, the best approach was to use and organize IRES promoters in different geometries [37]. This method led us to the successful expression of several multi-peptide proteins, such as the nicotinic receptors.

It is interesting to see now the progress in what was once called cellular surgery, first with nuclease approaches and now with CRISPR. In past years, we used nuclease-based techniques to produce cellular models (most of the time, unfortunately, based on cancer cells) that would express a single copy of the transgene, integrated into the cell genome at a single, neutral position [38]. This method was interesting because for comparisons of the molecular pharmacology of a receptor from different species, often from human and one or two rodent species, the comparison was more relevant because only the sequence of the receptors drove the differences between the pharmacological profiles. Indeed, it was integrated into the same cellular host—CHO or HEK cells—at an identical 'neutral' position, with a single copy of the gene, leading to a validity and accuracy in the data that was difficult to obtain whenever the transfection was less controlled.

When the enzymes have already been described/cloned, expression is easier in a host cell—often bacteria—but then the purification (of an active enzyme) often becomes the key. Typical examples of such purification strategies can be found for chymase [39], AANAT [13, 40], and indoleamine-2,3-dioxygenase [41].

Regarding other aspects of research the DD platform has conducted, we should mention work on already known targets that suddenly take on added interest because they turn out to be involved in an unexpected physiopathological situation. One example is the role of quinone reductase 2 beyond its presumed detoxifying role. The enzyme has been associated with cognitive processes on the one hand [42] and with melatoninergic systems on the other [43]. Aware of these observations, our attempt was to build a network around the notion that inhibitors of this enzyme could be interesting tools or drugs in understanding cognition and cognition deficits [24, 44], as well as better characterizing the MPTP Parkinson model in mice [45, 46]. We reported several examples in which we explored new pathways and found evidence for new proteins or new activities. For example, the observation that lysoPLD activity was present and active in an adipocyte culture medium led us to hypothesize that this medium contained a protein capable of catalyzing the breakdown of lyso-phosphatidylcholine. We reported this discovery [8], after having purified, characterized, and discovered alternative splicing forms [9], built the KO mice [23], and started a search for active inhibitors [12]. It is interesting to look at it from a time-frame perspective. Indeed, the initial observations were made in 1999 while our initial report was published in 2003 [8] and the last report on the compound, S32826, in 2008 [12]. Thus, it took about 10 years before all tools were in place and the program had sufficient experimental evidence to allow for a process to lead to an actual drug discovery program *per se*. Only in 2011 evidence in the literature has shown the probable implication of this target in metastasis [47]. The work on autotaxin also concerned an already known motility factor [48] that turned out to be an enzyme generating this motility factor, with a potential role in metastasis [47, 49].

Broadening the observation that N-myristoyltransferase was key to the maturation and delivery of oncoproteins, such as src, to the membrane, we became interested in the other proteins that were myristoylated [6] and sought to differentiate their cytosolic activity from the poorly described membrane-associated activity. These studies led us to wonder if there was a target for inhibitors that would turn out to be antiviral compounds (myristoylation of the membrane viral protein gag is key in the virus life cycle). Very early on, we became interested also in kinases and some of their modifying enzymes (e.g., NMT, see above). Indeed, we started our program by choosing to explore the main tyrosine protein kinase expressed in the HL60 cancer cell line [50, 51] and purification was the only option at a time when cloning was rather rare.

We still believe that following the expression of the target (enzyme) in bacteria, for instance, activity must be purified to homogeneity. Indeed, the further process of testing the activity should lead to unambiguous attribution to the target protein and not to a similar activity catalyzed by a bacterial endogenous enzyme. Therefore, much effort was often put into the purification process, even though the current literature reflects a lack of enthusiasm about obtaining a pure enzyme. Furthermore, the need for biophysical as well as structural data necessitates a pure product, in any case. Therefore, what is done at that stage serves at least three purposes: obtaining uniformity of the enzyme in the preparations; gaining the possibility of measuring unambiguously the relationship between molecules and their targets; and finally, achieving crystallogenesis, which requires the purest possible preparation to start with.

Considering receptors, the situation might be slightly more favorable to a less simplified system. Indeed, the main property of receptor binding is certainly that the binder is specific to the receptor; thus, considering membranes as an acceptable receptacle for receptor studies seems to be an adequate compromise. For instance, in a program linked to our historical involvement in melatonin receptor pharmacology, we had to find a way to check for the activity of agonist candidates in an *in vivo* model of depression that was a non-rodent and diurnal animal (melatonin being heavily involved as a master switch of the circadian rhythm as well as the circannual one) [52, 53]. Such models were not that common, especially at a time when the exact nature of the chronobiology was not understood. We then turned to a sheep model with the difficulty that, at that time, it was believed that two animals were known to be natural knockouts for one of the melatonin receptors (MT_2). Although this was clearly demonstrated for one strain of hamster [54], it was less clear for the sheep. Thus, we embarked on a challenge to finally clone, express, and characterize the MT_2 receptor from sheep, destroying this myth at the same time [55]. Such approaches became one of our interests in our multiple attempts to crystalize G-protein-coupled receptors (see also the structural biology section, below). In brief, a survey of the sequences of the receptors of a common family (e.g., melatonin) in various animals indicated variations of sequences with retention of specificity (towards melatonin). By measuring the thermal stability of the receptors, we can deduce the strongest structure that could be amenable to expression, solubilization, purification, and crystallogenesis attempts [56, 57], as anticipated a few years ago [58]. In other words, despite the apparent futility, cloning/expressing receptors from multiple sources might lead to findings of major importance. More recently, however, an attempt to clone the second melatonin receptor from the European hamster, previously reported as a natural knockout (as in the other hamster species), partially failed because of difficulty establishing the appropriate conditions to copy a particularly rich G-C region of the gene, as we had done for the sheep MT_2 receptor [55]. Finally, in our quest for stable versions of the melatonin receptors, we engaged in a series of cloning programs of these GPCRs from different animals, including bats, birds, snakes, and various mammals, most of which were not published (Guenin and Boutin, unpublished). Indeed, we ended up trying to characterize the melatonin receptors of the strangest mammal, the platypus. We did clone the ancestor of gpr50, a.k.a., Mel1c, and characterized its unique pharmacology; gpr50 has lost its melatonin-binding capacity in all mammals except for the platypus (Gautier et al., in press). Following the same line of work, we started a program aimed at validating the existence of a third melatonin-binding site [59], as reported earlier [60], to finally attempt and succeed in purifying it [43]. This effort led us to a series of studies demonstrating the key role of this enzyme in many different contexts [61, 62].

Of course, channels and receptors (as well as membrane-associated enzymes) require a system of expression in which the channel activity can be followed unambiguously because quite often, purification of these proteins is extremely difficult to achieve.

2.4. Testing the enzyme or the receptor (or else)

As noted, and as can be understood from the scheme in **Figure 1**, testing the enzyme or the receptor is the cornerstone of the whole process. Assaying a target involves several important requirements: the test should be robust, fast but reproducible, easy to handle and cheap and if possible should address only the activity that is targeted with minimal interference from the compounds in the assay ingredients. Several reviews have been published on this issue. For instance, the race for label-free solutions [63] or the use of instruments that measure directly the amount of product formed (or consumed) during the assay [64] are two perspectives on the never-ending moving/changing landscape that rises into view as soon as the screening process is involved. Books could be written on the way a screen must or can be done. Below are just a few examples of the choices we made.

Choosing the right test is a key decision that will influence the rest of the program. In the past, we spent some time trying to identify the best assay for our kinase program and evaluated the whole literature for the best possible options [65] before finally attempting to run our own original version [66]. We frequently found that the assay described for our target class was not fully adaptable to our instruments or presented potential interference with the assay component(s). Several dozens of assays were adapted from the literature and/or from the material we had in hand, such as the systematic use of HPLC [9, 39, 41, 67–69] and more recently, mass spectrometry [70]. Worth noting here is the use of a global technique such as NMR. Indeed, a feature of this method is of great interest for us: it has poor sensitivity but a high robustness [71] and can be used not only for screening purpose but also for monitoring poor-affinity target/compound interactions, as in the first step of the search for receptor ligands. In addition to its obvious use as an analysis technique, we have adapted this method in various frames, including a way to better trace enzymatic activity [72], use a fluorine-labeled spy molecule as a ligand for an enzyme (that screened compounds can chase) [73], or verify changes in a component of a reaction [74]. These techniques are all automatable and thus can be used with less staff power as long as the automate is running by itself—day and night—and the validation of the assay guarantees stability of the components over time.

When turning to non-enzymatic assays, such as receptor binding or protein-protein interaction, the constructs necessary to reveal the activity of the candidate compounds might be complex. For the receptor assays, where binding is the known first step, the functionality is the key information: e.g., agonists as well as antagonists are ligands in a binding assay, and only the functional assay—often cellular [75–77], but with exceptions [78]—thus should be able to distinguish between both entity types.

The recent evolution in understanding of receptor bias ligands has considerably changed our view of receptology. Indeed, for GPCR studies, compounds can be specific antagonists of a given signaling pathway (see, for example, a recent survey on the melatonin receptors [79]) but partial agonists in another measured pathway. Even if the bottom line is that an agonist should lead to the internalization of the receptor—which the antagonists should not—there will be exceptions and changes in paradigm(s) ([80], for instance, and Legros and Boutin [unpublished]).

Of course, in some cases, we had to develop and assess a completely new assay, such as when we addressed the difficult question of PPARγ ligands and had to use a new method of binding onto this soluble protein [81].

Globally, it is fair to say that four molecular target types cover most of the druggable biochemistry of living organisms: the enzymes, receptors, channels, and protein-protein interactions. In fact, our view is that a full spectrum of possible techniques should be available to play with and adapt to the current project, while validating as much as possible the potential biases of such techniques. We decided very early to double-check the results of a screen (i.e., validate the hits) by using an orthogonal assay (see Section 2.9), that is, an assay that does not have the same technical approach as the initial one.

2.5. Automatizing the assay

Automation is the capacity for an industrial laboratory to run literally hundreds or thousands of assays a day and be able to extract from this formidable amount of data a promising candidate that will fulfill at least some of the criteria for future development. It is thus important to have a decent number of automated stations without losing the capacity to understand and control the various parameters of such an assay.

We decided to go with small, independent stations that were not entirely automatized. One of the reasons for this choice was the fact that we could collaborate with the SIMM group that had all the capacities for running mammoth screen campaigns (over one million compounds). In addition, we believed—and still do—that some modularity is essential for the involvement of the technical personnel in these very repetitive tasks. Such modularity is more adaptive to numerous situations than a single, heavily integrated robot that will take weeks if not months to reconfigure for another assay, especially when the assays cover a very large spectrum of techniques. Indeed, we faced campaigns based on assays for widely different proteins and targets, including enzymes, receptors, protein-protein interactions, and channels, requiring being able to adapt the material at hand to the various approaches for screening these different target types.

Another aspect that is particularly important for us is repeatability of the screens. Indeed, we chose to run assays in independent duplicates at two different calendar dates and possibly with two different operators, leading to a higher level of robustness for the results, as long as both results were close to each other (see below).

2.6. Screening

Screening is the modern version of intelligently seeking the needle in the haystack. It concerns a test in which literally hundreds of thousands of compounds are evaluated, most of the time without any *a priori* information on their chemical structure or class (e.g., peptides, fragments, drug-like compounds, aptamers, toxins, natural extracts, natural compounds, etc.). Therefore, for cost constraint reasons, it may become important to screen in a smarter way [82]. This search has become a science in itself, a science that relies on chemical diversity. We view it as follows: the more diverse the compound library is, the more chemical space it covers, and the more successful we might be in finding one or several hits for a particular target.

In a given library of compounds, what are the chosen compounds that will lead to a new drug (i.e. active, specific, non-toxic, and patentable)? A perspective from some leading pharmaceutical companies was published in 2011 [83]. They gave their common view of the HTS programs, what they delivered, and what they failed to deliver. This particularly unusual publication (co-signed by the major pharmaceutical companies) exemplifies the reality of HTS expectations (too high) and of the quality/amounts of the results (the new drugs, too low). Nevertheless, as with the main progress in life science technologies in recent decades, the rise of HTS has led to plenty of new discoveries and approaches. We should not forget that all of these techniques accelerated discoveries, and even if those are not yet transformed into new drugs for the patient, they still add to the understanding of physiopathological processes. Mayr and Bojanic described the basic organization of an HTS laboratory—among other types—a few years back [84].

2.6.1. *High-throughput screening*

We embarked about 15 years ago on establishing a minimal HTS department in which a couple of screening robots together with an integrated analysis system permitted 'rapid' screening of several thousand compounds. The adaptability of the machine quickly became a problem: expanding our screening capacity—in terms of diversity of assays as well as number of compounds—would require several identical instruments running in parallel on which specialized personnel would apply their skills in an unvarying way. We chose something else for a time. We aimed at having small stations independent from one another to be able to treat or read between 40 and 50 384-well plates (~15,000 compounds). There are no general rules about how to arrange such a laboratory: it depends on the space, money, and personnel available. We felt that the whole process should be rigorously simple, with several key steps (go/no-go decisions) from the basic setup of the assay (and its validation with reference compounds) to the automation and test on a small scale of 10,000 compounds and finally both full-deck campaigns.

Figure 2 shows a series of typical examples of data obtained with this set of methods. In general, we screened about 10,000 compounds using the final conditions (set up previously) in two independent campaigns with the same compounds and different operators, if possible. The analysis of those data is what will permit moving forward to the full campaigns of 250,000 compounds, tested twice on the target. Without going too much into practical details, we found this methodology to be the most appropriate. Even if 2 or 3 out of 30 HTS campaigns turned out to be mute (no compound out of the HTS campaigns), the rest delivered several classes of compounds that could be pushed to the program downstream.

The figures show the repartition of the compounds according to their level of activity (left) while the graphs show the actual data where the results of the first test are plotted versus the second series of tests. The two tests are experimentally identical but run on a different day and if possible with a different operator. Because most of the compounds should be inactive, the Gaussian curves are centered to 0. The graphs should be aligned according to the diagonal of the rectangle because the data are theoretically identical, and should be massively located around 0. In **Figure 2A**, the first robotic setup led to a fat repartition of the compounds on the Gaussian curve, suggesting poor reproducibility, which is confirmed by the format of the correlation graph (or rather the lack thereof). In **Figure 2B**, with another setup, the data are more centered to the 0 and diagonal areas, respectively, in both figures, and in **Figure 2C**, the test was run first with a set of molecules, as in a feasibility attempt. We designated this process as a pre-HTS campaign. The data show a very good reproducibility of the tests, with compounds gathered along the diagonal of the graph.

2.6.2. *HTS system: factory or small business?*

It is the fashion to elaborate big systems that are very integrated and can run 'any' type of assays for any given number of compounds in a library. Unfortunately, despite beautiful examples of successful efforts with such machines, the issue of time frame in such situations is an elusive one. Indeed, moving on the same instrument from an enzymatic assay (e.g., with

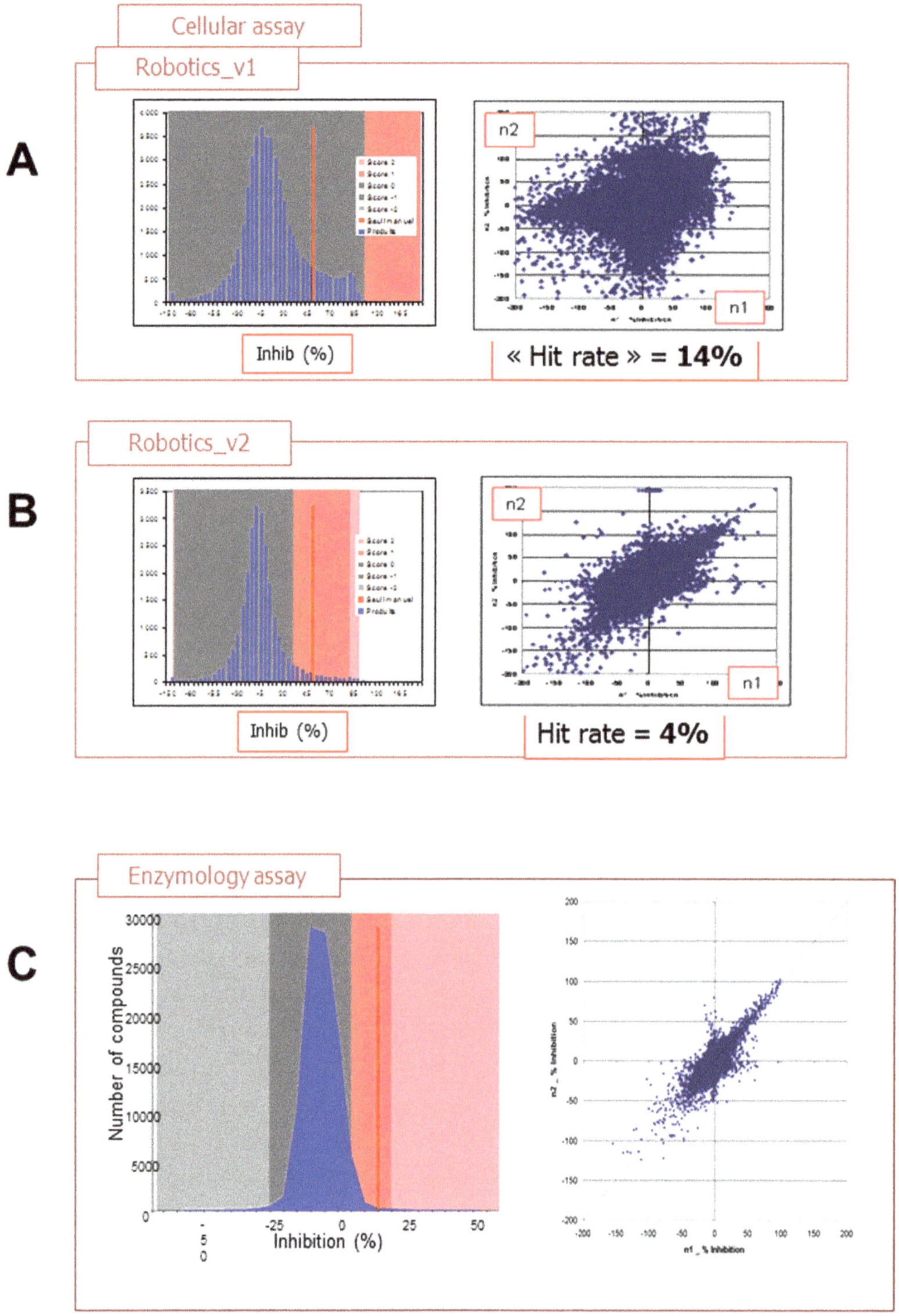

Figure 2. A typical and real example of the influence of the robotic setup on the quality of the screening results. The test was a cellular-based assay (*), comprising the detection of an intra-organelle color change potentially due to the tested compounds (see Jensen et al. for full description of the test [85]). A and B show cellular-based assay results; * note the use of differentiated primary cells; C shows an enzymatic assay. All results (whatever the biological sources) should resemble panel C. Poor results such as A and B, even if partially corrected by adapting robotics (between A and B), would lead to massive amounts of false positive hits.

fluorescent probes) to a cellular assay (e.g., with engineered cells) involves different instruments, setups, and prerequisites. One cannot honestly predict the length the preparation will require, and to a certain extent, the length of the global process (assessment + campaigns).

In the particular case of cellular assays, and as discussed elsewhere, the use of cancer cell lines brings difficulties, due to their genetic baggage, that is, to say the least, abnormal, leading to overexpression of many proteins. Alternatively, cells might be primary cells differentiated or not, the use of which leads to major variations from cells to cells, ultimately leading to massive false positive amounts (up to 14%, see **Figure 2**) and poor reproducibility from batches to batches. Finally one possible choice would be to work with differentiated stem cells, as their robustness is enhanced due to the current state of the art, with more and more publications describing works in this area. All these cells can be engineered with modern transfection techniques.

It is always possible for extreme cases to use different approaches. For instance, in a premodern time, we ran a HPLC assay for AANAT, ending with interesting hits despite the "low" number of compounds tested [67]. It is certainly an option whenever the available test involves extremely costly reagents or engineered fragile cells.

2.6.3. High-content screening (HCS) and its obligatory companion, functional genomic screening

High-content screening is a fast cellular-based approach that became possible in recent years, thanks to progress in imaging, computing, capturing, analyzing, and automating those processes. Moffatt et al. has summarized these approaches [86]. One also has to keep in mind that whatever the complexity of the engineered cell-based assay that is designed to identify compounds specific to given (cellular) pathways, it is probably less complex than the cellular metabolism. In other words, once the compound has been identified, one must check the *in situ* nature of its target. Treatment of siRNA libraries of the cellular systems and/or reverse pharmacology can be used to such an end. Saeidnia et al. [87] has reviewed the reverse pharmacology and possible solutions that are available.

The latest trend is to screen phenotypically engineered cells for the pathway in which the target is involved. If a compound is found, the validation process seems cumbersome to us. In fact, the deconvolution of the phenotype, to identify the actual target(s) of the hit compound(s), is a long process that is interesting, difficult, and expensive (in time and money). Cautions also have been published recently, warning scientists using such methodologies to be extremely careful in turning to these approaches because the number of biases is immense. We only very recently entered onto this path. In the meantime, we had serendipitously prepared the next steps by a very early attempt to industrialize our previous success in reverse pharmacology: the discovery of the third melatonin-binding site as quinone reductase 2 [43]. Nevertheless, this success has not been the rule. Several attempts done internally to find the target of given pharmacological agents have so far failed.

2.7. Screening what?

At the start of the year 2000, the question was, "How many compounds do you have in your library?" Without reference to the diversity of the compounds, some big players in the game had more than a million compounds available. Indeed, diversity is a complex problem that has been discussed at length by various authors (see Gillet et al., in particular [88, 89]). In the chemist community, it is often joked that there are as many definitions of diversity as individual chemists. Briefly, we chose to stay on the following path. Based on a definition of diversity that we found clear and attractive [90] and that gather all the basic concepts of diversity (and their measurement), we chose to base our own measure of diversity on the pharmacophore concept [91]. We felt that the more we wanted to pinpoint this diversity concept, the more we became lost in endless descriptors of the molecules [92]. Ultimately, we used the approach of Lepp [93] to establish a representative sub-library of compounds that can serve as a simplification of our complete library for pre-test purposes (see above) or to limit the number of compounds whenever the screening campaign uses a test that is either too expensive or cellular (i.e., "too" complex). Another way to define diversity is to measure the similarity between compounds, another approach that has also been discussed at length [94].

The diversity of the product collection that will be tested is indeed important and allows for anticipation of the discovery of new series on which the medicinal programs will be developed. Achieving diversity, however, will require the inclusion in the library of compounds with unusual or poorly documented structures.

A company like ours has a 60-year history of chemical synthesis of drug candidates. These molecules are still available in the compound collection and constitute an original source of diversity. To complete this panel while maintaining the largest diversity possible, we chose to integrate into the compound library natural pure products, extracts, peptides, and more generally 'drug-like' chemicals either synthesized internally or commercially available. We targeted having a total of about 250,000 compounds screened, systematically, for any targets of interest.

2.7.1. Natural compounds

A fundamental in this domain is certainly the belief that ethnopharmacology can identify interesting natural molecule(s) from traditional medicine (see Heinrich et al. for background in ethnopharmacology [95]). Ethnopharmacology focuses on a compendium of mixtures that medical practitioners in native populations prepared and gave to their patients, sometimes with outstanding success. The complexity of these approaches is immense. Indeed, besides the type of the plants used—not always easy to trace and not always easy to find in historical locations—there is the nature of the preparation, including the mixture of several different plants and associated products (of animal [including insects] or mineral origin). We tried to access the two main available sources of such compounds: pure compounds or extracts that need to be deconvoluted, usually by bio-directed strategies. We have reported our experiences with the latter in three publications [96–98] but rapidly abandoned these approaches for the following reasons: paucity of results; tediousness of the process; difficulty in repeating the exact same experiment, including trouble finding plants at the same location with the same properties; and last but not least, often difficulties with the structure identified, which turned out to be common or of a complexity beyond the reasonable feasibility of industrial production. It remains interesting to view those compounds as a mold of the target binding site and/or to use them as an inspiration for a future drug. At the other end of the spectrum, commercially available, pure compounds are hard to find in a decent quantitative supply. Often, compounds are available from vendors, but they are either common (flavonoids, coumarins, peptides, terpenoids, and alkaloids) or provided in minute quantities, with barely any reload possible. We therefore balanced our library with some of those pure compounds, as an internal control to assay, because often flavonoids—while poorly soluble—have turned out to be enzyme inhibitors (see, for example, [40, 99]).

In the interest of completeness, we add that one other path is to provide some biotech companies with a target. They screen the target with their proprietary sources of natural compounds (often as microorganisms, plants, and similar extracts to start with).

2.7.2. Peptide libraries

We became interested in peptide combinatorial libraries at the very beginning of this approach and studied several aspects of those libraries: numbers [100], quality control [101], and activity [102, 103]. For solid-phase synthesis approaches, the actual number of peptides in a given library is limited by the availability of amino acids on the resin, and that number is limited by the number of individual peptide repeats in the initial mixture, which is obviously by far the most complex one. The trick turned out to be the way syntheses were conducted, by having the last amino acids as a constant in each vessel (see Houghten et al. [104]). Regardless, these approaches are often interesting to follow, particularly when soluble or secreted targets are concerned.

2.7.3. Compound libraries

Despite the large diversity of compounds available for screening, whether through scientific collaboration, subcontracts, or vendors, the nature of the compounds is one of the most sensitive secrets of the pharmaceutical companies. As stated above, we attempted to complement our more than 60 years of internal chemical synthesis with compounds bought or synthesized with the greatest care to try to achieve the widest diversity of compounds and to be able, at the end of the screening process, to validate original molecules with great potential. This strategy is based on our capacity to analyze and understand chemical diversity and thus be able to predict what should be synthesized to fill in the gaps in this diversity picture.

2.8. Choosing the hits for further programs

The question here is, "Choosing among which hits and why?" In the industry, the answer is simple: to heal and to make a drug. For other scientists, the answer might be slightly different: understanding a pathway (such as those at the core of a pathology) or finding tools that permit the study of the pathology, the receptor, or the enzyme. In any case, the path from hits to lead and then from lead to candidate is particularly long and painful. Thus, the structure of the various candidates (often from two or three different families of compounds) must be chosen extremely carefully to avoid the various obstacles: chemistry difficulties, including that the drug will be synthesized at the ton level at the end; specificity towards the other proteins of the body (not less); pharmacokinetics (often the compound should be given orally);

and patentability. It is interesting to note that exceptional universities, such as the University of Michigan, have published their reflections on this subject [105]. On the other hand, one should realize that the hit rate of an *ab initio* screening is somewhere between 0.01 and 0.1%. For 250,000 molecules, that translates to 25 and 250 compounds. It looks like plenty to choose from, although the hope is that among those compounds, some are similar, suggesting a structure-activity relationship that enforces the results of the HTS.

Sometimes, as noted, researchers will choose compounds for their availability or their known lack of toxicity, despite other problems such as a lack of specificity. The purpose then is different: finding tools to validate a pathway or the engagement of a target in a given pathology (see Section 2.2). Examples like melatonin [106], curcumin [107], or resveratrol [108] are also interesting to note. Indeed, these compounds are fantastic tools to better understand a network of pathways involved in various pathologies, but none of them shows any type of specificity. To the contrary, they seem active in many pathological situations because they interfere with many targets.

A more recent approach has also involved the systematic use of chemoinformatics analyses with its formidable capacity of calculus and prediction [109, 110]. Starting from there, it is possible to rationalize the choice of the best hits: among others, the previous history of the compound in the earlier campaigns on other targets, similarity with known compounds from the literature, patentability, and accessibility to the chemistry (not too complicated to allow 'easy' generation of a large series of analogues).

2.9. Confirming the hit activity

Once hits have been identified, the process continues in validating the molecules in their recorded interaction with the targets. Genick and Wright [111] addressed this subject, among others, in their recent paper. Essentially, it comprises three aspects: biochemical validation, biophysical measurement, and structural data.

Our first step is towards an orthogonal confirmation of the activity of the compound. Obviously, whenever an enzyme is concerned, it is 'quite easy' to invent or copy an alternative assay that engages different physical parameters, going from the old, global, radioactive phosphocellulose paper-based detection assay [112] to a more specific radioactivity-based assay [113] for a kinase, for instance; trying to go from a protein-based phosphorylation assay [114] to a more specific peptide-based assay [66] or lastly, going from an antibody-based assay to a more specific ubiquitinated peptide-based assay [115]. There are multiple examples of such orthogonal assays, such as the use of HPLC, fluorescence polarization, mass spectrometry, and fluorescence resonance energy transfer (FRET) technology. We always felt that part of the reproducibility problem(s) was (were) due to the result of the poorly understood interferences between components of the assay, even sometimes the totally aspecific actions of the compound onto the target, for instance, by precipitating the protein rather than inhibiting it, with a similar effect in the assay (lack of activity in the presence of the compound). Compounds at the concentration used in the screening process—often 10 μM—tend to precipitate. The addition of dimethylsulfoxide (DMSO) as a compatible organic solvent limits this precipitation to a certain extent, but the presence of DMSO might affect the enzyme or the reactivity medium (not to mention the receptor, membrane-bound assay). This is also why we argue for work on purified targets to simplify, at least in this context, the environment of the protein.

For the receptor assay, it can be more complicated to find an alternative, often because of the uniqueness of the radioactive ligand used in the binding assay. We tried to circumvent this problem by developing options in this context, for example, in synthesizing other ligands, to have more than a single binder in our melatoninergic [116, 117] or MCH toolboxes [118]. If this goal is achievable for receptors that have been studied for decades (serotonin, adenosine, histamine, and melatonin), for other more recently studied receptors, it has been completely impossible, including the obvious case of orphan receptors for which ligands are not known and assays are built around receptor functionality. Thus, the study of such receptors has largely been done through efforts to de-orphanize them [119, 120] and to fully characterize them with all the tools of molecular pharmacology, as for gpr103 [121–124] or gpr50 [125, 126]. An easier alternative is to work with known ligands as peptides, as in our extensive work on melanin-concentrating hormone for which alterations in the natural sequence led to alternative ligands [118], agonists [127], or antagonists [28, 128]. Beyond the thrill of executing a *tour de force* design and the joy of manipulating peptides of short sequences, with their infinite possible variations, the work brought a panel of new tools that might ultimately contribute to understanding such integrated systems.

2.10. Structuring: what is the hit/target relationship at the atom level?

As noted, part of the validation is linked to the visualization of the molecular structure of the complex between the hit and the target. The key role of this approach has been reviewed numerous times (e.g., Scapin [129], Hu et al. [130], and Zheng et al. [131, 132]). It is now clear that the progression of the compounds from a hit to an elaborate drug will benefit immensely from structural biology data. We contributed also to a certain vision of how alternative methods will complete (and possibly compete with?) crystallography, particularly cryo-electronic microscopy [133].

We made the choice of an active and ambitious structural biology approach about 10 years ago. Creating efficient collaborations with some groups, our first attempts were to characterize the interactions between some of our compounds and a given target in neurogenerative diseases [134–136]. We then embarked on several kinase-related projects that ended with the discovery of powerful compounds [137–140]. However, we needed more freedom to operate and establish proof of concept of the importance of these approaches to complement our drug discovery programs. For this reason, we chose to install a dedicated laboratory inside a synchrotron (Soleil, St. Aubin, France) to gain full access not only to the beamlines but also to the vast scientific community behind this instrument. This choice led to several collaborative academic-oriented lines of research [136, 141] and to more internal research programs. In preparing the next steps of crystallization—the step involving the receptor and more generally membrane proteins—we assessed a series of methodologies for the solubilization and purification of functionally competent receptors [56, 57]. Furthermore, we also studied the impact of microfluidics on crystallization of proteins for structural biology studies [142, 143].

The companion science of structural biology is molecular modeling. It is key for discovery programs, either at the early stage (explaining and rationalizing the molecule-target relationship and even quantifying it) or at a later stage when new molecules, derived from a hit in the screening campaign, will be synthesized and need to be paused inside the structure of the target by calculation or co-crystallization. We have reported some examples of the use of those techniques for glucokinase [144], gpr103 [124], and rev-erbα [145].

2.11. "Biophysing": understanding and measuring the forces responsible for the relation between the molecule and its target

Many reviews have nicely summarized recent community perspectives on this aspect of compound characterization [146–148]. No doubt, the rise of all the physical biology methods affords more and more tools that are essential to a modern drug discovery program, particularly when trying to understand and measure the relationship between the compound—that is, the drug candidate or its ancestor—and its protein target.

From the seminal work—for us—of Shuman et al. on HIV proteases [149], we started to wonder if the complicated concepts of thermodynamics could be applied to the process of moving from hit to lead compounds. What would be the help of measuring the actual parameters of a target-compound association, even if the target were not a receptor but an enzyme? We became adopters of surface plasmon resonance (SPR) [150], calorimetric instruments, fast-flow machines to measure events of enzymatic activity that occur faster than a second [151], and native mass spectrometry to gain information on the minute conformational changes of proteins [152].

It is now clear that those tools have become part of ongoing studies for helping medicinal chemists better evaluate and thus better understand the impact of the minute modifications they make to their compounds. For instance, the use of calorimetry to determine the actual affinity of an inhibitor for its enzyme has proved to be accurate [134], while standard methodologies such as binding turned out to be cumbersome if not wrong [153]. Furthermore, the determination of the number of compounds and their nature associated with a given protein was also a key step in our understanding of quinone reductase 2 enzymatic behavior [70].

These "new" tools are increasingly reliable. "Structuring" and "biophysing" help give access to precise details on the structure of the co-crystal together with actual thermodynamics measures and thus the relationships at the atom level between the target and its ligand (at least, and for the moment, for enzymes); however, crystallization of the membrane-bound proteins (such as GPCRs) is still a challenge, despite recent major progress [154, 155]. These newer tools permit visualization and quantification of these interactions. The medicinal chemist can use this information as the basis for a synthesis strategy for the evolution of hits towards a series of compounds with *ad hoc* properties that are easier to predict and rationalize.

3. What next?

Research has always been a question of strategic and/or opportunistic decisions at a given time to explore areas that look promising for a better future. These decisions, at the industry level, are always difficult to make. Money, time, and energy go into anticipating what will be important—technology-wise—for the next decade of discovery.

Among the published reports that we attempted to explore were many approaches involving new, non-invasive techniques to better understand the role of a compound and its target inside a cell, the future of stem cells and of chemical proteins, and the modifications of proteins inside the cells.

3.1. Stem cells as expressing systems

Stem cells have been the new frontier for some time and remain so. One debate has been whether to target therapy with stem cells, directly (in cell therapy) or indirectly (by using the secretosome of differentiated stem cells) or to use the cells as hosts for a target that would then be expressed in an optimal environment, as opposed to the classical use as hosts of cancer cell lines that are either very derived from the original cell lines or comprise numerous nuclei with profoundly abnormal karyotypes. We chose the isolation, differentiation, production, and characterization of such stem cell-derived cardiomyocytes [156]. Potentially, these techniques open new roads to the use of natural hosts that would be a better context for the expression of targets in a natural environment. Furthermore, as demonstrated in several instances, stem cells can be derived from patients, and some can recapitulate the disease at the cellular level, leading to a possibly better understanding of the molecular cause(s) of a given disease [157, 158].

It might be important in the coming years or decades to be able to cope with the therapeutic use of such stem cells, despite initial concerns [159] and the extraordinary characteristics [160] of these cell types.

3.2. Chemical proteins

A boom in the area of chemical proteins followed the discovery—among others—of chemical ligation [161]. It became possible to synthesize enzymes chemically and measure their catalytic activity. After the chemical synthesis (by solid-phase synthesis) and use of ubiquitin, described for several decades, we chose a small enzyme (120 aa), calstabin, that we completely synthesized with our partner. We crystallized this enzyme and measured its catalytic activity. In doing so, we learned two important things: (1) such an approach is feasible, even though it led to small quantities of material, at least to start with, and the material was indistinguishable from the recombinant version and (2) the apparent mono-peak analysis of the result of the synthesis revealed, after further analyses, that the protein could be separated in two distinct peaks, one a fully refolded protein with catalytic activity and the other a denatured protein with no catalytic activity and no refolding [141]. These findings led us to consider that large peptides/proteins that are chemically synthesized and often described as being used in the literature (e.g., EPO, growth factors) might be a mixture of active and inactive substances if not appropriately characterized.

Our aim was and still is the validation of a process encompassing both the recombinant expression of pieces of a large protein—such as an antibody—that contained only natural amino acids and other pieces of the same protein, in which exotic amino acids were inserted. The fusion between those pieces would then be performed by chemical ligation(s). These approaches will open avenues to the incorporation of key functional groups in protein for derivatization with drugs (antibody-drug conjugates) or to incorporation into proteins of exotic chemical functions.

3.3. Ligases

Among the seminal studies of the *in cellulo* modifications of proteins are the numerous efforts of Alice Ting's group [162]. Using a modified ligase, it became possible to directly label target proteins in a cellular context. The label can be a fluorophore, radiolabeled compound, or NMR probe, for example, and the chemistry of the modification is the main limitation of this process. Coupling it with the power and resolution of magnifying instruments, including specialized beam lines in a synchrotron, can lead to the cartography of the protein inside a living cell. We began the process first by characterizing the enzymology beyond this ligase-catalyzed enzymatic reaction, using purified enzyme and reagents in an acellular context [163]. This technique will be adapted to intracellular processes with the goal of modifying a recombinant protein *in situ* and to allow labeling of a protein inside the cell to follow its fate.

4. Outside the box

Anticipating tomorrow's needs in modern research is a challenge that requires triangulating the many different areas necessary for drug discovery. It has thus been difficult to choose various avenues to make our efforts more successful, modern, and interesting and at the service of future trends and needs in drug discovery for therapies and cures. Choosing to enhance our capacities to incorporate new approaches is always a challenging but moderate risk, based on the way we perform these exploratory strategies. Indeed, one critical choice was to hire post-docs to scrutinize those ideas. In doing so, we not only identified and incorporated strong scientists but also could assign new technologies to categories such as 'dream', 'usable soon', 'needs more time', etc. Among the discoveries that we have published are the ligase use for *in cellulo* transformation of proteins [163], including antibodies; cellular imaging using large synchrotron instruments; synthetic proteins that can be as active as the recombinants [141]; and synthesis of proteins and peptides modified by ubiquitination the way it happens in the cell (as opposed to what was commercially available at that time) [115]. In addition, we started our first trials in thermodynamics, structural biology, new crystallization techniques, native mass spectrometry for structural biology approaches [152] and for target-molecule relationships, and the use of human stem cells as an alternative to rat cardiomyocytes in first culture, among other initiatives.

The engineering of cells and their use as therapeutic agents bring new challenges and new wonders almost daily. New challenges emerge because the necessary work to achieve therapies for tomorrow may not necessarily be what was done in the recent past. These challenges often require new approaches, particularly in the use of treatments with stem cells from the patient, or with cells that have been engineered to fulfill a task that only science fiction writers dreamed about in the 1950s. Just one example is the seminal paper by Schukur et al. [164] on the possibility of engineering a cell to produce a factor (such as tumor necrosis factor) following a native regulatory pathway in the patient in whom these cells will be grafted. The number of new technologies required to reach that end is just immense. If we do not prepare for such wonders, the industry will have an extremely complicated time reorienting to tomorrow's health-related demands.

5. Conclusions

The body of techniques developed and applied in the DD platform throughout the years has contributed to the introduction of several molecules on the market. The contribution of this platform concerned the initial steps of compound discovery that proceeded towards final molecules. Or else, the platform was involved in providing data on the biophysics of the interaction, most of the time, all steps of drug discovery contributed to the final results. Some findings have been published and showed the completeness of the approach that laid the foundations for the discovery and early clinical development of drug candidates [138, 139, 165].

There is obviously confusion between the use of research that is the replication of data obtained elsewhere (the role of the industry) and the de novo research programs that are developed in the pharmaceutical industry. The confusion is that work consisting of new research should not be done in the industry, but in academic institutions, while repeating published data should be done in the industry. In that way, by limiting the novelty of the industrial work, the novelty of the cure(s) found in such context might be limited, thus leading to a situation where alternate paradigms must be found. For instance, a way to access to novelty might be to fund biotechnology companies to explore new research areas and new ideas.

To echo arguments already made above, most of the published research is difficult (if not impossible) to repeat. And as noted, there has been a long debate in the scientific literature on the repeatability of data [166, 167]. Therefore, part of any efforts at clarity and repeatability should be sorting the reality from the fantasy in what we are reading. Furthermore, the key to success is often to be the one company that delivers first on something for the patients' benefit. Anyone coming in after the first- or second-place entry will be less rewarded. As mentioned in the introduction, research attrition in the pharmaceutical industry is around 90%, meaning that 9 out of 10 projects fizzle before reaching the clinic. In the meantime, the (discovery) show must go on, and the company must sustain this endeavor with internal and investor money or turn to other sources of innovation.

Finally, research is a never-ending dynamic process. If development of new techniques and new concepts ceases, such a drug discovery platform can rapidly become obsolete.

Author details

Jean A. Boutin[1,2]*, Olivier Nosjean[1,2] and Gilles Ferry[1]

*Address all correspondence to: jean.boutin@servier.com

1 Institut de Recherches SERVIER, Croissy-sur-Seine, France

2 Institut de Recherches Internationales SERVIER, Suresnes, France

References

[1] Gao G, Chen L, Huang C. Anti-cancer drug discovery: Update and comparisons in yeast, Drosophila, and zebrafish. Current Molecular Pharmacology. 2014;**7**:44-51

[2] O'Reilly LP, Luke CJ, Perlmutter DH, Silverman GA, Pak SC. *C. elegans* in high-throughput drug discovery. Advanced Drug Delivery Reviews. 2014;**69-70**:247-253

[3] Scudamore CL. Integrating pathology into human disease modelling—How to eat the elephant. Disease Models & Mechanisms. 2014;**7**:495-497

[4] Kamps MP, Buss JE, Sefton BM. Mutation of NH2-terminal glycine of p60src prevents both myristoylation and morphological transformation. Proceedings of the National Academy of Sciences of the United States of America. 1985;**82**:4625-4628

[5] Boutin JA, Ferry G, Ernould AP, Maes P, Remond G, Vincent M. Myristoyl-CoA:protein N-myristoyltransferase activity in cancer cells. Purification and characterization of a cytosolic isoform from the murine leukemia cell line L1210. European Journal of Biochemistry. 1993;**214**:853-867

[6] Boutin JA. Myristoylation. Cellular Signalling. 1997;**9**:15-35

[7] Boutin JA, Clarenc JP, Ferry G, Ernould AP, Remond G, Vincent M, Atassi G. N-myristoyl-transferase activity in cancer cells. Solubilization, specificity and enzymatic inhibition of a N-myristoyl transferase from L1210 microsomes. European Journal of Biochemistry. 1991;**201**:257-263

[8] Ferry G, Tellier E, Try A, Gres S, Naime I, Simon MF, Rodriguez M, Boucher J, Tack I, Gesta S, Chomarat P, Dieu M, Raes M, Galizzi JP, Valet P, Boutin JA, Saulnier-Blache JS. Autotaxin is released from adipocytes, catalyzes lysophosphatidic acid synthesis, and activates preadipocyte proliferation. Up-regulated expression with adipocyte differentiation and obesity. Journal of Biological Chemistry. 2003;**278**:18162-18169

[9] Giganti A, Rodriguez M, Fould B, Moulharat N, Coge F, Chomarat P, Galizzi JP, Valet P, Saulnier-Blache JS, Boutin JA, Ferry G. Murine and human autotaxin alpha, beta, and gamma isoforms: Gene organization, tissue distribution, and biochemical characterization. The Journal of Biological Chemistry. 2008;**283**:7776-7789

[10] Sun S, Wang R, Song J, Guan M, Li N, Zhang X, Zhao Z, Zhang J. Blocking gp130 signaling suppresses autotaxin expression in adipocytes and improves insulin sensitivity in diet-induced obesity. Journal of Lipid Research. 2017

[11] Boutin JA, Ferry G. Autotaxin. Cellular and Molecular Life Sciences. 2009;**66**:3009-3021

[12] Ferry G, Moulharat N, Pradere JP, Desos P, Try A, Genton A, Giganti A, Beucher-Gaudin M, Lonchampt M, Bertrand M, Saulnier-Blache JS, Tucker GC, Cordi A, Boutin JA. S32826, a nanomolar inhibitor of autotaxin: Discovery, synthesis and applications as a pharmacological tool. The Journal of Pharmacology and Experimental Therapeutics. 2008;**327**:809-819

[13] Ferry G, Loynel A, Kucharczyk N, Bertin S, Rodriguez M, Delagrange P, Galizzi JP, Jacoby E, Volland JP, Lesieur D, Renard P, Canet E, Fauchere JL, Boutin JA. Substrate specificity and inhibition studies of human serotonin N-acetyltransferase. The Journal of Biological Chemistry. 2000;**275**:8794-8805

[14] Ganguly S, Gastel JA, Weller JL, Schwartz C, Jaffe H, Namboodiri MA, Coon SL, Hickman AB, Rollag M, Obsil T, Beauverger P, Ferry G, Boutin JA, Klein DC. Role of a pineal cAMP-operated arylalkylamine N-acetyltransferase/14-3-3-binding switch in melatonin synthesis. Proceedings of the National Academy of Sciences of the United States of America. 2001;**98**:8083-8088

[15] Mozo J, Ferry G, Masscheleyn S, Miroux B, Boutin JA, Bouillaud F. Assessment of a high-throughput screening methodology for the measurement of purified UCP1 uncoupling activity. Analytical Biochemistry. 2006;**351**:201-206

[16] Mozo J, Ferry G, Studeny A, Pecqueur C, Rodriguez M, Boutin JA, Bouillaud F. Expression of UCP3 in CHO cells does not cause uncoupling, but controls mitochondrial activity in the presence of glucose. The Biochemical Journal. 2006;**393**:431-439

[17] Guigal N, Rodriguez M, Cooper RN, Dromaint S, Di Santo JP, Mouly V, Boutin JA, Galizzi JP. Uncoupling protein-3 (UCP3) mRNA expression in reconstituted human muscle after myoblast transplantation in RAG2−/−/gamma c/C5(−) immunodeficient mice. The Journal of Biological Chemistry. 2002;**277**:47407-47411

[18] Riquet FB, Rodriguez M, Guigal N, Dromaint S, Naime I, Boutin JA, Galizzi JP. In vivo characterisation of the human UCP3 gene minimal promoter in mice tibialis anterior muscles. Biochemical and Biophysical Research Communications. 2003;**311**:583-591

[19] Henderson LC, Gibert Y. Editorial: Validation techniques for therapeutic molecules in drug discovery. Current Topics in Medicinal Chemistry. 2017;**17**:2005

[20] Kaelin WG. Cell biology: Divining cancer cell weaknesses. Nature. 2006;**441**:32-34

[21] Chomarat P, Coge F, Guenin SP, Mailliet F, Vella F, Mallet C, Giraudet S, Nagel N, Leonce S, Ferry G, Delagrange P, Boutin JA. Cellular knock-down of quinone reductase 2: A laborious road to successful inhibition by RNA interference. Biochimie. 2007;**89**:1264-1275

[22] Kaelin WG. Molecular biology. Use and abuse of RNAi to study mammalian gene function. Science. 2012;**337**:421-422

[23] Ferry G, Giganti A, Coge F, Bertaux F, Thiam K, Boutin JA. Functional invalidation of the autotaxin gene by a single amino acid mutation in mouse is lethal. FEBS Letters. 2007;**581**:3572-3578

[24] Benoit CE, Bastianetto S, Brouillette J, Tse Y, Boutin JA, Delagrange P, Wong T, Sarret P, Quirion R. Loss of quinone reductase 2 function selectively facilitates learning behaviors. The Journal of Neuroscience. 2010;**30**:12690-12700

[25] Mailliet F, Ferry G, Vella F, Thiam K, Delagrange P, Boutin JA. Organs from mice deleted for NRH:quinone oxidoreductase 2 are deprived of the melatonin binding site MT3. FEBS Letters. 2004;**578**:116-120

[26] van Meeteren LA, Ruurs P, Stortelers C, Bouwman P, van Rooijen MA, Pradere JP, Pettit TR, Wakelam MJ, Saulnier-Blache JS, Mummery CL, Moolenaar WH, Jonkers J. Autotaxin, a secreted lysophospholipase D, is essential for blood vessel formation during development. Molecular and Cellular Biology. 2006;**26**:5015-5022

[27] Tanaka M, Okudaira S, Kishi Y, Ohkawa R, Iseki S, Ota M, Noji S, Yatomi Y, Aoki J, Arai H. Autotaxin stabilizes blood vessels and is required for embryonic vasculature by producing lysophosphatidic acid. The Journal of Biological Chemistry. 2006;**281**:25822-25830

[28] Della-Zuana O, Audinot V, Levenez V, Ktorza A, Presse F, Nahon JL, Boutin JA. Peripheral injections of melanin-concentrating hormone receptor 1 antagonist S38151 decrease food intake and body weight in rodent obesity models. Frontiers in Endocrinology. 2012;**3**:160

[29] Di CB, Maggio R, Aloisi G, Rivet JM, Lundius EG, Yoshitake T, Svenningsson P, Brocco M, Gobert A, De GL, Cistarelli L, Veiga S, De MC, Rodriguez M, Galizzi JP, Lockhart BP, Coge F, Boutin JA, Vayer P, Verdouw PM, Groenink L, Millan MJ. Genetic deletion of trace amine 1 receptors reveals their role in auto-inhibiting the actions of ecstasy (MDMA). The Journal of Neuroscience. 2011;**31**:16928-16940

[30] Arsenijevic D, Onuma H, Pecqueur C, Raimbault S, Manning BS, Miroux B, Couplan E, Alves-Guerra MC, Goubern M, Surwit R, Bouillaud F, Richard D, Collins S, Ricquier D. Disruption of the uncoupling protein-2 gene in mice reveals a role in immunity and reactive oxygen species production. Nature Genetics. 2000;**26**:435-439

[31] Tosini G, Owino S, Guillaume JL, Jockers R. Understanding melatonin receptor pharmacology: Latest insights from mouse models, and their relevance to human disease. BioEssays. 2014;**36**:778-787

[32] Charpentier E. CRISPR-Cas9: How research on a bacterial RNA-guided mechanism opened new perspectives in biotechnology and biomedicine. EMBO Molecular Medicine. 2015;**7**:363-365

[33] Jung D, Choi Y, Uesugi M. Small organic molecules that modulate gene transcription. Drug Discovery Today. 2006;**11**:452-457

[34] Uesugi M. Synthetic molecules that modulate transcription and differentiation: Hints for future drug discovery. Combinatorial Chemistry & High Throughput Screening. 2004;**7**:653-659

[35] Zhang M, Feng Y, Wang J, Zhao J, Li T, He M, Yang D, Nosjean O, Boutin J, Renard P, Wang MW. High-throughput screening for GPR119 modulators identifies a novel compound with anti-diabetic efficacy in db/db mice. PLoS One. 2013;**8**:e63861

[36] Li T, Lin GY, Zhong L, Zhou Y, Wang J, Zhu Y, Feng Y, Cai XQ, Liu Q, Nosjean O, Boutin JA, Renard P, Yang DH, Wang MW. W2476 ameliorates beta-cell dysfunction and exerts therapeutic effects in mouse models of diabetes via modulation of the thioredoxin-interacting protein signaling pathway. Acta Pharmacologica Sinica. 2017;**38**:1024-1037

[37] Allera-Moreau C, Chomarat P, Audinot V, Coge F, Gillard M, Martineau Y, Boutin JA, Prats AC. The use of IRES-based bicistronic vectors allows the stable expression of recombinant G-protein coupled receptors such as NPY5 and histamine 4. Biochimie. 2006;**88**:737-746

[38] Cabaniols JP, Ouvry C, Lamamy V, Fery I, Craplet ML, Moulharat N, Guenin SP, Bedut S, Nosjean O, Ferry G, Devavry S, Jacqmarcq C, Lebuhotel C, Mathis L, Delenda C, Boutin JA, Duchateau P, Coge F, Paques F. Meganuclease-driven targeted integration in CHO-K1 cells for the fast generation of HTS-compatible cell-based assays. Journal of Biomolecular Screening. 2010;**15**:956-967

[39] Ferry G, Gillet L, Bruneau V, Banales JM, Beauverger P, Coge F, Galizzi JP, Scalbert E, Okamoto T, Urata H, Boutin JA. Development of new assays and improved procedures for the purification of recombinant human chymase. European Journal of Biochemistry. 2001;**268**:5885-5893

[40] Ferry G, Ubeaud C, Dauly C, Mozo J, Guillard S, Berger S, Jimenez S, Scoul C, Leclerc G, Yous S, Delagrange P, Boutin JA. Purification of the recombinant human serotonin N-acetyltransferase (EC 2.3.1.87): Further characterization of and comparison with AANAT from other species. Protein Expression and Purification. 2004;**38**:84-98

[41] Ferry G, Ubeaud C, Lambert PH, Bertin S, Coge F, Chomarat P, Delagrange P, Serkiz B, Bouchet JP, Truscott RJ, Boutin JA. Molecular evidence that melatonin is enzymatically oxidized in a different manner than tryptophan: Investigations with both indoleamine 2,3-dioxygenase and myeloperoxidase. The Biochemical Journal. 2005;**388**:205-215

[42] Brouillette J, Quirion R. Transthyretin: A key gene involved in the maintenance of memory capacities during aging. Neurobiology of Aging. 2008;**29**:1721-1732

[43] Nosjean O, Ferro M, Coge F, Beauverger P, Henlin JM, Lefoulon F, Fauchere JL, Delagrange P, Canet E, Boutin JA. Identification of the melatonin-binding site MT3 as the quinone reductase 2. The Journal of Biological Chemistry. 2000;**275**:31311-31317

[44] Rappaport AN, Jacob E, Sharma V, Inberg S, Elkobi A, Ounallah-Saad H, Pasmanik-Chor M, Edry E, Rosenblum K. Expression of quinone reductase-2 in the cortex is a

muscarinic acetylcholine receptor-dependent memory consolidation constraint. The Journal of Neuroscience. 2015;**35**:15568-15581

[45] Janda E, Parafati M, Aprigliano S, Carresi C, Visalli V, Sacco I, Ventrice D, Mega T, Vadala N, Rinaldi S, Musolino V, Palma E, Gratteri S, Rotiroti D, Mollace V. The antidote effect of quinone oxidoreductase 2 inhibitor against paraquat-induced toxicity in vitro and in vivo. British Journal of Pharmacology. 2013;**168**:46-59

[46] Janda E, Isidoro C, Carresi C, Mollace V. Defective autophagy in Parkinson's disease: Role of oxidative stress. Molecular Neurobiology. 2012;**46**:639-661

[47] Samadi N, Bekele R, Capatos D, Venkatraman G, Sariahmetoglu M, Brindley DN. Regulation of lysophosphatidate signaling by autotaxin and lipid phosphate phosphatases with respect to tumor progression, angiogenesis, metastasis and chemo-resistance. Biochimie. 2011;**93**:61-70

[48] Stracke ML, Krutzsch HC, Unsworth EJ, Arestad A, Cioce V, Schiffmann E, Liotta LA. Identification, purification, and partial sequence analysis of autotaxin, a novel motility-stimulating protein. The Journal of Biological Chemistry. 1992;**267**:2524-2529

[49] Benesch MG, Tang X, Maeda T, Ohhata A, Zhao YY, Kok BP, Dewald J, Hitt M, Curtis JM, McMullen TP, Brindley DN. Inhibition of autotaxin delays breast tumor growth and lung metastasis in mice. The FASEB Journal. 2014;**28**:2655-2666

[50] Boutin JA, Ernould AP, Genton A, Cudennec CA. Partial purification and characterization of a new p36/40 tyrosine protein kinase from HL-60. Biochemical and Biophysical Research Communications. 1989;**160**:1203-1211

[51] Ernould AP, Ferry G, Barret JM, Genton A, Boutin JA. Substrate phosphorylation capacities of the major tyrosine protein kinase from the human promyelocytic cell line, HL-60. International Journal of Peptide and Protein Research. 1994;**43**:496-504

[52] Wood S, Loudon A. Clocks for all seasons: Unwinding the roles and mechanisms of circadian and interval timers in the hypothalamus and pituitary. The Journal of Endocrinology. 2016;**228**:X1

[53] Wood S, Loudon A. The pars tuberalis: The site of the circannual clock in mammals? General and Comparative Endocrinology. 2017;**S0016-6480**(17):30350-30357

[54] Weaver DR, Liu C, Reppert SM. Nature's knockout: The Mel1b receptor is not necessary for reproductive and circadian responses to melatonin in Siberian hamsters. Molecular Endocrinology. 1996;**10**:1478-1487

[55] Coge F, Guenin SP, Fery I, Migaud M, Devavry S, Slugocki C, Legros C, Ouvry C, Cohen W, Renault N, Nosjean O, Malpaux B, Delagrange P, Boutin JA. The end of a myth: Cloning and characterization of the ovine melatonin MT(2) receptor. British Journal of Pharmacology. 2009;**158**:1248-1262

[56] Logez C, Berger S, Legros C, Baneres JL, Cohen W, Delagrange P, Nosjean O, Boutin JA, Ferry G, Simonin F, Wagner R. Recombinant human melatonin receptor MT1 isolated in

mixed detergents shows pharmacology similar to that in mammalian cell membranes. PLoS One. 2014;**9**:e100616

[57] Logez C, Damian M, Legros C, Dupre C, Guery M, Mary S, Wagner R, M'Kadmi C, Nosjean O, Fould B, Marie J, Fehrentz JA, Martinez J, Ferry G, Boutin JA, Baneres JL. Detergent-free isolation of functional G protein-coupled receptors into nanometric lipid particles. Biochemistry. 2016;**55**:38-48

[58] Alkhalfioui F, Magnin T, Wagner R. From purified GPCRs to drug discovery: The promise of protein-based methodologies. Current Opinion in Pharmacology. 2009;**9**:629-635

[59] Paul P, Lahaye C, Delagrange P, Nicolas JP, Canet E, Boutin JA. Characterization of 2-[125I]iodomelatonin binding sites in Syrian hamster peripheral organs. The Journal of Pharmacology and Experimental Therapeutics. 1999;**290**:334-340

[60] Duncan MJ, Takahashi JS, Dubocovich ML. 2-[125I]iodomelatonin binding sites in hamster brain membranes: Pharmacological characteristics and regional distribution. Endocrinology. 1988;**122**:1825-1833

[61] Vella F, Ferry G, Delagrange P, Boutin JA. NRH:quinone reductase 2: An enzyme of surprises and mysteries. Biochemical Pharmacology. 2005;**71**:1-12

[62] Boutin JA. Quinone reductase 2 as a promising target of melatonin therapeutic actions. Expert Opinion on Therapeutic Targets. 2016;**20**:303-317

[63] Rocheville M, Jerman JC. 7TM pharmacology measured by label-free: A holistic approach to cell signalling. Current Opinion in Pharmacology. 2009;**9**:643-649

[64] Leveridge M, Buxton R, Argyrou A, Francis P, Leavens B, West A, Rees M, Hardwicke P, Bridges A, Ratcliffe S, Chung CW. Demonstrating enhanced throughput of RapidFire mass spectrometry through multiplexing using the JmjD2d demethylase as a model system. Journal of Biomolecular Screening. 2014;**19**:278-286

[65] Boutin JA. Tyrosine protein kinase assays. Journal of Chromatography. B, Biomedical Applications. 1996;**684**:179-199

[66] Boutin JA, Ernould AP, Ferry G, Genton A, Alpert AJ. Use of hydrophilic interaction chromatography for the study of tyrosine protein kinase specificity. Journal of Chromatography. 1992;**583**:137-143

[67] Ferry G, Boutin JA. High-capacity screening of arylalkylamine N-acetyltransferase inhibitors using a high-performance liquid chromatography system. Journal of Biomolecular Screening. 2000;**5**:361-368

[68] Thomas M, Sabatini M, Bensaude F, Mignard B, Ortuno JC, Caron I, Boutin JA, Ferry G. A microplate assay for the screening of ADAMTS-4 inhibitors. Matrix Biology. 2006;**25**:261-267

[69] Letellier MA, Guillard J, Caignard DH, Ferry G, Boutin JA, Viaud-Massuard MC. Synthesis of potential rho-kinase inhibitors based on the chemistry of an original heterocycle:

4,4-dimethyl-3,4-dihydro-1H-quinolin-2-one. European Journal of Medicinal Chemistry. 2008;**43**:1730-1736

[70] Antoine M, Marcheteau E, Delagrange P, Ferry G, Boutin JA. Characterization of cofactors, substrates and inhibitor binding to flavoenzyme quinone reductase 2 by automated supramolecular nano-electrospray ionization mass spectrometry. International Journal of Mass Spectrometry. 2012;**312**:87-96

[71] Shapiro MJ, Wareing JR. NMR methods in combinatorial chemistry. Current Opinion in Chemical Biology. 1998;**2**:372-375

[72] Ferry G, Ubeaud C, Mozo J, Pean C, Hennig P, Rodriguez M, Scoul C, Bonnaud A, Nosjean O, Galizzi JP, Delagrange P, Renard P, Volland JP, Yous S, Lesieur D, Boutin JA. New substrate analogues of human serotonin N-acetyltransferase produce in situ specific and potent inhibitors. European Journal of Biochemistry. 2004;**271**:418-428

[73] Assemat O, Antoine M, Fourquez JM, Wierzbicki M, Charton Y, Hennig P, Perron-Sierra F, Ferry G, Boutin JA, Delsuc MA. (1)(9)F nuclear magnetic resonance screening of glucokinase activators. Analytical Biochemistry. 2015;**477**:62-68

[74] Boutin JA, Marcheteau E, Hennig P, Moulharat N, Berger S, Delagrange P, Bouchet JP, Ferry G. MT3/QR2 melatonin binding site does not use melatonin as a substrate or a co-substrate. Journal of Pineal Research. 2008;**45**:524-531

[75] Luttrell LM, Maudsley S, Gesty-Palmer D. Translating in vitro ligand bias into in vivo efficacy. Cellular Signalling. 2017

[76] Luttrell LM, Maudsley S, Bohn LM. Fulfilling the promise of "biased" G protein-coupled receptor agonism. Molecular Pharmacology. 2015;**88**:579-588

[77] Maudsley S. G protein-coupled receptor biased agonism: Development towards future selective therapeutics. Mini Reviews in Medicinal Chemistry. 2012;**12**:803

[78] Audinot V, Fabry N, Nicolas JP, Beauverger P, Newman-Tancredi A, Millan MJ, Try A, Bornancin F, Canet E, Boutin JA. Ligand modulation of [35S]GTPgammaS binding at human alpha(2A), alpha(2B) and alpha(2C) adrenoceptors. Cellular Signalling. 2002;**14**:829-837

[79] Cecon E, Oishi A, Jockers R. Melatonin receptors: Molecular pharmacology and signalling in the context of system bias. British Journal of Pharmacology. 2017. DOI: 10.1111/bph.13950

[80] Boutin JA, Bonnaud A, Brasseur C, Bruno O, Lepretre N, Oosting P, Coumailleau S, Delagrange P, Nosjean O, Legros C. New MT(2) melatonin receptor-selective ligands: Agonists and partial agonists. International Journal of Molecular Sciences. 2017;**18**, pii: E1347

[81] Ferry G, Bruneau V, Beauverger P, Goussard M, Rodriguez M, Lamamy V, Dromaint S, Canet E, Galizzi JP, Boutin JA. Binding of prostaglandins to human PPARgamma: Tool assessment and new natural ligands. European Journal of Pharmacology. 2001;**417**:77-89

[82] Langer T, Hoffmann R, Bryant S, Lesur B. Hit finding: Towards 'smarter' approaches. Current Opinion in Pharmacology. 2009;**9**:589-593

[83] Macarron R, Banks MN, Bojanic D, Burns DJ, Cirovic DA, Garyantes T, Green DV, Hertzberg RP, Janzen WP, Paslay JW, Schopfer U, Sittampalam GS. Impact of high-throughput screening in biomedical research. Nature Reviews. Drug Discovery. 2011;**10**: 188-195

[84] Mayr LM, Bojanic D. Novel trends in high-throughput screening. Current Opinion in Pharmacology. 2009;**9**:580-588

[85] Jensen VK, Nosjean O, Dziegiel MH, Boutin JA, Sorensen MG, Karsdal MA, Henriksen K. A quantitative assay for lysosomal acidification rates in human osteoclasts. Assay and Drug Development Technologies. 2011;**9**:157-164

[86] Moffat JG, Vincent F, Lee JA, Eder J, Prunotto M. Opportunities and challenges in phenotypic drug discovery: An industry perspective. Nature Reviews. Drug Discovery. 2017;**16**:531-543

[87] Saeidnia S, Gohari AR, Manayi A. Reverse pharmacognosy and reverse pharmacology; two closely related approaches for drug discovery development. Current Pharmaceutical Biotechnology. 2016;**17**:1016-1022

[88] Gillet VJ. New directions in library design and analysis. Current Opinion in Chemical Biology. 2008;**12**:372-378

[89] Gillet VJ. Diversity selection algorithms. WIREs Computational Molecular Science. 2011;**1**:580-589

[90] Mount J, Ruppert J, Welch W, Jain AN. IcePick: A flexible surface-based system for molecular diversity. Journal of Medicinal Chemistry. 1999;**42**:60-66

[91] Makara GM. Measuring molecular similarity and diversity: Total pharmacophore diversity. Journal of Medicinal Chemistry. 2001;**44**:3563-3571

[92] Maldonado AG, Doucet JP, Petitjean M, Fan BT. Molecular similarity and diversity in chemoinformatics: From theory to applications. Molecular Diversity. 2006;**10**:39-79

[93] Lepp Z, Huang C, Okada T. Finding key members in compound libraries by analyzing networks of molecules assembled by structural similarity. Journal of Chemical Information and Modeling. 2009;**49**:2429-2443

[94] Jenkins JL, Glick M, Davies JW. A 3D similarity method for scaffold hopping from known drugs or natural ligands to new chemotypes. Journal of Medicinal Chemistry. 2004;**47**:6144-6159

[95] Heinrich M, Lardos A, Leonti M, Weckerle C, Willcox M. Best practice in research: Consensus statement on ethnopharmacological field studies—ConSEFS. Journal of Ethnopharmacology. 2018;**211**:329-339

[96] Bousserouel H, Litaudon M, Morleo B, Martin MT, Thoison O, Nosjean O, Boutin JA, Renard P, Sevenet T. New biologically active linear triterpenes from the bark of three new-caledonian Cupaniopsis species. Tetrahedron. 2005;**61**:845-851

[97] Litaudon M, Jolly C, Le CC, Cuong DD, Retailleau P, Nosjean O, Nguyen VH, Pfeiffer B, Boutin JA, Gueritte F. Cytotoxic pentacyclic triterpenoids from *Combretum sundaicum* and *Lantana camara* as inhibitors of Bcl-xL/BakBH3 domain peptide interaction. Journal of Natural Products. 2009;**72**:1314-1320

[98] Litaudon M, Bousserouel H, Awang K, Nosjean O, Martin MT, Dau ME, Hadi HA, Boutin JA, Sevenet T, Gueritte F. A dimeric sesquiterpenoid from a Malaysian Meiogyne as a new inhibitor of Bcl-xL/BakBH3 domain peptide interaction. Journal of Natural Products. 2009;**72**:480-483

[99] Boutin JA, Chatelain-Egger F, Vella F, Delagrange P, Ferry G. Quinone reductase 2 substrate specificity and inhibition pharmacology. Chemico-Biological Interactions. 2005;**151**:213-228

[100] Boutin JA, Fauchere AL. Combinatorial peptide synthesis: Statistical evaluation of peptide distribution. Trends in Pharmacological Sciences. 1996;**17**:8-12

[101] Boutin JA, Hennig P, Lambert PH, Bertin S, Petit L, Mahieu JP, Serkiz B, Volland JP, Fauchere JL. Combinatorial peptide libraries: Robotic synthesis and analysis by nuclear magnetic resonance, mass spectrometry, tandem mass spectrometry, and high-performance capillary electrophoresis techniques. Analytical Biochemistry. 1996;**234**:126-141

[102] Ferry G, Boutin JA, Atassi G, Fauchere JL, Tucker GC. Selection of a histidine-containing inhibitor of gelatinases through deconvolution of combinatorial tetrapeptide libraries. Molecular Diversity. 1997;**2**:135-146

[103] Boutin JA, Marande W, Petit L, Loynel A, Desmet C, Canet E, Fauchere JL. Investigation of S-farnesyl transferase substrate specificity with combinatorial tetrapeptide libraries. Cellular Signalling. 1999;**11**:59-69

[104] Houghten RA, Pinilla C, Blondelle SE, Appel JR, Dooley CT, Cuervo JH. Generation and use of synthetic peptide combinatorial libraries for basic research and drug discovery. Nature. 1991;**354**:84-86

[105] Dahlin JL, Walters MA. The essential roles of chemistry in high-throughput screening triage. Future Medicinal Chemistry. 2014;**6**:1265-1290

[106] Tordjman S, Chokron S, Delorme R, Charrier A, Bellissant E, Jaafari N, Fougerou C. Melatonin: Pharmacology, functions and therapeutic benefits. Current Neuropharmacology. 2017;**15**:434-443

[107] Shehzad A, Qureshi M, Anwar MN, Lee YS. Multifunctional curcumin mediate multitherapeutic effects. Journal of Food Science. 2017;**82**:2006-2015

[108] Tsai HY, Ho CT, Chen YK. Biological actions and molecular effects of resveratrol, pterostilbene, and 3′-hydroxypterostilbene. Journal of Food and Drug Analysis. 2017;**25**:134-147

[109] Xu J, Hagler A. Chemoinformatics and drug discovery. Molecules. 2002;**7**:566-600

[110] Humbeck L, Koch O. What can we learn from bioactivity data? Chemoinformatics tools and applications in chemical biology research. ACS Chemical Biology. 2017;**12**:23-35

[111] Genick CC, Wright SK. Biophysics: For HTS hit validation, chemical lead optimization, and beyond. Expert Opinion on Drug Discovery. 2017;**12**:897-907

[112] Radziejewski C, Miller WT, Mobashery S, Goldberg AR, Kaiser ET. Purification of recombinant pp60v-src protein tyrosine kinase and phosphorylation of peptides with different secondary structure preference. Biochemistry. 1989;**28**:9047-9052

[113] Barret JM, Ernould AP, Ferry G, Genton A, Boutin JA. Integrated system for the screening of the specificity of protein kinase inhibitors. Biochemical Pharmacology. 1993;**46**:439-448

[114] Cooper JA, Esch FS, Taylor SS, Hunter T. Phosphorylation sites in enolase and lactate dehydrogenase utilized by tyrosine protein kinases in vivo and in vitro. The Journal of Biological Chemistry. 1984;**259**:7835-7841

[115] Bacchi M, Fould B, Jullian M, Kreiter A, Maurras A, Nosjean O, Coursindel T, Puget K, Ferry G, Boutin JA. Screening ubiquitin specific protease activities using chemically synthesized ubiquitin and ubiquitinated peptides. Analytical Biochemistry. 2017;**519**:57-70

[116] Legros C, Matthey U, Grelak T, Pedragona-Moreau S, Hassler W, Yous S, Thomas E, Suzenet F, Folleas B, Lefoulon F, Berthelot P, Caignard DH, Guillaumet G, Delagrange P, Brayer JL, Nosjean O, Boutin JA. New radioligands for describing the molecular pharmacology of MT1 and MT2 melatonin receptors. International Journal of Molecular Sciences. 2013;**14**:8948-8962

[117] Legros C, Brasseur C, Delagrange P, Ducrot P, Nosjean O, Boutin JA. Alternative radioligands for investigating the molecular pharmacology of melatonin receptors. The Journal of Pharmacology and Experimental Therapeutics. 2016;**356**:681-692

[118] Audinot V, Lahaye C, Suply T, Beauverger P, Rodriguez M, Galizzi JP, Fauchere JL, Boutin JA. [125I]-S36057: A new and highly potent radioligand for the melanin-concentrating hormone receptor. British Journal of Pharmacology. 2001;**133**:371-378

[119] Rodriguez M, Beauverger P, Naime I, Rique H, Ouvry C, Souchaud S, Dromaint S, Nagel N, Suply T, Audinot V, Boutin JA, Galizzi JP. Cloning and molecular characterization of the novel human melanin-concentrating hormone receptor MCH2. Molecular Pharmacology. 2001;**60**:632-639

[120] Chartrel N, Alvear-Perez R, Leprince J, Iturrioz X, Reaux-Le GA, Audinot V, Chomarat P, Coge F, Nosjean O, Rodriguez M, Galizzi JP, Boutin JA, Vaudry H, Llorens-Cortes C. Comment on "Obestatin, a peptide encoded by the ghrelin gene, opposes ghrelin's effects on food intake". Science. 2007;**315**:766

[121] Le MO, Neveu C, Lefranc B, Dubessy C, Boutin JA, Do-Rego JC, Costentin J, Tonon MC, Tena-Sempere M, Vaudry H, Leprince J. Structure-activity relationships of a series of analogues of the RFamide-related peptide 26RFa. Journal of Medicinal Chemistry. 2011;**54**:4806-4814

[122] Chartrel N, Alonzeau J, Alexandre D, Jeandel L, Alvear-Perez R, Leprince J, Boutin J, Vaudry H, Anouar Y, Llorens-Cortes C. The RFamide neuropeptide 26RFa and its role in the control of neuroendocrine functions. Frontiers in Neuroendocrinology. 2011;**32**:387-397

[123] Neveu C, Lefranc B, Tasseau O, Do-Rego JC, Bourmaud A, Chan P, Bauchat P, Le MO, Chuquet J, Guilhaudis L, Boutin JA, Segalas-Milazzo I, Costentin J, Vaudry H, Baudy-Floc'h M, Vaudry D, Leprince J. Rational design of a low molecular weight, stable, potent, and long-lasting GPR103 aza-beta3-pseudopeptide agonist. Journal of Medicinal Chemistry. 2012;**55**:7516-7524

[124] Neveu C, Dulin F, Lefranc B, Galas L, Calbrix C, Bureau R, Rault S, Chuquet J, Boutin JA, Guilhaudis L, Segalas-Milazzo I, Vaudry D, Vaudry H, Santos JS, Leprince J. Molecular basis of agonist docking in a human GPR103 homology model by site-directed mutagenesis and structure-activity relationship studies. British Journal of Pharmacology. 2014;**171**:4425-4439

[125] Ould-Hamouda H, Chen P, Levoye A, Sozer-Topcular N, Daulat AM, Guillaume JL, Ravid R, Savaskan E, Ferry G, Boutin JA, Delagrange P, Jockers R, Maurice P. Detection of the human GPR50 orphan seven transmembrane protein by polyclonal antibodies mapping different epitopes. Journal of Pineal Research. 2007;**43**:10-15

[126] Sidibe A, Mullier A, Chen P, Baroncini M, Boutin JA, Delagrange P, Prevot V, Jockers R. Expression of the orphan GPR50 protein in rodent and human dorsomedial hypothalamus, tanycytes and median eminence. Journal of Pineal Research. 2010;**48**:263-269

[127] Audinot V, Beauverger P, Lahaye C, Suply T, Rodriguez M, Ouvry C, Lamamy V, Imbert J, Rique H, Nahon JL, Galizzi JP, Canet E, Levens N, Fauchere JL, Boutin JA. Structure-activity relationship studies of melanin-concentrating hormone (MCH)-related peptide ligands at SLC-1, the human MCH receptor. The Journal of Biological Chemistry. 2001;**276**:13554-13562

[128] Audinot V, Zuana OD, Fabry N, Ouvry C, Nosjean O, Henlin JM, Fauchere JL, Boutin JA. S38151 [p-guanidinobenzoyl-[des-Gly(10)]-MCH(7-17)] is a potent and selective antagonist at the MCH(1) receptor and has anti-feeding properties in vivo. Peptides. 2009;**30**:1997-2007

[129] Scapin G. Structural biology and drug discovery. Current Pharmaceutical Design. 2006;**12**:2087-2097

[130] Hu T, Sprague ER, Fodor M, Stams T, Clark KL, Cowan-Jacob SW. The impact of structural biology in medicine illustrated with four case studies. Journal of Molecular Medicine. 2018;**96**:9-19

[131] Zheng H, Handing KB, Zimmerman MD, Shabalin IG, Almo SC, Minor W. X-ray crystallography over the past decade for novel drug discovery—Where are we heading next? Expert Opinion on Drug Discovery. 2015;**10**:975-989

[132] Zheng H, Hou J, Zimmerman MD, Wlodawer A, Minor W. The future of crystallography in drug discovery. Expert Opinion on Drug Discovery. 2014;**9**:125-137

[133] Venien-Bryan C, Li Z, Vuillard L, Boutin JA. Cryo-electron microscopy and X-ray crystallography: Complementary approaches to structural biology and drug discovery. Acta Crystallographica Section F. 2017;**73**:174-183

[134] Calamini B, Santarsiero BD, Boutin JA, Mesecar AD. Kinetic, thermodynamic and X-ray structural insights into the interaction of melatonin and analogues with quinone reductase 2. The Biochemical Journal. 2008;**413**:81-91

[135] Pegan SD, Sturdy M, Ferry G, Delagrange P, Boutin JA, Mesecar AD. X-ray structural studies of quinone reductase 2 nanomolar range inhibitors. Protein Science. 2011;**20**:1182-1195

[136] Cassagnes LE, Rakotoarivelo N, Sirigu S, Perio P, Najahi E, Chavas LM, Thompson A, Gayon R, Ferry G, Boutin JA, Valentin A, Reybier K, Nepveu F. Role of quinone reductase 2 in the antimalarial properties of indolone-type derivatives. Molecules. 2017;**22**, pii: E210

[137] Sancier F, Dumont A, Sirvent A, Paquay de PL, Edmonds T, David G, Jan M, De MC, Coge F, Leonce S, Burbridge M, Bruno A, Boutin JA, Lockhart B, Roche S, Cruzalegui F. Specific oncogenic activity of the Src-family tyrosine kinase c-Yes in colon carcinoma cells. PLoS One. 2011;**6**:e17237

[138] Burbridge MF, Bossard CJ, Saunier C, Fejes I, Bruno A, Leonce S, Ferry G, Da VG, Bouzom F, Cattan V, Jacquet-Bescond A, Comoglio PM, Lockhart BP, Boutin JA, Cordi A, Ortuno JC, Pierre A, Hickman JA, Cruzalegui FH, Depil S. S49076 is a novel kinase inhibitor of MET, AXL, and FGFR with strong preclinical activity alone and in association with bevacizumab. Molecular Cancer Therapeutics. 2013;**12**:1749-1762

[139] Ferry G, Studeny A, Bossard C, Kubara PM, Zeyer D, Renaud JP, Casara P, de NG, Wierzbicki M, Pfeiffer B, Prudhomme M, Leonce S, Pierre A, Boutin JA, Golsteyn RM. Characterization of novel checkpoint kinase 1 inhibitors by in vitro assays and in human cancer cells treated with topoisomerase inhibitors. Life Sciences. 2011;**89**:259-268

[140] Petit P, Antoine M, Ferry G, Boutin JA, Lagarde A, Gluais L, Vincentelli R, Vuillard L. The active conformation of human glucokinase is not altered by allosteric activators. Acta Crystallographica. Section D, Biological Crystallography. 2011;**67**:929-935

[141] Bacchi M, Jullian M, Sirigu S, Fould B, Huet T, Bruyand L, Antoine M, Vuillard L, Ronga L, Chavas LM, Nosjean O, Ferry G, Puget K, Boutin JA. Total chemical synthesis, refolding, and crystallographic structure of fully active immunophilin calstabin 2 (FKBP12.6). Protein Science. 2016;**25**:2225-2242

[142] Gerard CJJ, Ferry G, Vuillard L, Boutin JA, Chavas LM, Huet T, Ferte N, Grossier R, Candoni N, Veesler S. Crystallisation using tubing microfluidics permits both in situ and ex situ X-ray diffraction. Acta Crystallographica. Section F, Structural Biology and Crystallization Communications. 2017;**73**:574-578

[143] Zhang S, Gerard CJJ, Ikni A, Ferry G, Vuillard L, Boutin JA, Ferte N, Grossier R, Candoni N, Veesler S. Microfluidic platform for optimization of crystallization conditions. Journal of Crystal Growth. 2017;**472**:18-28

[144] Mollica L, Theret I, Antoine M, Perron-Sierra F, Charton Y, Fourquez JM, Wierzbicki M, Boutin JA, Ferry G, Decherchi S, Bottegoni G, Ducrot P, Cavalli A. Molecular dynamics simulations and kinetic measurements to estimate and predict protein-ligand residence times. Journal of Medicinal Chemistry. 2016;**59**:7167-7176

[145] Westermaier Y, Ruiz-Carmona S, Theret I, Perron-Sierra F, Poissonnet G, Dacquet C, Boutin JA, Ducrot P, Barril X. Binding mode prediction and MD/MMPBSA-based free energy ranking for agonists of REV-ERBalpha/NCoR. Journal of Computer-Aided Molecular Design. 2017;**31**:755-775

[146] Folmer RH. Integrating biophysics with HTS-driven drug discovery projects. Drug Discovery Today. 2016;**21**:491-498

[147] Renaud JP, Chung CW, Danielson UH, Egner U, Hennig M, Hubbard RE, Nar H. Biophysics in drug discovery: Impact, challenges and opportunities. Nature Reviews. Drug Discovery. 2016;**15**:679-698

[148] Renaud JP, Delsuc MA. Biophysical techniques for ligand screening and drug design. Current Opinion in Pharmacology. 2009;**9**:622-628

[149] Shuman CF, Hamalainen MD, Danielson UH. Kinetic and thermodynamic characterization of HIV-1 protease inhibitors. Journal of Molecular Recognition. 2004;**17**:106-119

[150] Vaissiere A, Berger S, Harrus D, Dacquet C, Le MA, Boutin JA, Ferry G, Royer CA. Molecular mechanisms of transcriptional control by Rev-erbalpha: An energetic foundation for reconciling structure and binding with biological function. Protein Science. 2015;**24**:1129-1146

[151] Antoine M, Boutin JA, Ferry G. Binding kinetics of glucose and allosteric activators to human glucokinase reveal multiple conformational states. Biochemistry. 2009;**48**:5466-5482

[152] Stojko J, Fieulaine S, Petiot-Becard S, Van DA, Meinnel T, Giglione C, Cianferani S. Ion mobility coupled to native mass spectrometry as a relevant tool to investigate extremely small ligand-induced conformational changes. The Analyst. 2015;**140**:7234-7245

[153] Mailliet F, Ferry G, Vella F, Berger S, Coge F, Chomarat P, Mallet C, Guenin SP, Guillaumet G, Viaud-Massuard MC, Yous S, Delagrange P, Boutin JA. Characterization of the melatoninergic MT3 binding site on the NRH:quinone oxidoreductase 2 enzyme. Biochemical Pharmacology. 2005;**71**:74-88

[154] Liu X, Ahn S, Kahsai AW, Meng KC, Latorraca NR, Pani B, Venkatakrishnan AJ, Masoudi A, Weis WI, Dror RO, Chen X, Lefkowitz RJ, Kobilka BK. Mechanism of intracellular allosteric beta2AR antagonist revealed by X-ray crystal structure. Nature. 2017;**548**:480-484

[155] Zhang H, Qiao A, Yang D, Yang L, Dai A, de GC, Reedtz-Runge S, Dharmarajan V, Zhang H, Han GW, Grant TD, Sierra RG, Weierstall U, Nelson G, Liu W, Wu Y, Ma L, Cai X, Lin G, Wu X, Geng Z, Dong Y, Song G, Griffin PR, Lau J, Cherezov V, Yang H,

Hanson MA, Stevens RC, Zhao Q, Jiang H, Wang MW, Wu B. Structure of the full-length glucagon class B G-protein-coupled receptor. Nature. 2017;**546**:259-264

[156] Bedut S, Seminatore-Nole C, Lamamy V, Caignard S, Boutin JA, Nosjean O, Stephan JP, Coge F. High-throughput drug profiling with voltage- and calcium-sensitive fluorescent probes in human iPSC-derived cardiomyocytes. American Journal of Physiology. Heart and Circulatory Physiology. 2016;**311**:H44-H53

[157] Kujala K, Paavola J, Lahti A, Larsson K, Pekkanen-Mattila M, Viitasalo M, Lahtinen AM, Toivonen L, Kontula K, Swan H, Laine M, Silvennoinen O, Aalto-Setala K. Cell model of catecholaminergic polymorphic ventricular tachycardia reveals early and delayed afterdepolarizations. PLoS One. 2012;**7**:e44660

[158] Novak A, Barad L, Lorber A, Gherghiceanu M, Reiter I, Eisen B, Eldor L, Itskovitz-Eldor J, Eldar M, Arad M, Binah O. Functional abnormalities in iPSC-derived cardiomyocytes generated from CPVT1 and CPVT2 patients carrying ryanodine or calsequestrin mutations. Journal of Cellular and Molecular Medicine. 2015;**19**:2006-2018

[159] Cohen J. Surviving the cure. Science. 2017;**357**:122-125

[160] Gornalusse GG, Hirata RK, Funk SE, Riolobos L, Lopes VS, Manske G, Prunkard D, Colunga AG, Hanafi LA, Clegg DO, Turtle C, Russell DW. HLA-E-expressing pluripotent stem cells escape allogeneic responses and lysis by NK cells. Nature Biotechnology. 2017;**35**:765-772

[161] Kent S. Chemical protein synthesis: Inventing synthetic methods to decipher how proteins work. Bioorganic & Medicinal Chemistry. 2017;**25**:4926-4937

[162] Fernandez-Suarez M, Ting AY. Fluorescent probes for super-resolution imaging in living cells. Nature Reviews. Molecular Cell Biology. 2008;**9**:929-943

[163] Rouch A, Fould B, Jeantet E, Marcheteau E, Antoine M, Nosjean O, Ferry G, Boutin JA. On the acellular use of lipoic acid ligase for labeling proteins. Advances in Biochemistry and Biotechnology. 2017;**110**

[164] Schukur L, Geering B, Charpin-El HG, Fussenegger M. Implantable synthetic cytokine converter cells with AND-gate logic treat experimental psoriasis. Science Translational Medicine. 2015;**7**:318ra201

[165] Kotschy A, Szlavik Z, Murray J, Davidson J, Maragno AL, Le Toumelin-Braizat G, Chanrion M, Kelly GL, Gong JN, Moujalled DM, Bruno A, Csekei M, Paczal A, Szabo ZB, Sipos S, Radics G, Proszenyak A, Balint B, Ondi L, Blasko G, Robertson A, Surgenor A, Dokurno P, Chen I, Matassova N, Smith J, Pedder C, Graham C, Studeny A, Lysiak-Auvity G, Girard AM, Grave F, Segal D, Riffkin CD, Pomilio G, Galbraith LC, Aubrey BJ, Brennan MS, Herold MJ, Chang C, Guasconi G, Cauquil N, Melchiore F, Guigal-Stephan N, Lockhart B, Colland F, Hickman JA, Roberts AW, Huang DC, Wei AH, Strasser A, Lessene G, Geneste O. The MCL1 inhibitor S63845 is tolerable and effective in diverse cancer models. Nature. 2016;**538**:477-482

[166] Rosenblatt M. An incentive-based approach for improving data reproducibility. Science Translational Medicine. 2016;**8**:336ed5

[167] Jasny BR, Wigginton N, McNutt M, Bubela T, Buck S, Cook-Deegan R, Gardner T, Hanson B, Hustad C, Kiermer V, Lazer D, Lupia A, Manrai A, McConnell L, Noonan K, Phimister E, Simon B, Strandburg K, Summers Z, Watts D. Fostering reproducibility in industry-academia research. Science. 2017;**357**:759-761

10

Bioinformatics Discovery of Vertebrate Cathelicidins from the Mining of Available Genomes

José Manuel Pérez de la Lastra,
Cristina Garrido-Orduña, Andrés A. Borges,
David Jiménez-Arias,
Francisco Javier García-Machado,
Mercedes Hernández, Concepción González and
Alicia Boto

Abstract

Due to the worrying increase in antimicrobial resistance to conventional antibiotics, the search for alternatives is becoming increasingly important. Antimicrobial peptides (AMPs), originating from natural resources, have been recognised as a novel class of antibiotics. An advantage of peptides over antibiotics is that the resistance is more difficult to attain than for conventional antibiotics. With the increasing number of genomes sequenced and available in the public domain, one alternative methodology to obtain novel AMPs is to analyse genes and proteins from genomic databases to predict and identify amino acid sequences that share similarities and molecular features with natural bioactive antimicrobial peptides. In this chapter, we summarise some of our recent results on the production of antimicrobial peptides, particularly, how we managed to identify a family of antimicrobial peptides: cathelicidins, through bioinformatics tools, from the genomes of two lower vertebrates (a reptile and a bird) available in public databases. We hope that our preliminary investigation with these novel peptides could be useful for the design of future strategies that pursue the production of antimicrobial peptides through biotechnology.

Keywords: cathelicidin, antimicrobial, peptide, antibiotics, genome mining

1. Introduction

Conventional drugs for the treatment of human diseases can be classified as small molecules, proteins and peptides. The cost of goods, products quality and scalability are always major factors when considering the development of any new class of drugs. Generally, in the drug development process, small molecules are still preferred over peptides primarily due to their ease of production, simplicity of administration (as oral pill), and superior pharmacodynamics properties. In addition to stability and delivery, these factors have historically been seen as hurdles for peptide drug development versus their small molecule counterparts [1].

In the case of antibiotics, due to the worrying increase in antimicrobial resistance to conventional antibiotics, together with the long-term decline of investment by pharmaceutical companies, the search for alternatives is becoming increasingly important [2]. Traditionally, soil bacteria (especially actinomycetes), fungi and higher plants were main sources for drug discovery. However, no new class of antibiotics has been discovered since 1987 [3]. Antimicrobial peptides, originating from natural resources, have been recognised as a novel class of antibiotics [4]. Cationic antimicrobial peptides neutralise target pathogens through deleterious interactions with membrane components, which relies on the difference in lipid composition between normal eukaryotic and prokaryotic (or transformed eukaryotic) cell membranes [5]. Therefore, microbial resistance to antimicrobial peptides is rare. Moreover, peptide antimicrobials are active against both metabolically active and non-metabolising microorganisms, whereas most antibiotics have specific targets that define their mechanism of action and are active only against replicating microbes. Antimicrobials with novel *modi operandi* are consequently in high demand in a world faced with an increasing number of multidrug resistant pathogens, as well as a changing panorama of infections [4, 6].

Our emphasis in this chapter will be on the discovery of naturally occurring antimicrobial peptides for use in development of new antimicrobial drugs. Discovery of natural bioactive molecules is, of course, only the first step in the biodiscovery pipeline. The spectrum of available candidate peptide drugs is by far not limited to the human peptide pool. Through evolution, numerous peptides have evolved to exhibit their natural bioactivity outside of the producing organisms [5]. The cationic peptides polymyxin B and gramicidin S have been used in the clinic as topical over-the-counter medicines for a long time, and the cationic lantibiotic nisin is used as an antimicrobial food additive. In general, antimicrobial peptides in different species are surprisingly different. For example, magainins found in the skin of the frog *Xenopus laevis* were initially thought to be universal antimicrobial agents. However, it turns out that every frog investigated has its own peptide antibiotics [7]. It has been argued that that the immense diversity of cationic peptides arises from their antimicrobial function as well as the different pathogenic microbe challenges they face in each host organisms. We believe that nature still harbours a virtually infinite array of potential peptidic medications that await human pharmacological characterisation. Particularly, organisms living in germ-filled environments could be an abundant source of antimicrobials and can likely provide us with superior templates for use in development of new antimicrobial drugs to help solve the medical problems that exist today [8].

With the advent of facile genome sequencing, new antibiotics are being found by the techniques of genome mining, offering hope for the future [9]. The aim of this study is to illustrate the identification of novel antimicrobial peptides from exotic vertebrates through refined computational methods. Genome mining involves looking at the sequenced genome of organisms to determine if gene cluster involved in the production of new antimicrobial peptides can be found in these organisms. The cathelicidins are a family of antimicrobial peptides encoded in the genome of vertebrates. These peptides are characterised by being formed by a pre-propeptide, which in neutrophils is processed by the enzyme elastase to originate the active peptide. There is a great variability between the sequences of the active peptides of cathelicidins [10]. However, the pre-pro peptide is highly conserved, which is very useful for the mining of vertebrate genomes to identify putative genes of this family of antimicrobial peptides. The genes coding for cathelicidins typically consist of four exons, the fourth exon being the one that codes for the active peptide and, therefore, the least conserved. The number of cathelicidin genes is different among species. For example, cows have 11 genes, humans have only one, and sheep have eight [10, 11]. This structural and/or functional diversity within the cathelicidin family could reflect the spectrum of microbicide and immunomodulatory activities of cathelicidins in different species exposed to different microbial load [12].

We have previously described the characterisation of peptides derived from the genomes of mammals [13]. We here illustrate a simple method for the identification of two cathelicidin genes in the genome of lower vertebrates (birds and reptiles) living in different environments, and thus surrounded by different pathogens. We also perform the bioinformatic analysis of the corresponding active peptides to detect possible antimicrobial properties and describe the functional characterisation of the two identified cathelicidins against a panel of reference microorganisms. Finally, we describe our current attempt for the biotechnological production of these peptides in microalgae.

2. Materials and methods

2.1. Obtaining of the cathelicidin sequences

Access to the genomes of the different species studied was carried out in September 2012, through the genebank public databases (http://www.ncbi.nlm.nih.gov/genome). At these dates, different genomes were still assembled in contiguous, or contigs, that were accessible for tracing by nucleotide BLAST (http://blast.ncbi.nlm.nih.gov/Blast.cgi).

For the screening of animal genomes, a nucleotide sequence of 83 base pairs (bp) was used, based on a highly conserved region between bird cathelicidins, which corresponds to the following sequence:

cccaggctgtggactcctacaaccaacggcctgaggtgcagaatgccttccggctgctcagcgccgaccccgagcccggcccg

P R L W T P T T N G L R R M P S G C S A P T P S P A

The search for sequences homologous to this sequence was made using the BLAST application, using the values of the default parameters, which returned us the contiguous (contigs), or scaffolds, of genomic DNA where sequences homologous to our sequence and, therefore, probable coding genes for cathelicidins.

2.2. Prediction of cathelicidin genes

Once the different contigs of homology were obtained with this sequence, we proceeded to study if they contained genes corresponding to cathelicidins. For this, two types of programs were used: GenScan (http://genes.mit.edu/GENSCAN.html) and GeneMark (http://exon. gatech.edu/GeneMark/), with the default values of the different parameters. Both programs predict putative genes within these contigs or scaffolds of previously selected sequences. The criteria adopted for the identification of cathelicidins in these contigs was that the predicted genes contained four exons and that in addition the amino acid sequence of the first three exons was homologous to the already known cathelicidins, with a percentage of residue identity of more than one 30%, provided that the position of some key residues of the pre-pro-peptide, such as cysteines, essential for the maintenance of its structure, is preserved.

2.3. Prediction of antimicrobial peptides

The fourth exon of the predicted cathelicidins was then translated into amino acids and, to identify the possible cleavage site by the neutrophil elastase enzyme, the amino acid sequence of the fourth exon was subjected to the online Peptidecutter tool (http://web. expasy.org/ peptide_cutter/), taking as an active peptide that generated after the theoretical cut by this enzyme in its leftmost position, towards the C-terminal end.

2.4. Bioinformatic analysis of the cathelicidin sequences

The percentage of hydrophobicity and the Boman index of the derived cathelicidins were calculated by the ADP3 tool (http://aps.unmc.edu/AP/prediction/prediction_main.php). The Boman index estimates the potential of a protein to bind to another protein. Thus, if a protein has a high Boman index, it means that said peptide would be multifunctional and, once inside the cell, it would have more or less capacity to bind to several proteins and perform different functions within the cell, given its capacity to interact with a wide range of proteins. The antimicrobial activity of the peptides was evaluated in silico with the AMPA tool (http:// tcoffee.crg.cat/apps/ampa/do) described in [14] Torrent et al. and the APD3 tool (http://aps. unmc.edu/AP/prediction/prediction_main.php), described in [15], using the parameters that both have defined by default. The secondary structure of the peptides was calculated using the PSIPred tool (http://bioinf.cs.ucl.ac.uk/psipred/). The alpha-helicity of the regions present in the peptides was visualised in 2D by the helical projection tool available on the website http:// rzlab.ucr.edu/scripts/wheel/wheel.cgi.

2.5. Peptide synthesis

After performing the bioinformatic study, peptides were synthesised (Caslo, Lyngby, Denmark) on a 10 mg scale and with a purity of more than 90% (analysed by HPLC). To avoid degradation of peptides during storage, their N-terminal end was acetylated and their C-terminal end amidated. For the performance of the different assays, aliquots of each of the polypeptides (2 mg) were dissolved in pure water to a stock concentration of 100 μM.

2.6. Antimicrobial activity

The *in vitro* antimicrobial activity of the polypeptides was tested against the following pathogenic microbes, including bacteria and fungi: *Staphylococcus aureus* ATCC 6538, *Salmonella* sp. CECT 456, *Klebsiella pneumoniae* ATCC 23357, *Escherichia coli* ATCC 9637, *Bacillus cereus* ATCC 21772, *Proteus mirabilis* CECT 170, *Enterococcus faecalis* ATCC 29212, and *Candida albicans*. The minimum peptide concentration necessary to inhibit the growth of the tested microorganisms was evaluated by MIC assay, as described elsewhere [16]. Pathogenic microorganisms tested to evaluate the antimicrobial activity of the peptides were preserved at a temperature of −80°C in Luria-Bertani medium (LB) supplemented with 20% volume/volume glycerin. To determine the MIC, the peptides were solubilised in sterile milli-Q water to a final concentration of 100 μM, after which serial dilutions were carried out. 50 μl of each dilution of each polypeptide was mixed with 50 μl of the corresponding bacterial pointer suspension in Mueler-Hilton medium to a total volume of 100 μl in each well of a microplate. Thus, the effective concentrations to which the bacterial suspensions were subjected were 50, 25, 12.5, 6.5, 3.2, 1.6, 0.8, 0.4, 0.2 and 0.1 μM. Two replicates were carried out for each strain, concentration and peptide under test. As positive controls water was used in place of the specific polypeptide, and as negative controls each of the polypeptides was used without the corresponding bacterial suspension. In addition, two non-antimicrobial peptides were used as negative controls. Such peptides had a structure similar to the peptides of the invention (α-helix), but their sequence is totally different and shows no antimicrobial activity. The microplates were incubated at 37°C for 12–16 h with a shaking of 20 s prior to the measurement of the absorbance. To evaluate microbial growth, the optical density at 600 nm was measured using an EZ Biochrome plate reader. Each experiment was performed twice. As MIC, the lowest peptide concentration was taken at which no bacterial growth occurred at the end of the experiment.

2.7. Haemolytic activity

The haemolytic activity of the peptides is an indicator of the toxicity of peptides in eukaryotic cells, and a characteristic that is generally determined for those compounds that may come into contact with the human body. A lower percentage of haemolysis could be correlated with a lower cytotoxic activity of the peptide. Briefly, the haemolytic activity of the peptides was evaluated by determining the release of haemoglobin that is produced by contacting a solution comprising each of the peptides with a suspension of 10% volume from fresh human blood. Collection of blood samples was performed under aseptic conditions using a Vacutainer® K2E (Belliver, Great Britain) system with EDTA, and stored in Alsever medium at 4°C. When the assays were performed, blood was collected centrifuged at 6000 g for 5 min to separate the erythrocytes. After the erythrocytes were collected, they were washed three times with PBS buffer and resuspended in PBS buffer until a suspension containing 10% by volume of erythrocytes was obtained. In parallel, the peptides were solubilised in PBS buffer to obtain a battery of concentrations for each of them ranging from 12.5, 6.25, 3.13, 1.56, 0.78, 39, 0.2, 0.1,

0.05 and 0.02 μM. Three replicates were used for each peptide and concentration tested. Briefly, 50 μl of the 10% by volume erythrocyte suspension was mixed with 50 μl of the aliquots comprising each of the different concentrations of the peptide to be tested in each well of a 96-well plate, and the mixture for 45 min at 37°C under agitation. The plates were then centrifuged at 3500 g for 5 min, and 80 μl aliquots of the supernatant were transferred to 100-well flat bottom microplates, which were diluted with 80 μl of milli-Q water. The degree of haemolysis was determined from the absorbance at 540 nm with a plate reader. As a positive control for haemolysis assays, a PBS buffer solution containing 1% Triton X-100 (Sigma-Aldrich, Spain) was used. The percentage of haemolysis (H) was determined using the equation: $H = 100 \times [(Op - Ob)/(Om - Ob)]$ where Op is the optical density measured for one of the concentrations of the peptide tested; Ob is the optical density of the buffer solution; and Om is the optical density for the positive control with Triton X-100.

2.8. Molecular cloning of cathelicidins

Synthetic DNA (Genscript, Piscataway, NJ, USA) corresponding to amino acid sequence of the peptides was designed so that they contained the signal peptide from the Chlamydomonas aryl sulphatase protein, the codon optimisation for *C. reinhardtii* and they incorporated restriction sites for correct positioning into the multiple cloning sites (MCS) of the vector pChlamy_4. (Thermofisher, Madrid, Spain). For the transformation of the cyanobacteria *S. elongatus*, primers were designed to incorporate restriction sites for the correct positioning of the amplified inserts into the vector pSyn_6 (Thermofisher). The TAP and BG11 media and all restriction enzymes and primers were purchased from Thermofisher. The correct cloning of the inserts was verified by PCR (for colony screening) and by sequencing (Secugen, Madrid, Spain).

2.9. Transformation of microalga

For the cloning and transformation of the eukaryotic and prokaryotic microalga *C. reinhardtii* and *S elongatus*, we followed the recommendation of the manufacturer (Thermofisher). Antibiotics zeocin and spectinomycin were purchased from Thermofisher. The anti-V5 epitope antibody used for the immunodetection of recombinant peptides was purchased from Invitrogen.

3. Results

3.1. Identification of cathelicidins

Cathelicidins are found in varying numbers in numerous different species, including reptiles and birds. A remarkable degree of molecular diversity has been noted within this gene family. However, a well-conserved feature across evolutionary distant species is an N-terminal cathelin-domain. Using this domain to search into genome databases, we have found two novel cathelicidins from the genome mining of a reptile (painted turtle) and a bird (budgerigar). Predicted cathelicidins were identified by screening genome databases using the BLAST tool for DNA sequences. The painted turtle cathelicidin of 154 amino acids was found in contig number 974.21, whereas a bird cathelicidin of 151 amino acids was found in contig 900159920384 of the newly sequenced genomes of these species, which from September 2012 were available in the genome database (http://www.ncbi.nlm.nih.gov/genome/).

The complete sequence of cathelicidins from these two species was assembled by joining the four exons identified in abovementioned contigs using GeneScan and GeneMarK programs and located in the following positions:

Species	Exon	Begin	End	Length
Turtle	1	799	933	135
	2	2556	2663	108
	3	3485	3568	84
	4	4442	4579	138
Bird	1	125	298	174
	2	499	606	108
	3	712	792	81
	4	877	969	93

The DNA sequence thus assembled was translated into amino acids and the resulting protein was subjected to PSI-BLAST to confirm that this protein was indeed a cathelicidin (not shown). The cathelicidin of the painted turtle, thus obtained, had the following sequence:

LRKDVLSFRDFPAEIPDEPPLVTPTDPSRCRVGSNLGPQRMSLYCDMTSNPRQELKFMV-KETVCPVSENLNGTECDFRDNGVVRDCSGFFSTQQESPIVIINCNTVTKED-PHIRRSRSPRRSRWPRRWYLPGSYTLIAHGGGKGKGKGSRLQMA

Whereas for the bird, the sequence of the corresponding cathelicidin was the following:

MPSSWALVLVVLGGACALPAPAPLAYTQALAQAVASYNQRPEVQNSFRLLSADPEPAP-SIQLSSLQLLNFTIMETQCPARARIHPDACEFKEDGLVKDCSAPVPQHGGPVLGVTCVD-STADPVRVKRFWPLLVTAIRTVAAGVSMFKSSKG

The coding sequence of exon 4 (in blue) is that which corresponds to the active peptide, while the remaining portion corresponds to the conserved pre-pro-peptide.

The amino acid sequence of exon 4 from both reptile and bird cathelicidin was then subjected to the prediction of the cut site for neutrophil elastase and it generated the following antimicrobial peptides:

Cc_SP-37: SPRRSRWPRRWYLPGSYTLIAHGGGKGKGKGSRLQMA

Mm_KR-26: KRFWPLLVTAIRTVAAGVSMFKSSKG

3.2. Bioinformatic analysis of peptides

Peptides Cc_SP-37 and Mm_KR-26 were subjected to *in silico* analysis of their antimicrobial activity using several bioinformatic tools. For example, the online tool APD3 calculated the different parameters related to the possible antimicrobial activity of the peptides. The APD database has a unique peptide prediction program. For example, the program will calculate select properties of the peptide (e.g., net charge, length, percentage of hydrophobic residue and amino acid composition). The *in silico* structural analysis of the peptides indicated that both of them were alpha helical and had a positive net charge. However, the cathelicidin Mm_KR-26, from the bird, had a lower net charge, higher hydrophobicity and lower Boman index than the cathelicidin Cp_SP-37, from the reptile (**Table 1**).

To predict and calculate the regions of the protein with possible antimicrobial activity, the AMPA bioinformatics tool was used, which predict antimicrobial regions on any protein by assigning an antimicrobial index to each residue (**Figure 1**).

The AMPA algorithm also uses an antimicrobial propensity scale to generate an antimicrobial profile by means of a sliding window system. The probability values displayed correspond to misclassification probability that is the probability to find the predicted stretch in a non-antimicrobial protein. Using this tool, a single stretch, spanning residues 2–15, was found for the turtle cathelicidin Cc_SP-37, which confirmed the possible antimicrobial character of the predicted cathelicidin. No stretch was found for the bird cathelicidin Mm_KR-26 (**Figure 2**).

Peptide	Specie	Net charge	Hydroph	Boman index
Cp_SP-37	*Chrysemys picta bellii*	+9	24%	2.59 kcal/mol
Mm_KR-26	*Melopsittacus undulatus*	+5	50%	0.65 kcal/mol

Table 1. Structural analysis of genome-derived cathelicidins from painted turtle (*Chrysemys picta bellii*) and budgerigar (*Melopsittacus undulatus*).

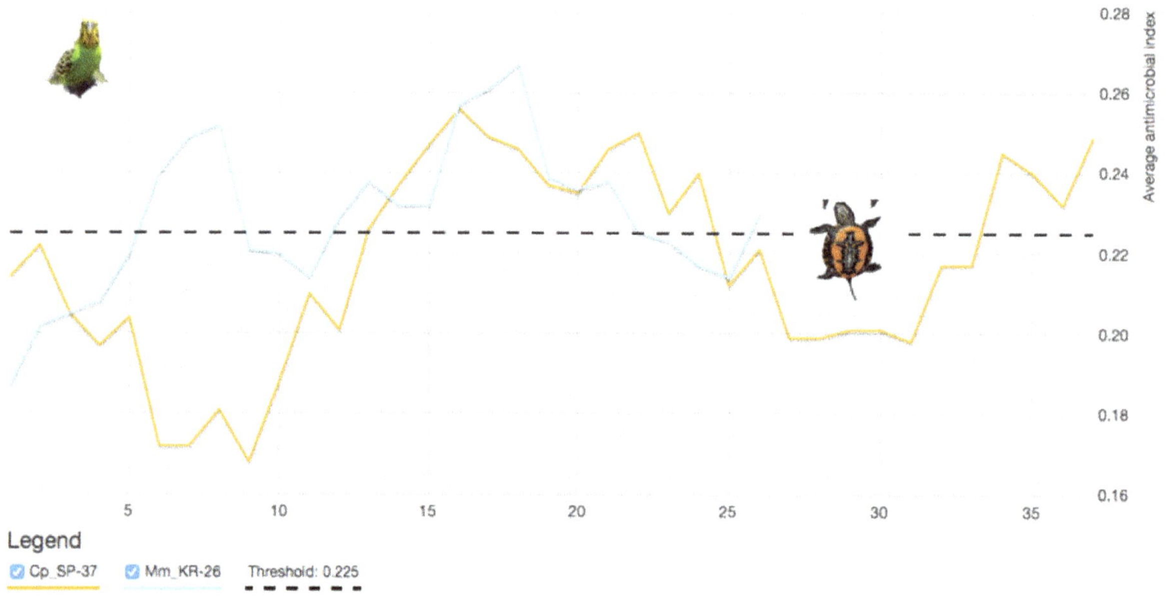

Figure 1. Graphical result of the in silico study of the cathelicidin sequences Mm_KR-26 (blue line) and Cp_SP-37 (yellow line), using the AMPA bioinformatic tool. The calculated average antimicrobial index is represented along the amino acid sequences. The threshold value of this index is indicated by a dashed line.

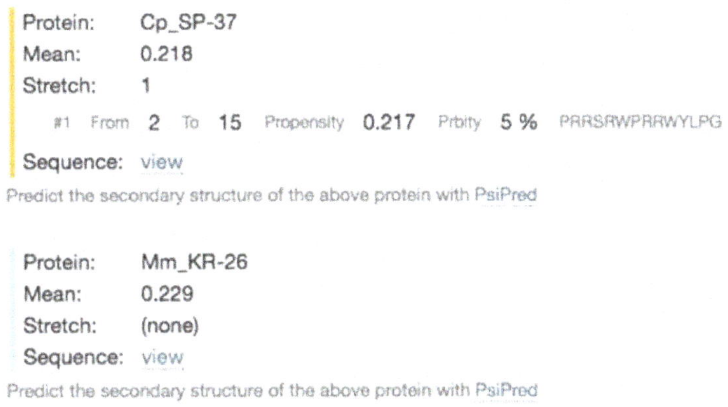
Protein: Cp_SP-37
Mean: 0.218
Stretch: 1
#1 From 2 To 15 Propensity 0.217 Prbity 5 % PRRSRWPRRWYLPG
Sequence: view
Predict the secondary structure of the above protein with PsiPred

Protein: Mm_KR-26
Mean: 0.229
Stretch: (none)
Sequence: view
Predict the secondary structure of the above protein with PsiPred

Figure 2. Result of the in silico study of the cathelicidin sequences, using the AMPA bioinformatic tool. The antimicrobial stretches are shown with a mean and a propensity and probability value.

The secondary structure of the bird and turtle cathelicidins was then computed with the PSIPred tool, which for the bird cathelicidin Mm_KR-26, predicted a single helical region comprised between residues 2 and 23 (**Figure 3**). However, no helical portion was predicted for the turtle cathelicidin Cc_SP-37 (not shown).

To further study the amphipathic character of the helices predicted by the PSI-Pred tool, these residues were represented in helical projection (**Figure 3**). For the helix of the peptide Mm_KR-26, comprised between the residues 2 and 23, it was observed that the two positively charged residues (R12 and K22) were disposed towards the same side, thus generating an amphipathic helix, characteristic of the antimicrobial peptides, with a hydrophobic moment of 4.37 units at 14.1°C.

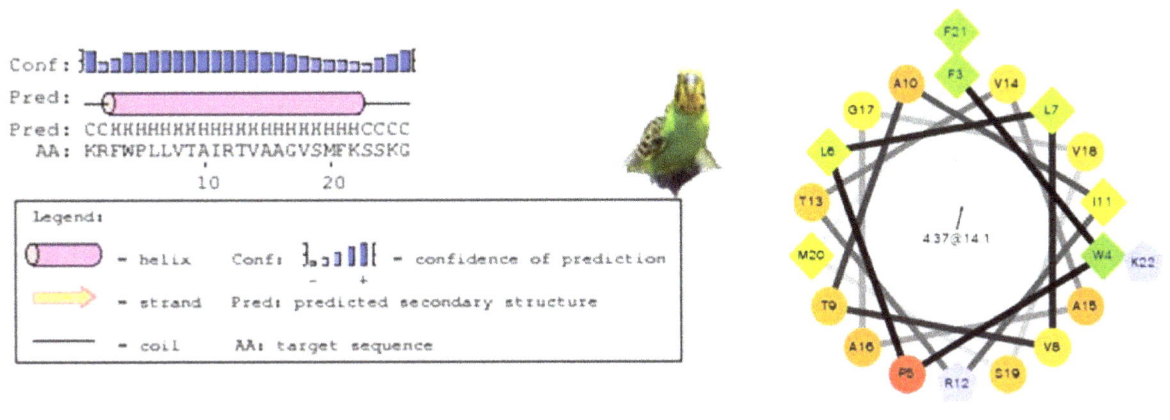

Figure 3. Result of the in silico study of the cathelicidin Mm_KR-26, using the PSIPred bioinformatic tool for the prediction of the secondary structure. The predicted helical content of the bird cathelicidin Mm_KR-26 was then subjected to a helical projection and calculation of the hydrophobic moment, using the on line viewer available at http://rzlab.ucr.edu/scripts/wheel/wheel.cgi. Hydrophilic residues are presented as circles, hydrophobic residues as diamonds, potentially negatively charged as triangles, and potentially positively charged as pentagons. Hydrophobicity is colour-coded: the most hydrophobic residue is green, and the amount of green is decreasing proportionally to the hydrophobicity, with zero hydrophobicity coded as yellow. Hydrophilic residues are coded red with pure red being the most hydrophilic (uncharged) residue, and the amount of red decreasing proportionally to the hydrophilicity. The potentially charged residues are light blue. The scalar value of the hydrophobic moment of the helix and the angle of its direction are shown inside the helix.

3.3. Antimicrobial activity of peptides

For the analysis of the antimicrobial activity of cathelicidins, we used the minimal inhibitory concentration assay over a panel of different microorganisms of reference (**Table 2**). For simplicity, we show some figures with the microorganisms *B. cereus, E. coli, E. faecalis, C. albicans, P. corrugata and Salmonella* sp. In these experiments, it was found that both the bird peptide Mm_KR-26 and the painted turtle Cc_Sp-37 were particularly effective at a low dose to inhibit the growth of *B. cereus,* with MIC values of 1.6–3.1 and of 3.1–6.3 μM, respectively. However, both peptides were not effective, at the higher dose tested, to inhibit the growing of *S. aureus* and *P. mirabilis* and both were not very effective against *C. albicans,* with MIC values of 25–50 μM (**Table 2**).

To visualise the relative efficacy of the inhibition of the growing of microorganism, we estimated the percentage of inhibition of the growing of microorganisms at different concentrations of peptide, as well as the effective concentration of peptide to inhibit at 50% the growing of the microorganism, the EC_{50} values. **Figures 4** and **5** (top and bottom) show these values obtained with a few representative microorganisms for the bird peptide Mm_KR-26 and the painted turtle Cc_Sp-37, respectively.

As can be seen from the results shown in **Figure 4**, the cathelicidin Mm_KR-26 was particularly effective against *E. faecalis,* which required less concentration of peptide for inhibition of the growth of this microorganism, (with an EC_{50} value of 1.3 μM) and, in less extent, against *C. albicans* with an EC_{50} value of 34.6 μM (**Figure 4**).

As can be seen from the results shown in **Figure 4**, the cathelicidin Mm_KR-26 was particularly effective against *E. faecalis,* which required less concentration of peptide for inhibition of the growth of this microorganism, (with an EC_{50} value of 1.3 μM) and, in less extent, against *C. albicans* with an EC_{50} value of 34.6 μM (**Figure 4**).

Similarly, the painted turtle peptide Cc_SP-37 was particularly effective against *E. faecalis,* which required less concentration of peptide for inhibition of the growth of this microorganism, (with

Reference microorganism	Mm_KR-26	Cc_SP-37	Kanamycin
S. aureus (ATCC6538)	>50 μM	>50 μM	0.8–1.6 μg/ml
Salmonella sp. *(CECT456)*	3.1–6.3 μM	12.5–25 μM	0.4–1.6 μg/ml
K. pneumoniae (ATCC23357)	1.6–3.1 μM	3.1–6.3 μM	0.4–0.8 μg/ml
E. coli (ATCC9637)	3.1–6.3 μM	6.3–12.5 μM	0.4–1.6 μg/ml
B. cereus (ATCC21772)	1.6–3.1 μM	3.1–6.3 μM	0.8–3.1 μg/ml
P. mirabilis (CECT170)	>50 μM	>50 μM	0.4–0.8 μg/ml
E. faecalis (ATCC29212)	0.8–1.6 μM	6.3–3.1 μM	0.4–0.8 μg/ml
C. albicans	25–50 μM	25–50 μM	–
P. corrugata	6.3–12.5 μM	25–50 μM	–

Table 2. Minimum inhibitory concentration of the bird peptide Mm_KR-26 and the painted turtle Cc_Sp-37 compared with the antibiotic kanamycin.

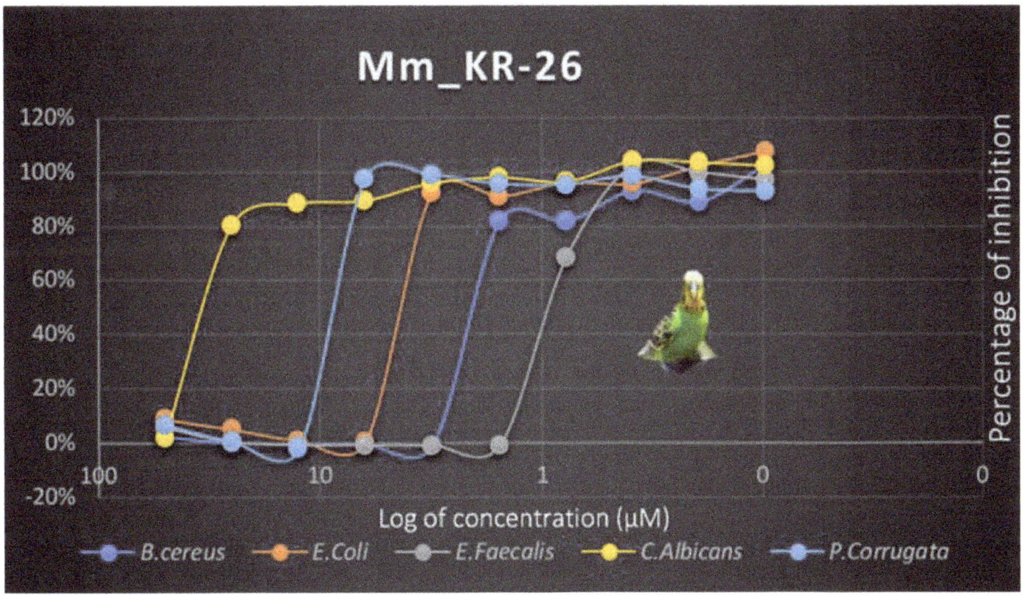

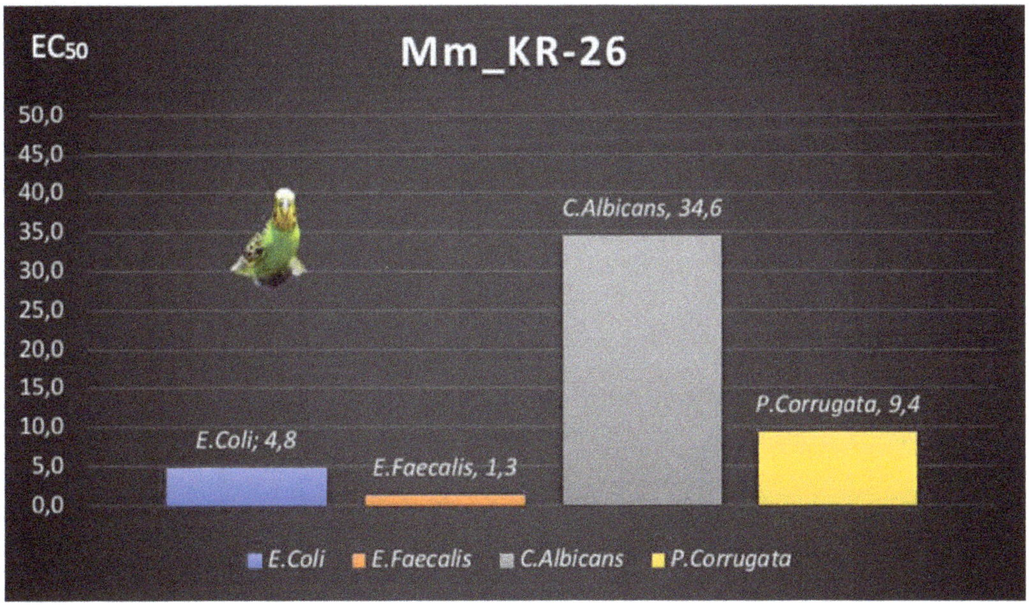

Figure 4. Analysis of the in vitro relative antimicrobial activity of the bird peptide Mm_KR-26 against a panel of representative microorganisms, showed as the percentage of inhibition (top) and calculating the effective dose for the inhibition at 50% (EC50), showed bottom.

an EC_{50} value of 5.7 μM) and, in less extent, against *C. albicans* and *P. corrugata* with EC_{50} values of 46.8 and 40.8 μM, respectively (**Figure 5**).

For both cathelicidin peptides, we tested the haemolytic activity at concentrations ranging from 12.5 to 0.2 μM, concentrations at which the peptides were able of inhibiting the growth of pathogenic microorganisms. The haemolytic activity of both peptides was always less than 35%, indicating that the peptides at these concentrations do not show toxicity for human erythrocytes (data not shown).

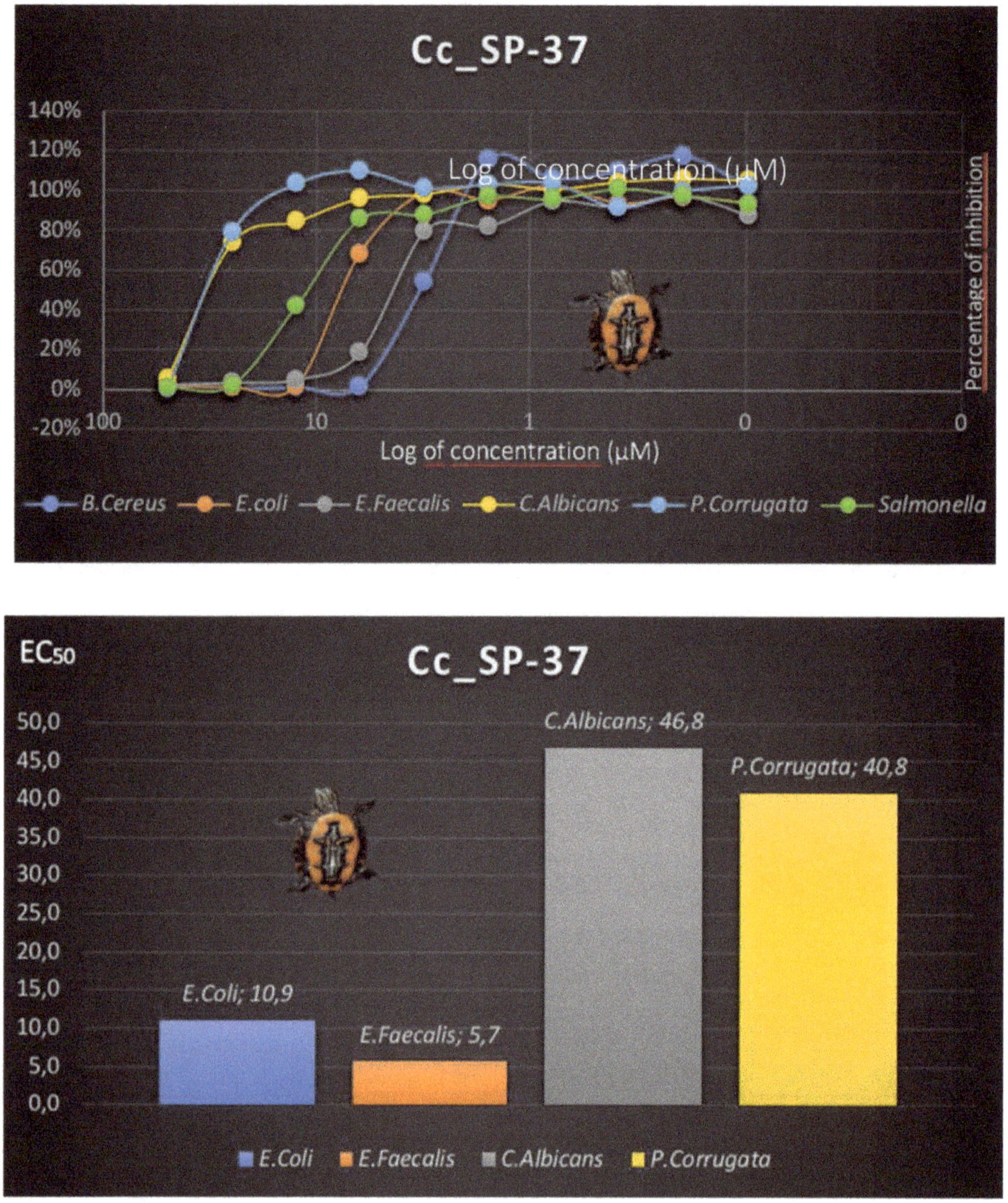

Figure 5. Analysis of the in vitro relative antimicrobial activity of the painted turtle peptide Cc_SP-37 against a panel of representative microorganisms, showed as the percentage of inhibition (top) and calculating the effective dose for the inhibition at 50% (EC50), showed bottom.

Once we tested the antimicrobial activity of the peptides, we next initiated the recombinant production of peptides in the eukaryotic microalga *Chlamydomonas reinhardtii* and in prokaryotic cyanobacteria *Synechococcus elongates,* given the advantages of using these microalga as biofactories [17]. For the eukaryotic microalga, in order to obtain a secreted product, we considered the introduction of the signal peptide of the aryl sulphatase, as previously described [18], and the synthetic DNA with the codon optimisation for this particular microalga. We also added restriction sites for the correct cloning of the synthetic DNA into the vectors pChlamy_4 and pSyn_6. Both expression systems, prokaryotic and eukaryotic microalga have strong promotors and can introduce 6xHis tags for the purification of the recombinant proteins (**Table 3**).

Vector features	pChlamy_4	pSyn_6
Promoter	HSP70-rbcs2 (strong, endogenous)	psbA1 (strong, endogenous)
Selection	Bleomycin/Zeocin	Spectinomycin
Epitope tags	TEV-cleavable N-terminal 6His, or C-terminal V5-6His	
Gene integration	Stable (random)	Stable (targeted)
Growth media	TAP	BG-11

Table 3. Comparison of the microalga vectors pChlamy_4 and pSyn_6 (Thermofisher) used for the recombinant expression of cathelicidin antimicrobial peptides into the microalga *C. reinhardtii and S. elongatus,* respectively.

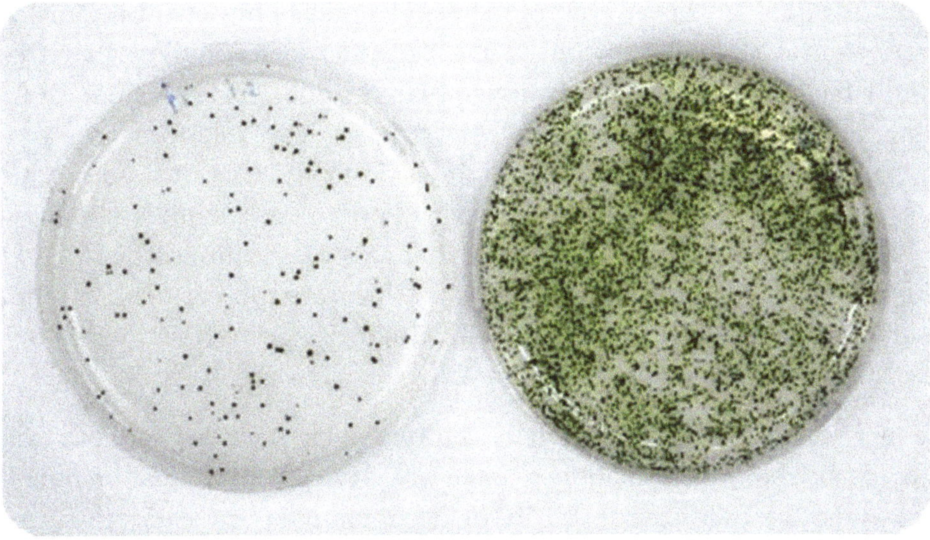

Figure 6. Transformed cyanobacteria *S. elongatus* growing in BG-11 agar plates containing spectinomycin (5 μg/ml). Negative control with no insert (left) and containing the bird cathelicidin peptide Mm_KR-26.

Using the commercially available kits for microalga expression, two microalga (*C. reinhardtii and S. elongatus*) were transformed for the recombinant expression of the bird and painted turtle cathelicidins. As an example, **Figure 6** shows the transformation of *S. elongatus* with the DNA coding for the bird cathelicidin peptide Mm_KR-26.

Current experiments are underway in order to optimise the recombinant production of these cathelicidins in a higher culture volume and to study the yield of the peptide production using microalga as biofactories.

4. Discussion

Currently, approximately 15 therapeutic agents based on AMP peptides are found in clinical trials of anti-infective or anti-inflammatory indications, generally limited to topical applications

[19]. One of the main questions to bring this type of molecules to the clinical application refers to their toxicity. To date, most clinical trials focus on topical use. Although, many peptides have activity on eukaryotic membranes, this activity is much lower compared to prokaryotes. This may be due to the absence of negatively charged lipids on the surface of eukaryotic membranes, the lower membrane potential in most cells and the presence of cholesterol in eukaryotes. However, despite the large number of peptides described in various organisms (more than 2000) and the advances to take advantage of its clinical potential, there is currently no peptide approved for use in humans by the Food and Drug Administration (FDA) [20].

One of the most widely used strategies for the biotechnological production of proteins and recombinant peptides is their expression in microorganisms, such as *E. coli* or yeast. Among the advantages of these expression systems is the well-known physiology of these microorganisms and the existence of specific and well-characterised strains to achieve high levels of expression, the existence of numerous protocols for the transformation of *E. coli* and/or yeasts and the availability of vectors that contain a great diversity of promoters and selection markers, and so on [21]. However among the disadvantages presented by this antimicrobial peptide, production system is, obviously, the potential susceptibility that the producing microbes could have to the harmful antimicrobial peptides, in case these are exposed to. Another disadvantage, in case the peptide is trapped as insoluble form in inclusion bodies, implies the need to further purify these peptides from the extract, and, according to the potential use of the peptides, also the removal of endotoxins. Synthetic biology techniques facilitate the availability of the genetic material that codes for antimicrobial peptides with the codon optimisation of the host and it also allows the incorporation of signal peptides, epitopes for the detection of the final product, or the inclusion of appropriate targets for proteolytic enzymes, tags or tails to facilitate purification [22].

An alternative for an expression system of antimicrobial peptides without contaminating endotoxins could be the transformation of eukaryotic cells from animal or human origin. In this case, it may not be necessary to purify or decontaminate the extracts, since the culture would be free of pathogens. However, the cost of producing recombinant proteins would be considerably higher than using conventional microorganisms. Therefore, the economic yield of these clean expression systems is lower than the microbial ones [23].

We here propose that a production system based on microalga could be an alternative to the conventional fermentation system, which uses bacteria or yeast and/or mammalian cells [24]. First, the antimicrobial peptide is less likely to be toxic to this production system. Second, this production system differs from the others due to the greater volume of scaling that these cultures allow, since it can be spread over large areas, in microalgae production systems. This fact makes these production systems very profitable. Although they can be less efficient, the cost/benefit ratio could be higher for the large-scale production of these peptides. Another advantage of these green production systems is that some microalgae are considered generally regarded as safe (GRAS). Hence, in these cases, depending on the type of application expected for the antimicrobial peptides, purification processes may not be necessary, for example, applications for cosmetics, topical medicines, pesticides for agriculture, food conservation, and so on.

There are already numerous tools for the efficient transformation microalgae. For example, in the case of the microalga *Chlamydomonas reinhardtii*, it is possible to transform the three genomes: nuclear, chloroplastic and mitochondrial. Once transformed, microalgae can be grown in photobioreactors, in controlled conditions and free of pathogens. The microalga used as biofactories of recombinant drugs, on the other hand, could also be grown under controlled conditions to avoid escaping into the environment and to improve the biosecurity of the final product [25].

5. Conclusions

Antimicrobial peptides, originating from natural resources, have been recognised as a novel class of antibiotics. We have shown that genome mining is an effective method for finding new antimicrobial peptides, such as cathelicidins, from the genomes of a turtle and a bird. The derived peptides were tested for their *in vitro* antimicrobial activity showing that these antimicrobial peptides were particularly effective against bacterial growth, both Gram+ (*E. faecalis*) and Gram− (*E. coli*). In addition, these peptides had low haemolytic activity in human erythrocytes, which makes them suitable for use in different formulations and/or pharmaceutical, cosmetic and/or phytosanitary compositions, among others. Using synthetic constructions, current experiments are underway to produce these peptides as recombinant chimeric proteins in eukaryotic microalga and cyanobacteria. We hope that our preliminary investigation with these novel peptides could be useful for the design of future strategies that pursue the production of antimicrobial peptides through biotechnology in order to provide novel treatment opportunities based on antimicrobial peptides.

Acknowledgements

This work was supported by the Spanish Ministry of Economy, Industry and Competitiveness (MINECO), project SAF2013-48399-R. C. Garrido-Orduña is a recipient of the research assistant program of the Spanish "Fondo de Garantía Juvenil". We are grateful to our students of Master thesis who spent some time in our lab during the project: C. Lidia Borges, David Tejera, Crismarys Hernández, Elisa González, Antonia Cionfrini and Jonay Ayoze Vega.

Author details

José Manuel Pérez de la Lastra*, Cristina Garrido-Orduña, Andrés A. Borges, David Jiménez-Arias, Francisco Javier García-Machado, Mercedes Hernández, Concepción González and Alicia Boto

*Address all correspondence to: jm.perezdelalastra@csic.es

Institute of Natural Products and Agrobiology (IPNA), Spanish Research Council (CSIC), Avda. Astrofísico Fco. Sánchez, San Cristóbal de La Laguna, Santa Cruz de Tenerife, Spain

References

[1] Kaspar AA, Reichert JM. Future directions for peptide therapeutics development. Drug Discovery Today. 2013;**18**:807-817

[2] Joerger RD. Alternatives to antibiotics: Bacteriocins, antimicrobial peptides and bacteriophages. Poultry Science. 2003;**82**:640-647

[3] Cars O, Hedin A, Heddini A. The global need for effective antibiotics—Moving towards concerted action. Drug Resistance Updates. 2011;**14**:68-69

[4] Zasloff M. Antimicrobial peptides of multicellular organisms. Nature. 2002;**415**:389-395

[5] Peschel A, Sahl HG. The co-evolution of host cationic antimicrobial peptides and microbial resistance. Nature Reviews Microbiology. 2006;**4**:529

[6] Zasloff M. Antimicrobial Peptides: Do they have a Future as Therapeutics? In: Harder J, Schröder JM, editors. Antimicrobial Peptides. Birkhäuser Advances in Infectious Diseases. Cham: Springer International Publishing; 2016. pp. 147-154

[7] Barra D, Simmaco M. Amphibian skin: A promising resource for antimicrobial peptides. Trends in Biotechnology. 1995;**13**:205-209

[8] Yoo WG, Lee S, Lee MR, Yun MR, Kwon T, Kim DW. Genome-wide identification of antimicrobial peptides in the liver fluke, Clonorchis sinensis. Bioinformation. 2015;**11**:17

[9] Wang P, Hu L, Liu G, Jiang N, Chen X, Xu J, et al. Prediction of antimicrobial peptides based on sequence alignment and feature selection methods. PLoS One. 2011;**6**:e18476

[10] Bals R, Wilson JM. Cathelicidins-A family of multifunctional antimicrobial peptides. Cellular and Molecular Life Sciences. 2003;**60**:711-720

[11] Zanetti M. Cathelicidins, multifunctional peptides of the innate immunity. Journal of Leukocyte Biology. 2004;**75**:39-48

[12] Lehrer RI, Ganz T. Cathelicidins: A family of endogenous antimicrobial peptides. Current Opinion in Hematology. 2002;**9**:18-22

[13] Pérez de la Lastra JP, Garrido-Orduña C, Borges CL, Borges AA, Boto A. Antimicrobial activity of cathelicidins of mammals from avian, aquatic and terrestrial environments. In: Mendez-Vilas, editor. Antimicrobial research: Novel bioknowledge and educational programs. Formatex; 2017. pp. 9-18

[14] Torrent M, Di Tommaso P, Pulido D, Nogués M, Notredame C, Boix E, Andreu D. AMPA: An automated web server for prediction of protein antimicrobial regions. Bioinformatics. 2012;**28**:130-131

[15] Wang G, Li X, Wang Z. APD3: The antimicrobial peptide database as a tool for research and education. Nucleic Acids Research. 2016;**44**:D1087-D1093

[16] Wiegand I, Hilpert K, Hancock RE. Agar and broth dilution methods to determine the minimal inhibitory concentration (MIC) of antimicrobial substances. Nature Protocols. 2008;**3**:163-175

[17] Wijffels RH, Kruse O, Hellingwerf KJ. Potential of industrial biotechnology with cyanobacteria and eukaryotic microalgae. Current Opinion in Biotechnology. 2013;**24**(3): 405-413

[18] Rasala BA, Lee PA, Shen Z, Briggs SP, Mendez M, Mayfield SP. Robust expression and secretion of Xylanase1 in Chlamydomonas reinhardtii by fusion to a selection gene and processing with the FMDV 2A peptide. PLoS One. 2012;**7**(8):e43349

[19] Wimley WC, Hristova K. Antimicrobial peptides: Successes, challenges and unanswered questions. The Journal of Membrane Biology. 2011;**239**:27-34

[20] Kang SJ, Park SJ, Mishig-Ochir T, Lee BJ. Antimicrobial peptides: Therapeutic potentials. Expert Review of Anti-Infective Therapy. 2014;**12**(12):1477-1486

[21] Terpe K. Overview of bacterial expression systems for heterologous protein production: From molecular and biochemical fundamentals to commercial systems. Applied Microbiology and Biotechnology. 2006;**72**(2):211

[22] Welch M, Villalobos A, Gustafsson C, Minshull J. You're one in a googol: Optimizing genes for protein expression. Journal of the Royal Society Interface. 2009;**6**(Suppl 4):S467-S476

[23] Wurm FM. Production of recombinant protein therapeutics in cultivated mammalian cells. Nature Biotechnology. 2004;**22**(11):1393-1398

[24] Potvin G, Zhang Z. Strategies for high-level recombinant protein expression in transgenic microalgae: A review. Biotechnology Advances. 2010;**28**(6):910-918

[25] Boto A, Pérez de la Lastra JM, González CC. The road from host-defense peptides to a new generation of antimicrobial drugs. Molecules. 2018;**23**:311

Permissions

All chapters in this book were first published in DDCM, by InTech Open; hereby published with permission under the Creative Commons Attribution License or equivalent. Every chapter published in this book has been scrutinized by our experts. Their significance has been extensively debated. The topics covered herein carry significant findings which will fuel the growth of the discipline. They may even be implemented as practical applications or may be referred to as a beginning point for another development.

The contributors of this book come from diverse backgrounds, making this book a truly international effort. This book will bring forth new frontiers with its revolutionizing research information and detailed analysis of the nascent developments around the world.

We would like to thank all the contributing authors for lending their expertise to make the book truly unique. They have played a crucial role in the development of this book. Without their invaluable contributions this book wouldn't have been possible. They have made vital efforts to compile up to date information on the varied aspects of this subject to make this book a valuable addition to the collection of many professionals and students.

This book was conceptualized with the vision of imparting up-to-date information and advanced data in this field. To ensure the same, a matchless editorial board was set up. Every individual on the board went through rigorous rounds of assessment to prove their worth. After which they invested a large part of their time researching and compiling the most relevant data for our readers.

The editorial board has been involved in producing this book since its inception. They have spent rigorous hours researching and exploring the diverse topics which have resulted in the successful publishing of this book. They have passed on their knowledge of decades through this book. To expedite this challenging task, the publisher supported the team at every step. A small team of assistant editors was also appointed to further simplify the editing procedure and attain best results for the readers.

Apart from the editorial board, the designing team has also invested a significant amount of their time in understanding the subject and creating the most relevant covers. They scrutinized every image to scout for the most suitable representation of the subject and create an appropriate cover for the book.

The publishing team has been an ardent support to the editorial, designing and production team. Their endless efforts to recruit the best for this project, has resulted in the accomplishment of this book. They are a veteran in the field of academics and their pool of knowledge is as vast as their experience in printing. Their expertise and guidance has proved useful at every step. Their uncompromising quality standards have made this book an exceptional effort. Their encouragement from time to time has been an inspiration for everyone.

The publisher and the editorial board hope that this book will prove to be a valuable piece of knowledge for researchers, students, practitioners and scholars across the globe.

List of Contributors

Yu-Chen Lo
Department of Bioengineering, Stanford University, Stanford, CA, USA

Jorge Z. Torres
Department of Chemistry and Biochemistry, University of California, Los Angeles, CA, USA

Charles J. Malemud
Department of Medicine, Division of Rheumatic Diseases, Case Western Reserve University School of Medicine/University Hospitals Cleveland Medical Center, Cleveland, Ohio, USA

John J. Bowling, William R. Shadrick and Elizabeth C. Griffith
Department of Chemical Biology and Therapeutics, St. Jude Children's Research Hospital, Memphis, TN, United States

Richard E. Lee
Department of Chemical Biology and Therapeutics, St. Jude Children's Research Hospital, Memphis, TN, United States Department of Pharmaceutical Sciences, University of Tennessee Health Science Center, Memphis, TN, United States

Desam Nagarjuna Reddy and Abdul Jabbar Al-Rajab
Centre for Environmental Research and Studies, Jazan University, Jazan, Saudi Arabia

Gowkanapalli Ramachandra Reddy
Department of Polymer Science and Technology, College of Science, Sri Krishnadevaraya University, Anatapur, AP, India

Yu-Chen Lo
Department of Bioengineering, Stanford University, The United States

Ren Gui and Hiroshi Honda
Department of Bioengineering, Northwestern Polytechnic University, The United States

Jorge Z. Torres
Department of Chemistry and Biochemistry, University of California, Los Angeles, The United States

Domokos Gerő
Institute of Pathophysiology, Semmelweis University Medical School, Budapest, Hungary University of Exeter Medical School, Exeter, UK

Abdulkarim Najjar and Wolfgang Sippl
Department of Pharmaceutical Chemistry, Martin-Luther University of Halle-Wittenberg,Halle (Saale), Germany

Fidele Ntie-Kang
Department of Pharmaceutical Chemistry, Martin-Luther University of Halle-Wittenberg,Halle (Saale), Germany Department of Chemistry, University of Buea, Buea, Cameroon and Department of Pharmaceutical Chemistry, Martin-Luther University of Halle-Wittenberg, Halle, Germany

Sudhakar Pola and Venkata Narasimha Kadali
Department of Biotechnology, Andhra University, Visakhapatnam, India

Gilles Ferry
Institut de Recherches SERVIER, Croissy-sur-Seine, France

Jean A. Boutin and Olivier Nosjean
Institut de Recherches SERVIER, Croissy-sur-Seine, France Institut de Recherches Internationales SERVIER, Suresnes, France

José Manuel Pérez de la Lastra, Cristina Garrido-Orduña, Andrés A. Borges, David Jiménez-Arias, Francisco Javier García-Machado, Mercedes Hernández, Concepción González and Alicia Boto
Institute of Natural Products and Agrobiology (IPNA), Spanish Research Council (CSIC), Avda. Astrofísico Fco. Sánchez, San Cristóbal de La Laguna, Santa Cruz de Tenerife, Spain

Index

Ingram Content Group UK Ltd.
Milton Keynes UK
UKHW050758130323
418479UK00003B/37

9 781639 871698